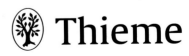

Ultrasonic Energy for Cutting, Coagulating, and Dissecting

Wolfgang Feil, M.D.
Professor
Academic Hospital Manager
Chairman, Surgical Departments
Evangelical Hospital Vienna
Vienna, Austria

Michel Degueldre, M.D., Ph.D.
Professor
Centre Hospitalier Universitaire St. Pierre
Department of Gynecology and Obstetrics
Brussels, Belgium

Dietrich Löhlein, M.D.
Professor
Klinikum Dortmund GmbH
Surgical Clinic
Dortmund, Germany

Bernhard Dallemagne, M.D.
Clinic St. Joseph
Surgery Service
Liege, Belgium

Minna Kauko, M.D., Ph.D.
North Karelian Central Hospital
Department of Obstetrics and Gynecology
Joensuu, Finland

Bruno Walther, M.D.
Associate Professor
Lund University Hospital
Department of Surgery
Lund, Sweden

With contributions by
E-G Achilles, S. Amaya Alarcon, G. Bates, D.C. Broering, J. Burgos, F. Ciampaglia, M. Degueldre, R. Eyb,
W. Feil, M. Gagner, P. Gertsch, P.C. Guilianotti, C. Haglund, T. Heier, A. D'Hoore, W.B. Inabnet, R. Jancovici,
M. Kauko, X. de Kerangal, L. Lang-Lazdunski, C. Lanzi, G. Lesti, H. Löppönen, F. Lozano Moreno, D. Maguire,
O.J. McAnena, H. Mignot, H.R. Nürnberger, R. Perunovic, F. Pons, C. Power, F. Psalmon, F. Quenet, T. Reck,
X. Rogiers, C.M.S. Royston, A.L. Sardellone, J. Scholler, P.C. Sedman, J. Sirén, N. Steventon, E.C. Tsimoyiannis,
J. Vandromme, P. Voutilainen, B. Walther, D. Zacharoulis

442 illustrations
26 tables

Thieme
Stuttgart · New York

Library of Congress Cataloging-in-Publication Data
Ultrasonic energy for cutting, coagulating, and dissecting /
Wolfgang Feil ... [et al.].
  p. ; cm.
Includes bibliographical references.
ISBN 1-58890-065-7 (alk. paper)—ISBN 3-13-127521-9 (alk.
paper)
1. Ultrasonics in surgery.
[DNLM: 1. Surgical Instruments. 2. Ultrasonic Therapy—in-
strumentation. 3. Dissection—instrumentation. 4. Hemosta-
sis, Surgical—instrumentation. 5. Laparoscopy—methods.
WO 162 U47 2005] I. Feil, W.
  RD33.7.U47 2005
  617'.07543—dc22   2004017014

Important note: Medicine is an ever-changing science undergoing continual development. Research and clinical experience are continually expanding our knowledge, in particular our knowledge of proper treatment and drug therapy.
Insofar as this book mentions any dosage or application,
readers may rest assured that the authors, editors, and publishers have made every effort to ensure that such references are in accordance with **the state of knowledge at the
time of production of the book.**
Nevertheless, this does not involve, imply, or express any
guarantee or responsibility on the part of the publishers in
respect to any dosage instructions and forms of applications
stated in the book. **Every user is requested to examine
carefully** the manufacturers' leaflets accompanying each
drug and to check, if necessary in consultation with a physician or specialist, whether the dosage schedules mentioned
therein or the contraindications stated by the manufacturers differ from the statements made in the present book.
Such examination is particularly important with drugs that
are either rarely used or have been newly released on the
market. Every dosage schedule or every form of application
used is entirely at the user's own risk and responsibility. The
authors and publishers request every user to report to the
publishers any discrepancies or inaccuracies noticed.

Some of the product names, patents, and registered designs
referred to in this book are in fact registered trademarks or
proprietary names even though specific reference to this
fact is not always made in the text. Therefore, the appearance of a name without designation as proprietary is not to
be construed as a representation by the publisher that it is in
the public domain.

© 2005 Georg Thieme Verlag,
Rüdigerstrasse 14, 70469 Stuttgart, Germany
http://www.thieme.de

Thieme New York, 333 Seventh Avenue,
New York, NY 10001 USA
http://www.thieme.com

Typesetting by primustype Hurler GmbH, Notzingen
Printed in Germany by Druckhaus Götz, Ludwigsburg

ISBN 3-13-127521-9 (GTV)
ISBN 1-58890-065-7 (TNY)   1 2 3 4 5

Preface

Surgical technique fundamentally consists of cutting and hemostasis. Ancient civilizations used sharp instruments made of stone, and later of metal, to make surgical incisions. The principle of employing specifically designed tools to cut tissue has not changed significantly since; the scalpel and scissors that are indispensable tools in the modern operating room today are little more than the result of refinements in production and application techniques.

In ancient times, as far as we can tell from existing records, hemostasis was accomplished with compresses made of plant material. Surgical wounds, in particular those incurred in amputations following battle injuries, were controlled with tourniquets. Later, wounds were cauterized with red-hot iron to stop bleeding.

The two main principles of hemostasis—ligation and cauterization by heat—are still valid today, whereby technical improvements in controlling bleeding have been represented by surgical ligation, and, more recently, by the use of clips or rows of staples.

Hemostasis through the application of heat experienced a renaissance with the introduction of electrocoagulation. Here, high-frequency (HF) electrical power is passed through the patient and focused at the tip of an active electrode. The electrical density at the tip leads to the release of thermal energy in the immediate vicinity, which then can be used to cauterize blood vessels.

HF surgery is not free of risks; tissues can be damaged by heat and electrical current. The significance of the risks and related complications in HF surgery are particularly evident in laparoscopic surgery.

By using ultrasound as a source of energy, an alternative method for cutting and hemostasis during surgery was introduced—without the risk of electrical injury, and with significantly lower thermal stress to tissues.

The initial motivation for the development of this new technology was the desire to develop a safe and less complicated method for surgical hemostasis. As it turns out, the result is a significant paradigm shift. Today, ultrasound is used not only for hemostasis; rather, multifunctional instruments offer the possibility of performing procedures while sparing tissues, conserving blood, and reducing complications. Incision, dissection, and hemostasis can now be dealt with in a single procedure.

This book deals with the fundamentals of the technique; it traces the technical evolution, examines the technical requirements for successful use, and above all discusses the continuous development of the system and its practical uses in various areas of surgery.

Renowned surgeons from throughout Europe and the USA pass on their experience with ultrasound dissection and hemostasis in a practice-oriented survey.

This book is intended to further the successful spread of the method and initiate ideas and projects for the development of further technical and practical improvements.

We would like to thank all of the authors and staff for their important and outstanding contributions. Many thanks also to the colleagues at Thieme Publishers and Johnson & Johnson for their cooperation.

And finally, a special thank-you to my family for their understanding and support.

Vienna, Summer 2004   Wolfgang Feil

List of Contributors

Eike-Gert Achilles, MD
University Hospital Hamburg
Department of Hepatobiliary Surgery
Hamburg, Germany

Santiago Amaya Alarcon, MD
Professor
Facultad de Medicina de Alcalá de Henares
Madrid, Spain

Grant Bates, BSc, BM, BCh, FRCS
Oxford Radcliffe Hospitals NHS Trust
Radcliffe Infirmary
Department of Otolaryngology
and Head & Neck Surgery
Oxford, England

Dieter C. Broering, MD
University Hospital Hamburg Eppendorf
Department of Hepatobiliary Surgery
Hamburg, Germany

Jesus Burgos, PhD
Ramon y Cajal Hospital
Facultad de Medicina de Alcalá de Henares
Madrid, Spain

Michel Degueldre, MD, PhD
Professor
Centre Hospitalier Universitaire St. Pierre
Department of Gynecology and Obstetrics
Brussels, Belgium

R. Eyb, MD
Supervising Physician
Donauspital
Department of Orthopedic Surgery
Vienna, Austria

Michel Gagner, MD, FACS
New York Presbyterian Hospital
Weill Medical College of Cornell University
Department of Surgery
New York, USA

Philippe Gertsch, MD, FRCS
Professor
Primario Servicio di Chirurgia
Ospedale San Giovanni
Bellinzona, Switzerland

Pier Cristoforo Guilianotti
Ospedale Della Misericordia
Department of General Surgery
Grosseto, Italy

Caj Haglund, MD, PhD
Associate Professor
Helsinki University Central Hospital
Department of Surgery
Hus, Helsinki, Finland

Tore Heier
Diakonhjemmet Hospital
Surgical Department
Oslo, Norway

André D'Hoore, MD
University Clinics Gasthuisberg
Department of Abdominal Surgery
Leuven, Belgium

William B. Inabnet, MD
New York Presbyterian Hospital
Section of Endocrine Surgery
New York, USA

René Jancovici, MD
Professor
Hôpital d'Instruction des Armées Percy
Department of Thoracic and General Surgery
Clamart, France

Minna Kauko, MD, PhD
North Karelian Central Hospital
Department of Obstetrics and Gynecology
Joensuu, Finland

Loïc Lang-Lazdunski
Hôpital d'Instruction des Armées Percy
Department of Thoracic and General Surgery
Clamart, France

Giovanni Lesti, MD
Professor
Department of Surgery
Hospital „Renzetti"
Lanciano, Italy

Heikki Löppönen, MD, PhD
Oulo University Hospital
Department of Otorhinolaryngology
Oulo, Finland

Francisco Lozano Moreno, MD
Hospital Don Benito-Villanueva
Orthopedic Surgery Service
Don Benito (BA), Spain

Donal Maguire, MD, FRCSI
University College Hospital
Galway, Ireland

Oliver J. McAnena, MCh, FRCSI
University College Hospital
Galway, Ireland

Hubert Mignot
Centre Hospitalier Général
Saintes, France

Hartwig-Richard Nürnberger, MD
Klinikum Dortmund GmbH
Surgical Clinic
Dortmund, Germany

Radoslav Perunovic, MD, MSci
KBC „Dr Dragisa Misovic" University Hospital
Surgical Ward
Belgrade, Serbia

Colm Power, FRCSI
University College Hospital
Galway, Ireland

François Psalmon
Clinique de la Marche
Guéret, France

François Quenet, MD
CRLC Val d'Aurelle
Paul-Lamarque
Montpellier, France

Thomas Reck, MD
Professor
Surgical Clinic
Krankenhaus der Bundesknappschaft
Püttlingen, Germany

Xavier Rogiers, MD
Professor
Department of Hepatobiliary Surgery
University Hospital Hamburg Eppendorf
Hamburg, Germany

Christopher M.S. Royston
Hull Royal Infirmary
Hull, UK

Josef Scholler, MD
Donauspital
Department of Gynecology and Obstetrics
Vienna, Austria

Peter Charles Sedman
Hull Royal Infirmary
Hull, UK

Jukka Sirén, MD, PhD
Department of Gastroenterological
and General Surgery
Helsinki University Central Hospital
Meilahti Hospital
Helsinki, Finland

Nicholas Steventon
Oxford, UK

Evangelos C. Tsimoyiannis, MD, FACS
Department of Surgery
G. Hatzikosta General Hospital
Ioannina, Greece

Jean Vandromme, MD
Centre Hospitalier Universitaire St. Pierre
Department of Gynecology and Obstetrics
Brussels, Belgium

Petri Voutilainen
Selkämeri Hospital
Kristiinankaupunki, Finland

Bruno Walther, MD
Associate Professor
Lund University Hospital
Department of Surgery
Lund, Sweden

Dimitris Zacharoulis, MD
University of Thessaly
Larisa, Greece

Contents

1 UltraCision: System and Instruments

W. Feil

The UltraCision system utilizes ultrasonic energy to enable hemostatic cutting and/or coagulation of soft tissue. The system consists of an ultrasonic generator (Fig. 1.1), a footswitch, an optional hand-switching adapter, a hand piece, and a variety of open and minimally invasive instruments.

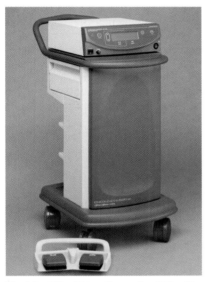

Fig. 1.1   UltraCision Generator 300 with cart.

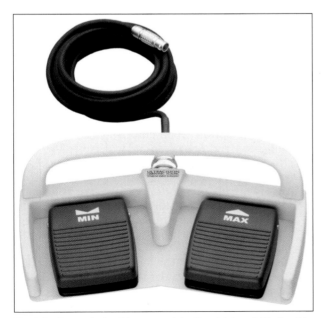

Fig. 1.2   Footswitch with two pedals: the right pedal is fixed to level 5; the left pedal can be changed from levels 1 to 5, but preferably is set to level 2 or 3.

The UltraCision instruments vibrate longitudinally at 55 500 Hz. This ultrasonic vibration enhances the blade's cutting ability and coagulates blood vessels as tissues are incised. Hemostasis occurs when tissues are coupled with the instrument. This coupling causes collagen molecules within the tissue to vibrate and become denatured, thus forming a coagulum.

The UltraCision system is indicated for soft tissue incisions when bleeding control and minimal thermal injury are desired. The instruments can be used as an adjunct to or substitute for electrosurgery, lasers, or steel scalpels.

The generator is connected to a regular power supply. It supplies the hand piece with electrical energy and facilitates the selection of power levels, system monitoring, and system diagnosis. The footswitch (Fig. 1.2) has two pedals to activate the ultrasound application. For the left pedal, ultrasound energy can be chosen from five levels (25 to 100 µm longitudinal extension of vibration) on the generator. The right pedal is set to level 5 (100 µm) solely.

Generator

There are two types of generators: first and second generation.

The first-generation generator (Fig. 1.3) is connected to the local alternating current supply. The electrical connector and the cooling air source connector from the silicon tube are connected to the generator. The electrical connector provides the power supply for the ultrasonic transducer in the hand piece and allows continuous monitoring of ultrasonic function by the generator's electronics. Irregularities of ultrasonic vibration in any part of the system will result in an acoustic signal and immediate shutdown of the system.

After switching the system on, the device performs a brief system test and is then ready for use. The standby mode on the generator is intended for use during assembly or during the change of assembled instruments.

The second-generation generator (Fig. 1.4a) provides only one connector for the cable leading to the hand piece.

The generator delivers two power levels: minimum (Min) and maximum (Max). The minimum power level may be adjusted by the user from level 1 to level 5. The maximum power level is always level 5. With all instruments except the ball coagulator, use a higher generator power level for higher tissue cutting speed,

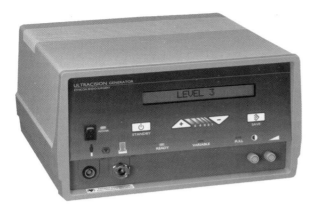

Fig. 1.**3**   First-generation generator.

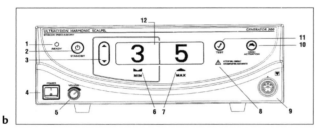

a

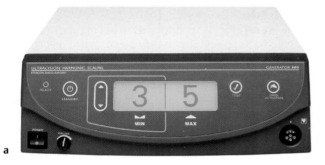

b

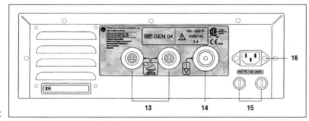

c

Fig. 1.**4 a** Second-generation generator (Generator 300). **b** Operation of the Generator 300 (front panel). **c** Operation of the Generator 300 (back panel).

and a lower generator power level for greater coagulation. For the ball coagulator, higher generator power levels will provide greater coagulation. The amount of energy delivered to the tissue and resultant tissue effects are a function of many factors, including the power level selected, instrument characteristics, grip force (when applicable), tissue tension, tissue type, pathology, and surgical technique.

The front panel (Fig. 1.**4 b**) of the generator has all the controls needed for the practical use of the system.

1) **Ready:** When this indicator is green, the system is ready for activation.
Note: In the Ready mode, for self-diagnostic purposes, the system sends a low-amplitude signal to the blade, causing the blade to vibrate slightly. This vibration does not pose a risk to the user.

2) **Standby:** Push this button to enter or exit the Standby mode. In Standby mode, all power is removed from the hand piece. Both the footswitch and hand switch are disabled. Upon power-up, the system defaults to Standby. The system is ready for TEST in the Standby mode. When the generator is on standby, the indicator is orange.

3) **Increase/Decrease Power:** Push this button to increase or decrease the minimum (Min) power setting to the desired level (from 1 to 5). The level chosen will be shown on the graphic display. The power level may be adjusted when the generator is in the Ready or Standby modes.

4) **Power:** This switch controls the main electrical power to the generator.

5) **Volume:** Turn this knob to adjust the volume of the activation tones. A tone will sound demonstrating the volume level selected.

6) **Min:** Indicates the user-settable minimum power level setting. When this power level is activated, the Min indicator will flash. On power-up the system defaults to Min level 3. Refer to the instruments' package inserts for the recommended Min power level.

7) **Max:** Indicates the maximum power level setting (level 5). When this power level is activated, the Max indicator will flash.

8) **Alarm Indicator:** This red indicator only appears if a system alarm occurs in response to a component or generator problem.

9) **Hand Piece Receptacle:** This receptacle is used to connect the hand piece to the generator.

10) **Hand Activation:** When the indicator is green, hand activation on the hand switching adapter is enabled. To disable the Hand Activation mode, press the button. Upon power-up, the system defaults to Hand Activation mode disabled.
Note: If the footswitch is installed, the footswitch is always enabled.

11) **Test:** Pressing this button initiates the Test mode. This mode is used during troubleshooting. The generator will emit a tone when the Test mode is active and "test in progress" will appear on the display.

12) **Graphic Display:** In the Ready or Standby modes, this display indicates the minimum (user-settable level 1 to 5) and maximum (level 5) power levels. If a system or component problem exists, error codes will appear on this display.
The back panel of the generator (Fig. 1.**4 c**) bears connectors and fuse holders.

13) **Footswitch Receptacles:** For the user's convenience, identical receptacles allow connection of one or two footswitch assemblies. If only a single footswitch is to be used, it may be connected to either receptacle.

14) **Potential Equalization Terminal:** This terminal provides a means for connection to a Potential Equalization Conductor.

15) **Fuses:** Refer to the "replacement parts" drawings in the back of the manual for additional fuse locations and fuse type.

16) **Power Cord Receptacle:** This receptacle is used to attach the power cord to the generator. For power cord requirements, refer to the manual's chapter 10, System Specifications.

Audible Signals: The generator delivers audible tones to signal activation, test, and alarm states. The user may choose from three activation tone pitches.

Silicon Tube/Cable and Hand Piece with Ultrasonic Transducer

The hand piece contains an acoustic transducer that converts the electrical energy supplied by the generator to mechanical motion. The transducer is connected to an ultrasonic wave guide/amplifier that amplifies the motion produced by the transducer and relays it to the instrument.

There are three types of silicon tubes/cables connecting the instruments and the generator. The 3 m long silicon tube of the basic equipment has two at-

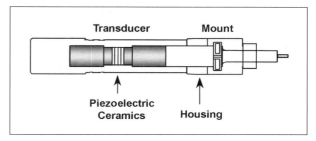

Fig. 1.**5**   Hand piece with ultrasonic transducer.

tachments for connection to the first-generation generator (Fig. 1.**5**). The silicon tube carries the air stream for cooling the ultrasound system and holds the electric supply for the ultrasonic transducer, which is situated in the hand piece at the other end of the silicon tube.

> Editor's tip: The silicon tube can be secured to the drapes with the two clamps. In every case, ensure when fixing the silicon tube to the operating table that no adhesive materials are used and that the cooling air stream is not reduced through kinking.

The hand piece contains the ultrasonic transducer and the ultrasonic amplifier (Fig. 1.**6**). Electrical energy is converted to ultrasonic energy through a piezoelectric ceramic system.

The 3 m long silicon cable of the revised system (Fig. 1.**7 a**) connects to the electric plug of the first-generation generator and has a stopcock to deactivate

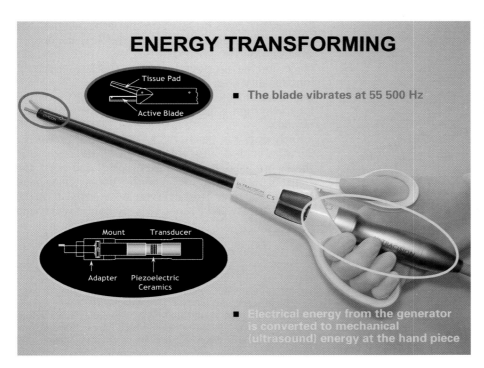

Fig. 1.**6**   Electrical energy is converted into ultrasonic vibration in a Piezoelectric ceramic system. Energy is transferred to the blade systems by an acoustic mount coupled to the housing of the hand piece.

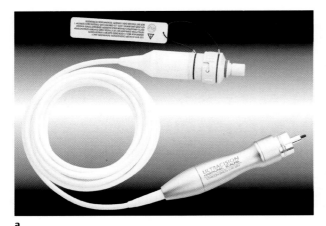

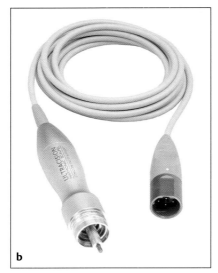

Fig. 1.**7a**   Silicone tube with one connector for the generator, and a stopcock to deactivate the cooling air supply on one side and the acoustic mount with the ultrasonic transducer on the other side. **b** Silicon cable for the Generator 300.

the cooling air supply when the old generator is used. The new cable is slim and supple, thus promoting ergonomic surgical work.

The revised cable and hand piece provide major benefits and will replace the standard equipment stepwise.

The new cable (Fig. 1.**7b**) bears only one connector for the Generator 300 and may also be used with the hand-activation adapter. The silicon cable, either with or without the hand piece, is removed from the sterile tray (if provided) and connected to the generator (Fig. 1.**8**). The second-generation generator is compatible only with the new metal hand piece; the first-generation generator is compatible with both the standard silicone cable and hand piece and the new slim cable without the need for air cooling.

The appropriate adapter (if necessary) is then assembled, the blade system is screwed onto the attachment and is fixed with the torque wrench.

Blade Wrench

The blade wrench (Fig. 1.**9**) is designed as a torque wrench to ensure secure fixation of the screw connection between the blade system and the ultrasonic transducer. The adapter must always be secured to the hand piece first, and the blade system subsequently. If assembled incorrectly, the silicon rings on the instruments can be damaged. The blade system is tightened with the blade wrench.

Test Tip

The test tip (Fig. 1.**10**) serves to check the functionality of the ultrasonic scalpel when the first-generation generator is used. The test tip is screwed on instead of a blade, and the ultrasound system is checked for correct functionality. (Fig. 1.**11**).

When using the Generator 300 the testing procedure for the system is performed with the instrument attached.

Each time the generator is activated after exiting Standby, hold the instrument in the air (if coagulating shears are used, open the clamp arm) and press the "Min" or "Max" power level on the footswitch or hand switching adapter. "Test in Progress" will appear on the graphic display and a rapid, two-tone pulse will sound

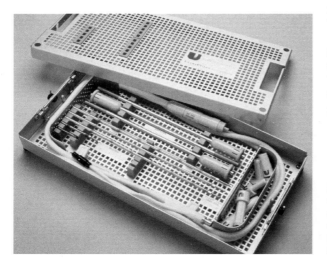

Fig. 1.**8**   The sterile tray carries the silicone tube (3 m) or cable with hand piece and ultrasonic transducer, the blade wrench and the test tip. In some countries, where reusable blades are offered, the tray contains a laparoscopic 10 mm blade system (three blades and sheaths), adapters, and an HS2 blade with adapter for open surgery.

while the test occurs. During this five-second period, a system check is being performed.

If the system is operating properly, the activation tone corresponding to the power level activated will be heard when the check is complete. Stop activation, position the instrument on tissue, and resume activation. If the system is not operating properly, an error code will appear.

The footswitch or hand switch must be pressed until the system check is complete. If the switch is released prematurely, the check will reinitiate at the next activation.

The Hand Activation button on the generator control panel must be illuminated for the hand switch to be active. To deactivate the hand switch, press the Hand Activation button (if the Hand Activation button is not illuminated, the hand switch will be inactive).

If the hand switch will not turn off during operation, press the button corresponding to the power level opposite that being activated to turn it off. An alarm will sound. Release the button to silence the alarm. Place the generator on Standby and replace the hand switch, or continue using the footswitch after deactivating the hand switch.

If the system senses a generator, hand piece, or instrument fault during use, an audible alarm (a tone with long pulses) will sound and a visual alarm indicator will appear on the control panel.

Editor's tip: Close and longer contact of the working blade with metallic material (e.g., clamps) results in ultrasonic coupling, which may cause damage to the blade. Such damage is not necessarily detectable with the naked eye. When a damaged blade is activated the generator will emit a continuous alarm sound. The damaged blade should be dismounted and the proper generator function documented with the Test Tip or with the testing procedure of the Generator 300. Ultrasonic coupling also will produce audible frequencies, which are harmless but may well be uncomfortable.

The Blades

The mechanical motion from the acoustic amplifier advances to the instrument, transmitting ultrasonic energy which enables hemostatic cutting and/or coagulation of tissue.

Editor's comment: One of the surgeons' most frequently asked questions is about the design of the sickle-like blades. When the prototype generator was built, the system was connected to a conventional rectangular dissecting hook familiar from laparoscopic cholecystectomy, but the ultrasonic wave forces caused immediate breakage of those instruments. Further development with specific

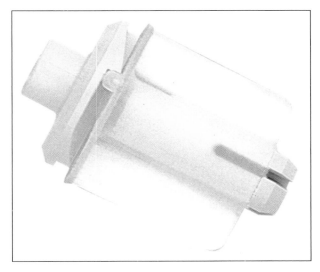

Fig. 1.9   The blade wrench is used to securely tighten the blade to the coupling mount.

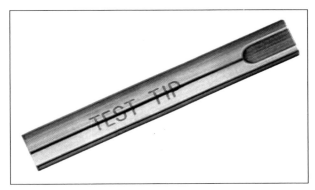

Fig. 1.10   The test tip is used to check the system prior to attachment of a blade, or to check generator function when a defective blade causes a system error.

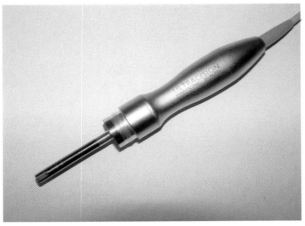

Fig. 1.11   Test tip attached to revised hand piece.

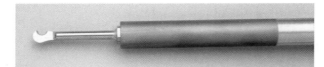

Fig. 1.**12** The first "Laparosonic Dissecting Hook" was designed in 1991.

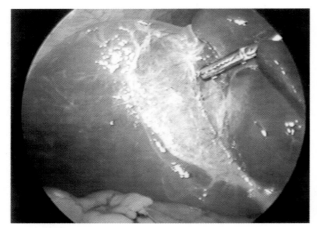

Fig. 1.**13** The first human laparoscopic cholecystectomy was performed by Joe Amaral in 1991.

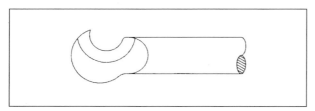

Fig. 1.**14** The former HS2 blade is designed like a sharp sickle.

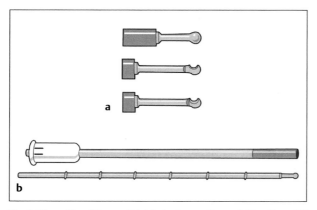

Fig. 1.**15 a** The 10 mm SH blade is configured like the HS2 blade with a 40° open angle; the 10 mm DH blade presents a more dull blade surface with a 60° open angle. **b** The active blade is covered by a protecting sheath. The silicone rings at the "nodes" affix the blade to the sheath without energy losses.

consideration of the mechanical forces of the ultrasound wave led to the refined instrument (Fig. 1.**12**) used for the first laparoscopic cholecystectomy conducted by Joe Amaral in 1991 (Fig. 1.**13**).

The shape of the former HS2 blade (Fig. 1.**14**) reflects the original blade design and is used for open surgery. The same design is also used for the 10 mm SH blade (Fig. 1.**15 a**). The silicone rings are fixed on those positions of the blade where the amplitude of the mechanical vibration wave is zero. At these points the blade is guided in the protection sheath (Fig. 1.**15 b**).

A variety of 5 mm blades for open and laparoscopic surgery (Fig. 1.**16 a, b**) offer surgical preparation and dissection opportunities for all purposes. The basic design corresponds to the original 10 mm blades; the active working blade with silicone rings is covered by a protective sheath. In the case of the 5 mm blades, these two components cannot be taken apart.

Editor's comment: The black covering sheath of the 5 mm blades is not completely attached to the working blade. This is visible at the tip of the instrument, where fluid and debris can enter the narrow channel between blade and sheath. This space is obviously not accessible for cleaning procedures.

The 5 mm blades for laparoscopic surgery (working length 32 cm) are offered in four tip configurations (Fig. 1.**17 a–d**). The sharp (SH) blade presents with a sharp inner side perfectly suited for quick cutting. The dissecting (DH) blade is a little more open and less sharp—a perfect tool for a more blunt dissection and cutting. The coagulation ball is suited for hemostasis in parenchymatous organs (e.g., the liver) if frank, venous bleeding is pouring from the liver bed during cholecystectomy. The HS blade shape was constructed in a shorter version specifically for harvesting the mammarian vessels for coronary bypass operations, but it has proved to be suitable for other purposes as well.

For open surgery the SH and DH blades come in 10 and 14 cm sizes (Fig. 1.**18 a–c**), as do HS blades (Fig. 1.**19 a, b**). With the 14 cm long version, an additional rubber grip extension is provided for ergonomic handling (Fig. 1.**20**).

Additionally, the new 5 mm HF blade has been introduced (Fig. 1.**21 a, b**). Compared to the standard curved HS blade, the tip is more pointed and sharp and the side margin is also sharper. This blade is a perfect tool for quick cutting as well as dissection of smaller vessels, providing sufficient hemostasis.

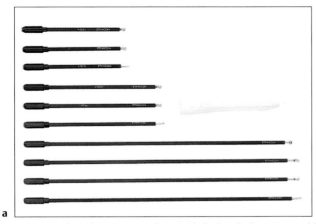

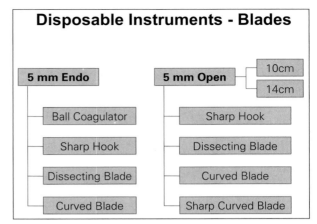

Disposable Instruments - Blades

5 mm Endo	5 mm Open	
		10cm
		14cm
Ball Coagulator	Sharp Hook	
Sharp Hook	Dissecting Blade	
Dissecting Blade	Curved Blade	
Curved Blade	Sharp Curved Blade	

Fig. 1.**16 a, b** The 5 mm single-use blade family for open and laparoscopic surgery.

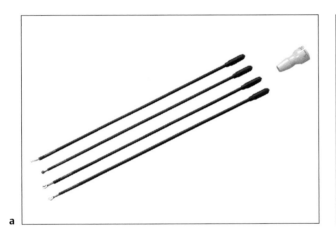

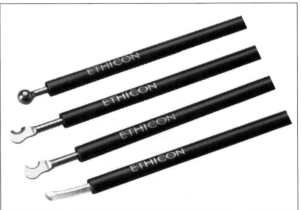

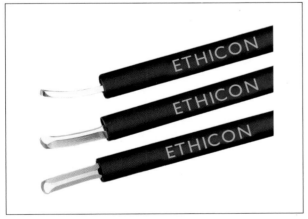

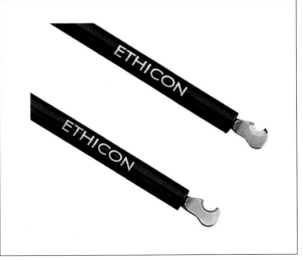

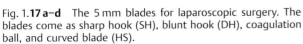

Fig. 1.**17 a–d** The 5 mm blades for laparoscopic surgery. The blades come as sharp hook (SH), blunt hook (DH), coagulation ball, and curved blade (HS).

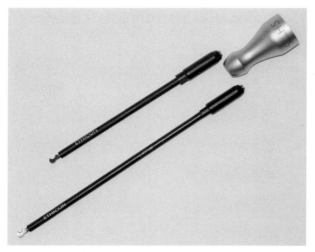

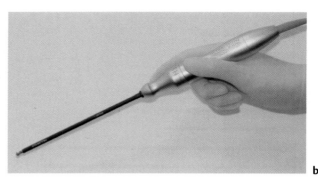

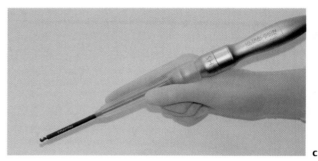

Fig. 1.**18 a–c**   The 5 mm SH and DH blade in 10 and 14 cm for open surgery connected to the standard hand piece.

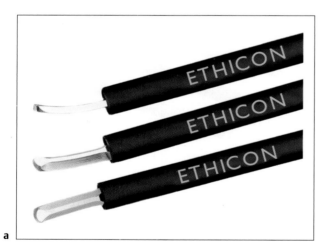

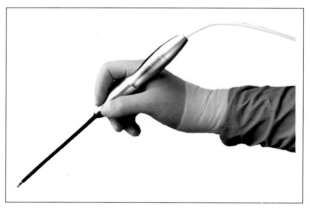

Fig. 1.**19 a, b**   The 5 mm HS blade in 10 and 14 cm suitable for open surgery.

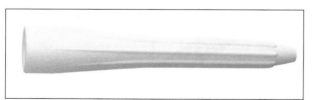

Fig. 1.**20**   Rubber grip extension for the 1 cm long 5 mm blades in open surgery.

The Shears

UltraCision shears of 5 and 10 mm size are offered for open and laparoscopic surgery, using different types of handles (Fig. 1.**22**). The latest development is the 5 mm shears with the curved blade tip (Fig. 1.**23**).

Editor's comment: Blades are perfect instruments for cutting. As it is necessary to press vessel walls together in order to achieve hemostasis with the activated blade, a counterpart to the blade is a prerequisite. Usually this counterpart is provided by the surrounding or underlying tissue (e.g., liver bed, soft tissue). Surgical experience with the first

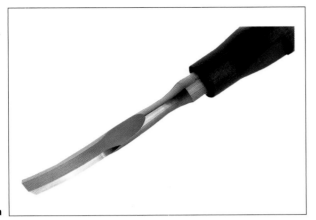

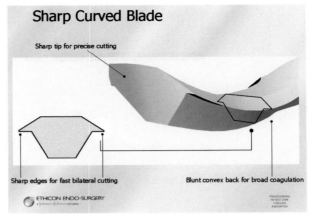

a

b

Fig. 1.**21 a**   The 5 mm HF blade for open surgery. **b** Design of the sharp curved HF blade, with a sharp edge used for flat, bilateral cutting.

blades showed clearly that such a regional tissue counterpart is absent in most cases of major surgery (e.g., transection of the mesentery). In this situation it is obviously necessary to provide a permanent local counterpart to the blade—the Teflon pad of the shears.

The first type of shears were the 10 mm LCS shears with the regular "pistol grip" (Fig. 1.**24**). These were followed by the 10 mm CS shears for open surgery (Fig. 1.**25**). The CS or LCS shears consist of a CS or LCS grip housing (tissue pad length 10 or 15 mm), a CS or LCS multifunction blade (active blade length of 10 or 15 mm), a CS/LCS adapter and a safety cotter pin (Fig. 1.**26**). The CS system for open surgery has a working length of 20 cm; the LCS for laparoscopic and open surgery has a working length of 33 cm.

The CS/LCS adapter is screwed onto the hand piece, and the multifunction blade is then affixed to the hand piece using the blade wrench. The active blade side is correctly positioned to the tissue pad and the security splint is then removed.

The multifunction blade has three sides: sharp, blunt, and flat (Fig. 1.**27**). The multifunction blade can be attached and fixed in three positions in the grip housing against the tissue pad. The blunt side of the blade is marked by a superficial hole.

Editor's comment: The ultrasound energy is propagated longitudinally in the active blade. At the nodes, the extension of the sinus wave is zero; this is where silicone rings are applied to guide the active blade in the protective sheath. In the middle, between the nodes, the longitudinal extension of the mechanical wave is at its maximum.

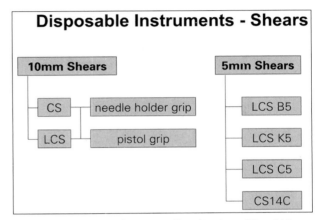

Fig. 1.**22**   UltraCision shears are offered in sizes of 5 and 10 mm for open and laparoscopic surgery, using different handles.

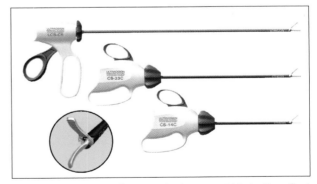

Fig. 1.**23**   The 5 mm shears with the curved-blade tip reflect the latest engineering development of the technique and provide instruments for both open and laparoscopic surgery.

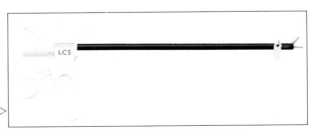

Fig. 1.**24**   The 10 mm LCS shears with pistol grip for laparo- ▷ scopic surgery.

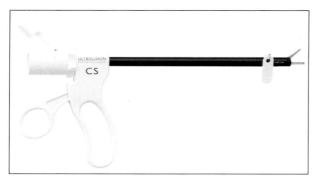

Fig. 1.**25**   The 10 mm CS shears with pistol grip for open surgery.

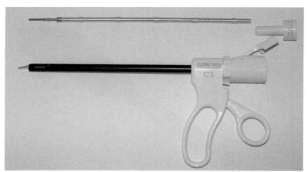

Fig. 1.**26**   The CS/LCS shears consist of a grip house assembly with security splint, working blade, and CS/LCS adapter.

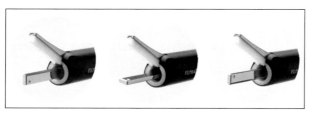

Fig. 1.**27**   UltraCision CS/LCS shears. Three types of blade configuration: sharp side, flat, and blunt.

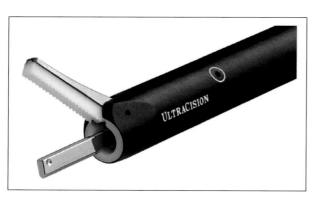

Fig. 1.**28**   The active blade of the CS/LCS shears vibrates 55 500 times per second.

The blade of the CS/LCS multifunction instrument vibrates axially with a frequency of 55 500 Hz (Fig. 1.**28**). An extension of this vibration between 25 µm (level 1) and 100 µm (level 5) can be selected on the generator. The ultrasound effect in the tissues is dependent on the setting of the device (levels 1 to 5), the type of tissue, the mechanical pressure against the Teflon-coated tissue pad, and the choice of blade side.

The lateral width of tissue exposed to ultrasound energy is dependent upon blade configuration. The sharp blade is designed for cutting tissues. Hemostasis occurs only to a very limited extent with this setting and is adequate only in the smallest blood vessels (Fig. 1.**29**). The width of the outermost lateral coagulation zone is 0.25 to 1 mm.

The blunt blade serves for both coaptation and coagulation and for tissue cutting. The extent of each of these functions depends on the setting and operation of the device and on the tissue (Fig. 1.**30**). The width of the lateral coagulation zone is 0.75 to 1.50 mm.

The flat side is suitable for hemostasis by means of coagulation (Fig. 1.**31**). The width of the lateral coagulation zone is up to 2 mm.

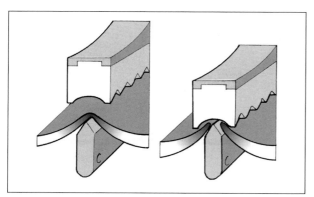

Fig. 1.**29**   When cutting tissue with the sharp blade of the CS/LCS shears, the lateral coagulation zone is 0.25 to 1.0 mm.

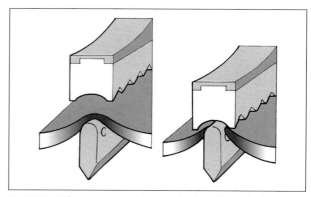

Fig. 1.**30**   When cutting tissue with the blunt blade of the CS/LCS shears, the lateral coagulation zone is 0.75 to 1.5 mm.

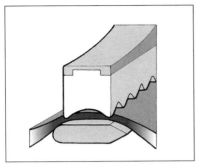

Fig. 1.**31** During coagulation with the flat side, the zone of necrosis corresponds to the thickness of the tissue pad (2 mm) of the CS/LCS shears.

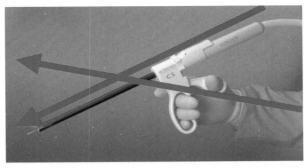

Fig. 1.**32** The "pistol grip" is at times not ergonomic because of the diverting axes between the forearm axis and the instrument axis. Additionally, elevation of the shoulder is needed frequently to bring the instrument into a working position.

Editor's comment: In laparoscopic surgery the use of an instrument with a pistol grip is not uncommon. Thus, the LCS shears were widely accepted; however, reflections to improve ergonomics were proposed by the surgical community. The problem of ergonomics with the pistol grip became obvious with the CS shears. The combination of the pistol grip, unusual in open surgery, with the relatively heavy hand piece and thick silicone cable standing out of the instrument raised serious complaints in terms of handling (Fig. 1.**32**).

Another problem with the pistol grip of the 10 mm CS/LCS shears is the fact that the blade itself is not rotatable. Occasionally, ridiculous anatomical positions of the surgeon's arm and upper body occurred because of this.

Another problem arose with the LCS shears in laparoscopic surgery due to the fact that, in certain situations, the tip of the instrument was hidden by the shaft. This problem was aggravated by the straight blade tip configuration (Fig. 1.**33**).

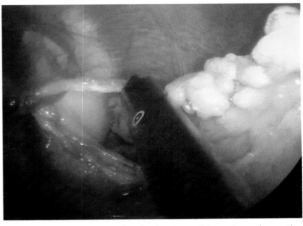

Fig. 1.**33** Laparoscopic fundoplication. Dissection along the greater curvature with LCS shears. Reduced sight to the tip.

These ergonomic complaints, especially in open surgery, led to the development of the "needle-holder grip" for the LCS (Fig. 1.**34**) and CS (Fig. 1.**35**) shears. In this way, the problem of diverted axes was eliminated (Fig. 1.**36**).

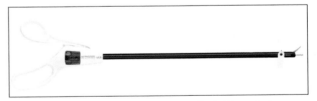

Fig. 1.**34** 10 mm LCS shears with "needle-holder grip."

Editor's comment: Most surgeons using the standard CS/LCS shears have chosen the blunt side of the blade for the majority of preparation and dissection work (more than 85 % of the time). The sharp and the flat side were infrequently used. The next step of instrument development was the 5 mm straight shears.

The 5 mm straight shears (Fig. **37 a**, **b**) present with one blade shape most likely resembling the blunt side of the CS/LCS blade. Not only the blade but also the whole tip of the instrument (including the Teflon pad) is rotatable. Accordingly, the bias of the pistol grip is minimized.

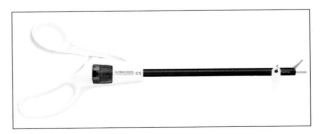

Fig. 1.**35** 10 mm CS shears with "needle-holder grip."

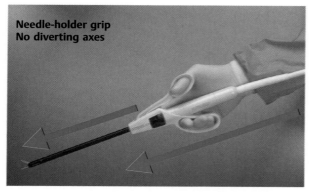

Fig. 1.**36** Improved ergonomics using the "needle-holder grip." The diversion between the forearm axis and the instrument axis is avoided. Only minor shoulder elevation by the surgeon is needed to bring the instrument into the desired position.

Editor's comment: The development of the 5 mm shears was the big step toward ergonomic instruments, leaving the somewhat clumsy 10 mm instruments aside. The next major issue was the development of a curved blade able to satisfactorily withstand the extreme forces of the ultrasound wave without shattering.

The new series of 5 mm shears offer instruments for open (Fig. 1.**38**; Fig. 1.**39**) and laparoscopic surgery (Fig. 1.**40**).

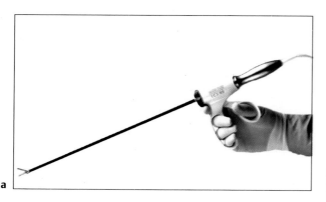
a

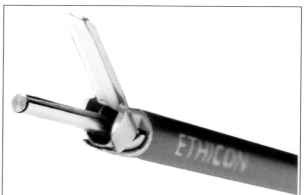
b

Fig. 1.**37 a, b**   5 mm straight shears. The tip of the instrument including the Teflon pad is rotatable.

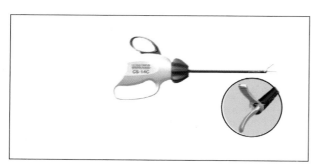

Fig. 1.**38**   The new 5 mm LCS C14 shears for open surgery.

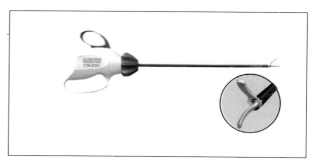

Fig. 1.**39**   The new 5 mm LCS C23 shears for open surgery.

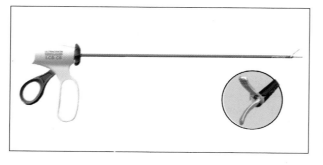

Fig. 1.**40**   The new 5 mm LCS C5 shears for laparoscopic surgery.

The Hand-Activated Blade

When using the Generator 300 the hand-activation adapter may be used (Fig. 1.**41**). The hand-activation adapter allows the user to activate the system either in minimum (Min) or maximum (Max) modes, depending upon which button is pressed. The hand activations are communicated to the microprocessor. The adapter may be used with a regular sharp blade, for example (Fig. 1.**42**).

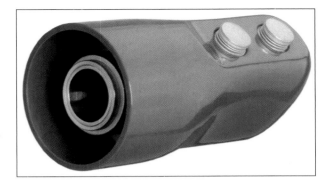

Fig. 1.**41** The new adapter for hand activation of the blades together with the Generator 300.

Fig. 1.**42** The new hand-activated system with an attached HF 105 blade.

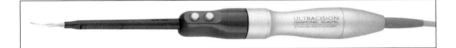

2 Principles of Ultrasonic Energy for Cutting and Coagulation

W. Feil

In minimally invasive video-endoscopic surgery, the technique of dissecting without blood loss is of paramount importance. The range of possible indications was significantly influenced by the reliability of the technology employed for dividing tissues while securing hemostasis. Thick and/or adipose structures with numerous blood vessels (greater omentum, mesentery of the large and small intestine, regional lymph drainage areas) have particularly poor accessibility for video-endoscopic hemostasis. Safe video-endoscopic division of these anatomical structures usually exceeds the capacity of both high frequency current techniques and video-endoscopic suturing. Ultrasound dissection technology (UltraCision) was developed as an alternative process.

UltraCision was conceived primarily for video-endoscopic surgery in order to dispense with the considerable disadvantages and risks associated with current high-frequency (HF) technology. UltraCision also facilitates new methods of extremely gentle surgical dissection techniques without blood loss.

The rationale of UltraCision is atraumatic surgical dissection and hemostasis that is gentle to the tissues, using direct application of ultrasound (Table 2.1). Electrical energy is converted into mechanical energy by the generator in the hand piece through a piezoelectric crystal system. The blade or tip of the instrument being used vibrates axially with a constant frequency of 55 500 Hz. The longitudinal extension of the vibration can be varied between 25 and 100 μm in five levels (see Chapter 1). The energy liberated as an ultrasound wave is directly applied to the tissue.

UltraCision yields four possible effects: cutting, cavitation, coaptation, and coagulation. These effects can be applied to the tissue solely or in synergic combination. The synergic expression of these four effects depends upon the type of tissue (each with its specific water content), level selection on the generator (extension of longitudinal vibration), application time of energy, type and handling of the active instruments, and tension and/or pressure to the tissue.

Table 2.**1** Limitation of indications in videoscopic surgery

Insufficient instruments for exact anatomical preparation
Unsatisfactory equipment for sufficient hemostasis (electrosurgery, laser, loops, sutures, clips, staplers, etc.)
Frequent instrument changes
Exploding costs

Premises for the Development of New Ultrasonically Activated Instruments

In surgery, it is possible to divide smaller and larger blood vessels between ligatures during dissection or to control them by transfixion in the event of active bleeding. In addition, high-frequency electrical coagulation (HF cautery) has been used in all branches of surgery for decades to deal with even the smallest sources of bleeding. HF cautery is used for cutting tissue as well as for hemostasis.

The techniques of tissue division and hemostasis familiar from open surgery cannot be used in the usual way in video-endoscopic surgery. This problem has led to various compromise solutions and has, hitherto, appreciably narrowed the range of indications of video-endoscopic surgery.

The "cautery hook" that is used mainly for laparoscopic cholecystectomy is suitable for dissection and division of anatomically distinct planes (i.e., non-infected cholecystectomy). The "hook", however, rapidly proves to be an inadequate instrument when local operating conditions are difficult, or when the range of indications of one's own video-endoscopic repertoire is being extended, especially as regards hemostasis.

Classical surgical dissection technique (forceps, scissors) can be used in video-endoscopic surgery up to the point at which clamps have to be applied and ligatures or transfixion placed under "open" conditions because of bleeding or for preliminary hemostasis. These situations can take place in a comparable manner in video-endoscopic surgery but are more difficult. Placing clips, suture loops, or transfixion sutures, or using stapling devices, even when the surgeon possesses the appropriate expertise, is often tedious, time-consuming, cost-intensive, and surgically unsatisfactory.

These limited technical possibilities prevented an extension of the range of indications of video-endoscopic surgery, but, on the other hand, they did stimulate the development of new technologies, such as UltraCision.

The problem of frequent instrument changes in "classic" videoscopic surgery is abolished by the implementation of the multipurpose instruments (e.g., CS and LCS shears) that enhance single-step preparation, hemostasis, and dissection.

The concept of ultrasound dissection was first developed for videoscopic surgery. General acceptance of this new technology rapidly enhanced the practical use of UltraCision in all fields of surgical activity, thus launching a variety of new instruments. Here, the contributions of surgeons exerted an influence on the development of new instruments, especially their ergonomics.

Arguments from the surgical community led to the development of more ergonomic handles and new instrument shapes. The arguments that led to the fitting of shear handles mainly originated in Europe and focused on the previously overlooked fact that the average glove size of a European surgeon is 7¹/₂ (Japan 7 and US 8).

> Editor's tip: The somewhat clumsy handling of the 10 mm CS shears in open surgery, which caused serious complaints among surgeons, has now been eliminated by the implementation of the new 5 mm CS shears.

Surgeons frequently complained about the need for a foot switch in open surgery, especially when using a blade. This led to the development of the hand-activated blade, which has been introduced to the surgical community only recently.

The argument of hand activation for the shears is still seen as controversial, and must be classified as a work in progress.

Ultrasonic Energy

The ultrasonically activated scalpel relies on the mechanical propagation of sound from an energy source. These waves are then conducted to an active blade element.

Sound waves are longitudinal mechanical pressure waves that propagate in solids, liquids, or gases. Longitudinal mechanical waves cover a large range of frequencies, with audible sound waves being confined to those frequencies that can stimulate the human ear and the corresponding part of the brain to the sensation of hearing: 20 to 20 000 cycles per second. A longitudinal wave with a frequency below 20 cycles per second, such as an earthquake wave, is called infrasonic; one whose frequency is above the audible range is called ultrasonic (Fig. 2.1).

Ultrasonic waves may be produced by applying electromagnetic energy to either piezoelectric (also termed electrostrictive) or magnetostrictive transducers, which create mechanical vibrations in response to electric or magnetic fields, respectively. When ultrasonic waves are applied at low power levels, no tissue effect occurs, as is the case with the waves used for diagnostic ultrasound imaging. Higher sound wave power levels and power densities, however, can be harnessed to produce surgical cutting, coagulation, and dissection of tissues.

UltraCision is an ultrasonic surgical instrument for cutting and coagulating tissue, operating at an ultrasonic frequency of 55 500 cycles per second (55.5 kHz). UltraCision is composed of a generator, hand piece, and blade. The hand piece houses the ultrasonic transducer, which consists of a stack of piezoelectric ceramics sandwiched under pressure between two metal cylinders (Fig. 2.2). The transducer is attached to a mount, which is then attached to the blade extender and blade.

The generator is a microprocessor-controlled, high-frequency switching power supply that drives the acoustic system in the hand piece with AC current. This results in vibration of the transducer at its natural harmonic frequency of 55.5 kHz. The microprocessor senses changes in the acoustic system to control power delivery and alert the user to system faults. The mechanical vibration established in the hand piece is con-

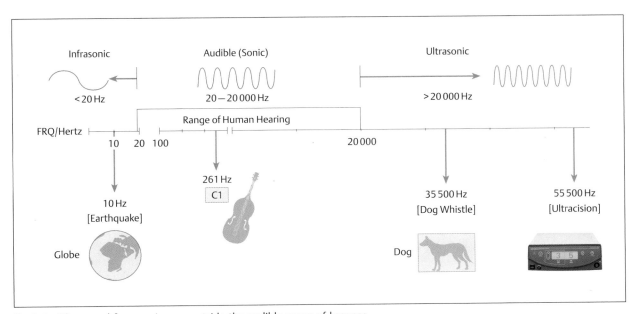

Fig. 2.**1**   Ultrasound frequencies are outside the audible range of humans.

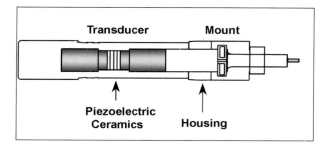

Fig. 2.**2**   Hand piece with ultrasonic transducer.

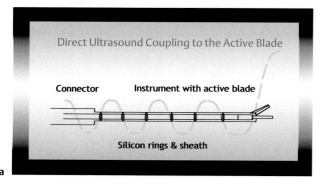

Fig. 2.**3**   The transducer is attached to a mount that is then attached to the blade extender and blade.

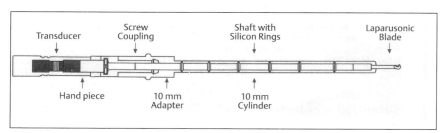

a

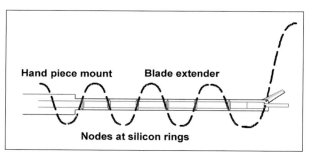

b

Fig. 2.**4 a**   Propagation of the ultrasound wave from the acoustic mount to the blade tip. **b** At the nodes, silicone rings attach the active vibrating blade to a protective sheath without energy losses.

the mechanical vibration wave is zero. At those points the blade is guided by the protection sheath (Fig. 2.**4 a, b**). The active vibrating blade is attached to the overtube without any mechanical wave energy losses, as the molecular movement is zero at these places.

Four Qualities of Action: Cutting, Cavitation, Coaptation, Coagulation

The basic mechanism for coagulating bleeding vessels ultrasonically is similar to that of electrosurgery or lasers. Vessels are coapted by tamponading, and sealed with a denatured protein coagulum. The manner in which protein is denatured, however, is completely different for each of these modalities. Electrosurgery and lasers form the coagulum by heating tissues to denature the protein. The former uses electric current, whereas the latter uses light energy.

With the new technology of UltraCision, coupling of the tissue with a mechanical ultrasound wave provokes molecular tissue alterations that completely differ from the local tissue damage produced by conventional cutting and/or coagulating devices, like laser or HF cautery.

Cutting

Cutting with UltraCision is completely different from cutting with an HF cautery device. With electrosurgery, cutting is achieved by extreme local heat produced by focused electric density, which causes the tissue to vaporize and disrupt. Cutting with UltraCision is more comparable to cutting with a regular cold steel scalpel. With UltraCision the blade is moved not only by the surgeon's hand but also by the propagated mechanical ultrasound wave.

ducted to a blade via an extender, to make the system the appropriate length depending upon the surgical application. The extender and blade shaft are housed in a protective sheath in a variety of diameters for laparoscopic and open surgery (Fig. 2.**3 a, b**). The entire system vibrates harmonically at a frequency of 55.5 kHz with a maximum longitudinal displacement of 100 µm.

The wave propagates as a sine wave from the acoustic mount to the tip of the blade. Silicone rings are fixed at the positions of the blade where the amplitude of

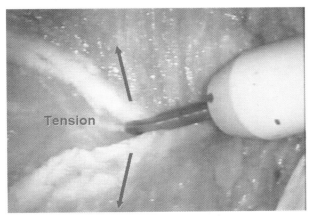

Fig. 2.**5**　Laparotomy by midline incision. Quick cutting of the prestretched fascia with the HS2 blade.

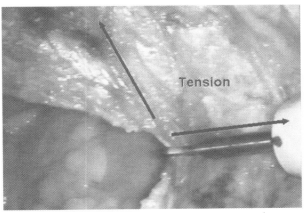

Fig. 2.**6**　Laparotomy by midline incision. Cutting of the (pre)peritoneum. Stretching and tension controls cutting speed.

Editor's tip: The effect of cutting can be explained by the "rubber band phenomenon." If the blade of a scalpel is applied to an unstretched rubber band, it will retreat because of its elasticity. However, if this rubber band is stretched close to its elastic limit, a light touch of the blade is enough to cut through it.

By using tension and/or pressure, the tissue is rapidly stretched beyond its elastic limit by the high-frequency vibration and is cut smoothly by a sharp blade or instrument tip. In order to enhance ultrasonic cutting, it is appropriate to prestretch the tissue (Figs. 2.**5**, 2.**6**).

The same tension has to be established to cut tissue in laparoscopic cholecystectomy. A dissecting blade can be used that is similar to the cautery hook familiar from HF surgery (Fig. 2.**7 a**).

When using a blade for cholecystectomy, the HC blade gives excellent performance of tissue dissection and cutting. It is possible to load up the tissue and cut it under visual control even with a relatively blunt instrument, like the HC blade (Fig. 2.**7 b**).

Editor's tip: It takes some experience to find the appropriate tension in order to cut tissue properly without bleeding. For obvious reasons it is recommended to practice this in open surgery.

Cutting speed depends on various factors: generator level, tissue condition, and blade sharpness. Ultrasonically activated blade cutting works with appropriate velocity with relatively blunt blades (Fig. 2.**7 c**), but functions very rapidly when the blade has a sharp edge.

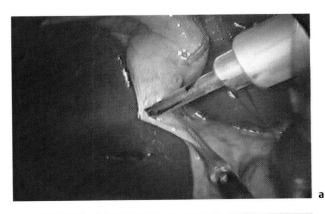

a

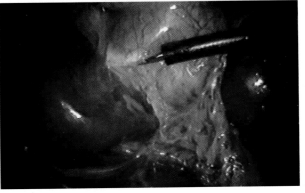

b

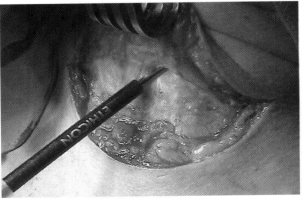

c

Fig. 2.**7 a**　Laparoscopic cholecystectomy with an UltraCision ▷ 10 mm dissection blade system. Cutting is achieved by application of energy and appropriate tension to the tissue. **b** Laparoscopic cholecystectomy with a 5 mm HC blade. Loading up the tissue and cutting it with the side of the activated blade. **c** Thyroid surgery: quick cutting of the soft tissue with a (relatively) blunt HC blade is enhanced by additional tension to the tissue.

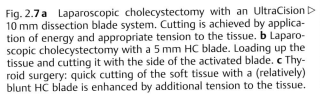

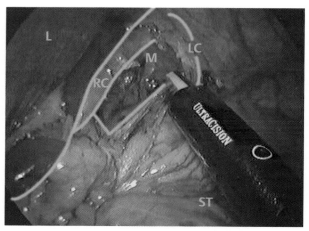

Fig. 2.**8**   Laparoscopic fundoplication with UltraCision LCS multifunctional shears. Application of energy in combination with pressure and tension to the tissue allows precise and hemostatic cutting with minimal tissue damage. *L* liver *RC* and *LC* right and left crus of the diaphragm. *M* mediastinum, *ST* stomach.

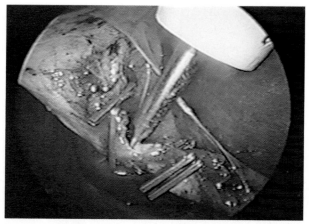

Fig. 2.**9**   Laparoscopic cholecystectomy with UltraCision 10 mm dissection blade. Cutting between applied clips is not harmful to either clips or cystic duct.

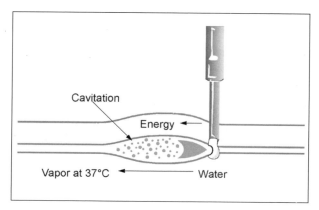

Fig. 2.**10**   Cavitation by application of ultrasound to the tissue causes dissection of tissue planes by water vaporization at body temperature.

Cutting with the shears follows the same physical premises. In laparoscopic fundoplication, cutting is achieved with the multifunctional shears (Fig. 2.**8**). Tissue tension is controlled by applying more or less pressure to the grip of the instrument and/or performing more or less tension to the tissue itself by pulling, pushing forward, or rotating the instrument in the appropriate direction.

Cutting with UltraCision is not restricted to tissue alone. It is also possible to cut other material, such as sutures, which can be easily cut using the dissecting blade. This can be beneficial in certain situations in video-endoscopic surgery, thereby avoiding the need for disposable scissors.

> Editor's tip: UltraCision must not be used for cutting bone, cartilage, metal, or other hard substances; otherwise blades may overheat and/or break. In order to prevent this, the system will immediately shut off in such situations and warn the surgeon by producing a continuous beeping sound.

Cutting with UltraCision is possible in the vicinity of metal clips or even staple rows, as long as these are merely touched rather than totally impacted in the jaws of the UltraCision shears. For example, it is feasible to cut the cystic duct between clips without any hazard to either clips or duct (Fig. 2.**9**).

Cavitation

Cavitation describes the formation and appearance of vapor bubbles in flowing liquids when the velocity is altered. If the pressure falls below the vapor pressure of a liquid whose flow is accelerating, vapor bubbles then form in the liquid. With subsequent deceleration, the pressure rises again, causing condensation. These large alterations of volume cause vigorous surges of pressure that lead to sound radiation and damage to solid bodies. Cavitation occurs, for example, in turbines, valves, and ship propellers.

When UltraCision is used, the cavitation occurs the other way around by means of high-frequency vibration of a solid body. The vibration is transmitted to the tissues and there leads to rapid volume changes of the tissue and cell fluid. This in turn leads to the formation of vapor bubbles at body temperature. In the parenchyma, cells explode while in connective tissue; the bubble formation leads to the dissection of tissue planes (Fig. 2.**10**).

Cavitation is associated with the presence of water and is therefore employed predominantly in tissues with a high water content. On the other hand, the cutting is preferred in tissues with extremely low water content (e.g., fascia). In laparoscopic cholecystectomy (Fig. 2.**11**), the cavitation leads to a separation of the planes of dissection. When additional pressure is used, coaptation is achieved additionally.

Cavitation to dissect tissue planes is of benefit especially in anatomically inaccessible regions or in the vicinity of vulnerable structures. The cavitation process is not

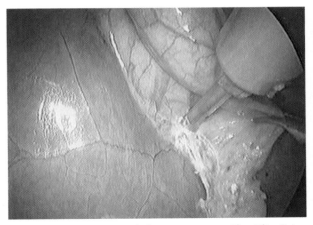

Fig. 2.**11** Laparoscopic cholecystectomy with UltraCision 10 mm dissection blade system. Cavitation is achieved by application of energy without pressure to the tissue causing dissection of tissue planes. Concomitant pressure will cause coaptation of underlying vessels.

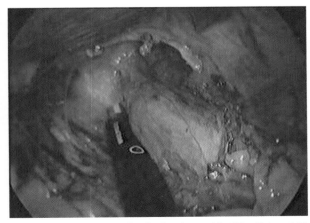

Fig. 2.**13** Laparoscopic fundoplication with UltraCision LCS multifunctional shears. Cavitation is used to separate tissue planes thus allowing blunt and gentle dissection along avascular anatomical planes. *M* mediastinum, *E* esophagus.

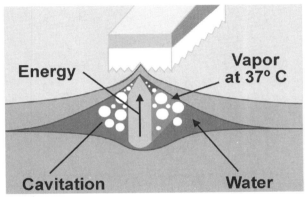

Fig. 2.**12** Cavitation and shears. Low pressure parallel to the active blade causes fluid to vaporize at low temperature. Cavitation causes separation of tissue planes.

only observed when using blades but also with the various shears. When using the shears, cavitation affects tissue on both sides parallel to the active blade (Fig. 2.**12**). In preparation for laparoscopic fundoplication (Fig. 2.**13**), exposure of the esophagus with the UltraCision LCS shears takes place in plain view, without any bleeding.

Cavitation results not only in the formation of gas bubbles at body temperature but also in desiccation of the tissue, as intra- and intercellular water is vaporized due to the repetitive exhaustive mechanical pressure changes induced by the ultrasound wave coupled with the tissue. This vaporization of water at local temperature dries the tissue out, and the induced tissue alterations lead to other effects of UltraCision—coaptation and coagulation (Fig. 2.**14 a**).

Cavitation is a side effect of the ultrasound-induced action that runs coincidentally with cutting, coaptation, and coagulation. Thus cavitation enhances visualization in the operative field by separating anatomical planes and initiates subsequent hemostasis by inducing tissue changes that set water free by mechanical alteration.

Cavitation as a side effect becomes apparent whenever ultrasonically activated blades are used (Fig. 2.**14 b**);

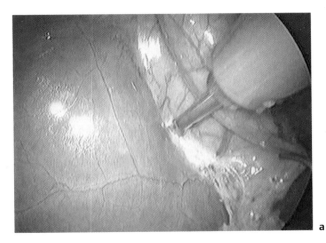

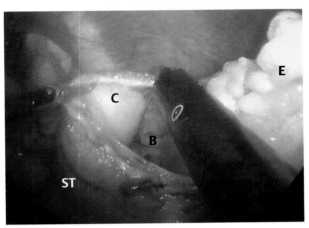

Fig. 2.**14 a** Cavitation helps to separate anatomical planes. In laparoscopic cholecystectomy the visceral peritoneum is elevated, and thus the dissection plane to the liver bed is opened. Cutting of an already coapted vessel (*V*) without bleeding can be done with the sharp edge of the blade by application of energy and concomitant tension. **b** Cavitation (*C*) as side effect when the omentum is dissected from the greater curvature in laparoscopic fundoplication. *B* bursa omentalis, *ST* stomach, *E* esophagus.

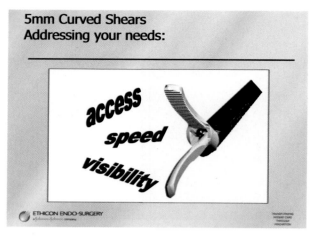

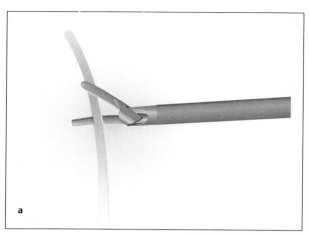

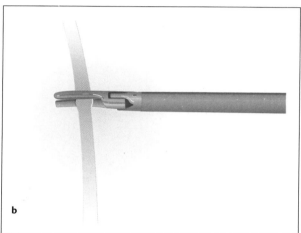

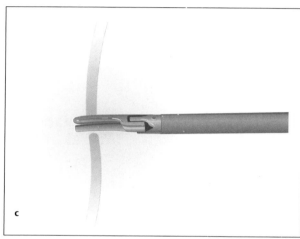

Fig. 2.15 a–c   Pressure and coaptation are the keywords for controlling bleeders. Application of ultrasound energy to the tissue, with exertion of pressure at the same time, leads to sealing of superficial vessels, which can then be divided without bleeding.

gas bubbles form and extremely small water drops are set free. The amount and size of the gas bubbles and the intensity of the resulting "fog" depends mainly on the tissue condition and the local tissue water content.

> Editor's tip: Using ultrasonically activated instruments causes formation of a "fog" that may reduce visibility in laparoscopic surgery. Leaving the valve of one port slightly open and thus producing a continuous refreshing air stream in the body cavity eliminates this problem. If appropriate, the use of a suction device close to the action field of the activated blade also gives excellent results.

Coaptation

Coaptation means the adherence and/or welding together of tissues. When ultrasound and pressure are used on tissue at the same time, there is disruption of the tertiary hydrogen bonds in proteins. This fragmentation of protein compounds causes the collagen molecules to collapse and leads to the adherence of collagen molecules at low temperature (body temperature up to max. 63 °C). The tissue is transformed into a sticky coaptate.

When coaptation is achieved and concomitant pressure is applied to the tissue (e.g., by pressing two vessel walls together), it is possible to seal these vessel walls by mechanically induced tissue alteration alone (Fig. 2.15 a–c). This tissue alteration consists of cavitation and of changes in the molecular structure of the tissue proteins—namely collapse and defragmentation of proteins at a temperature below 63 °C.

Coaptation and pressure are the keywords of UltraCision for the preliminary control of vessels in surgical preparation. Regional application of ultrasound energy to the tissue and concomitant pressure to the tissue seals (coaptates) the vessel walls together before transection. The effect of UltraCision is modified by level (from 1 to 5), shape of the active blade, tissue tension/pressure, and application time of energy.

Coagulation

When the locally applied energy acts for longer periods, there is also a rise in temperature leading to the thermally induced release of water vapor (63 to 100 °C) and later to coagulation at a maximum temperature of 150 °C.

Secondary heat arises from friction and causes protein denaturation (>63 °C) depending on exposure time (coupling of tissue with ultrasound energy). In practice, the transition between coaptation and coagulation is fluent. For coagulation (Fig. 2.**16**), the ultrasound energy is applied to the tissue together with pressure for longer periods (i.e., a few seconds). The additional thermal effect causes coagulation (denaturing) of proteins as well as coaptation (fragmentation).

The tissue changes induced by coagulation with UltraCision are not comparable with tissue changes caused by other coagulating devices like electrosurgery and/or laser.

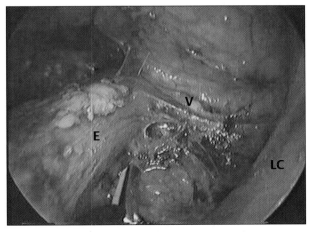

Fig. 2.**16**   Laparoscopic fundoplication with the UltraCision LCS multifunctional   shears. Application of energy in combination with pressure allows preliminary hemostasis, and then tissue transection. Atraumatic preparation of the distal esophagus (*E*) is achieved with no risk of thermal necrosis or bleeding. The coagulated venous plexus (*V*) aside the esophageal wall can be transected without any bleeding now. *LC* left crus of the diaphragm.

> Editor's comment: In practice there is a fluent transition between coaptation and coagulation that is mainly determined by the exposure time to ultrasonic energy. When ultrasonic energy is coupled with tissue this energy has to be transformed anyway and production of heat is one essential modality. Hence prolonged exposure time of the tissue with energy causes a local temperature rise and thus produces coagulation. If the exposure time is short, coaptation occurs instead since the temperature remains low.

In surgical practice all four effects (cutting, cavitation, coaptation, and coagulation) are applied simultaneously or consecutively. When using a blade, it is essential to have a local counterpart to be able to obtain pressure for sufficient hemostasis (Fig. 2.**17 a**). Cavitation is a frequent side effect, offering better visualization only under certain conditions (Fig. 2.**17 b**). The tissue can also be loaded on the blade (Fig. 2.**17 c**) and can be cut securely under full vision just by twisting the blade to the cutting edge (Fig. 2.**17 d**).

Synergy: The Principle of Practical Use

The four effects of UltraCision can always be used both as single functions and in any chosen modified synergistic combination (Fig. 2.**18**). The effect of the applied ultrasound energy on the tissue is dependent upon the following parameters:

● Control of ultrasound effect
● Type of tissue (parenchyma, connective tissue)
● Water content of the tissue

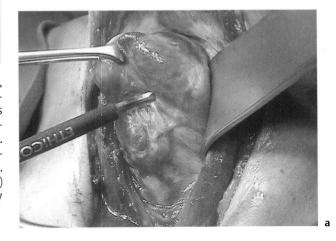

a

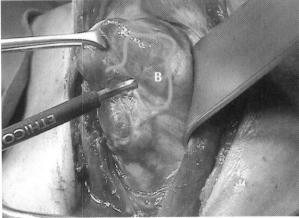

b

Fig. 2.**17**   Thyroid resection with the HC blade. **a** Coagulation of a vessel by obtaining pressure and applying energy. **b** Bubble formation (*B*) by cavitation separates fibrous capsule of the thyroid.

Fig. 2.**17 c, d** ▷

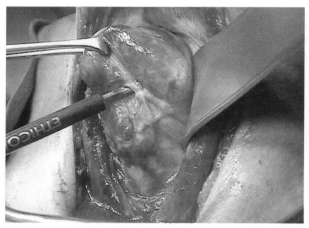
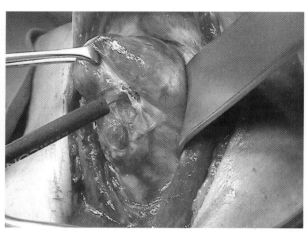

c   d

Fig. 2.**17 c**   Loading up the coapted/coagulated vessels and applying more energy to securely weld the vessels. **d** Twisting the blade to the cutting edge and transecting the sealed vessels.

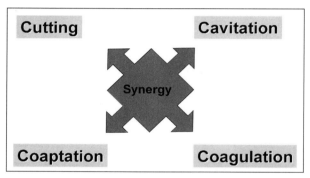

Fig. 2.**18**   Synergy of the four UltraCision effects: cutting, cavitation, coaptation, coagulation.

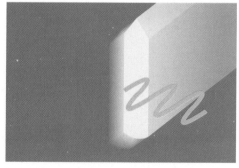

Fig. 2.**19**   Extension of the active blade tip at level 1 (approx. 25 µm).

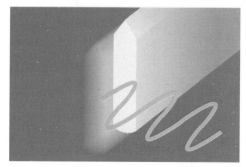

Fig. 2.**20**   Extension of the active blade tip at level 5 (approx. 100 µm).

- Setting of the device (variation of amplitude at five levels)
- Type of instrument used
- Operation of the instrument used
- Exertion of tension and/or pressure on the tissue
- Duration of energy effect on the tissue

The amplitude of the axial vibration of the tip of the instrument can be set on the generator at five levels, from level 1 to level 5.

At level 1 (Fig. 2.**19**), the axial amplitude of vibration (deflection of tip of instrument in its longitudinal axis) is 25 µm. The frequency of the ultrasound energy (55.5 kHz) is not affected by this setting.

At level 5 (Fig. 2.**20**), the amplitude of the vibration of the tip of the instrument is 100 µm. The vibration frequency remains 55.5 kHz.

> Editor's comment: The difference between level 1 and level 5 can be explained with an example: If you are cutting a slice from a loaf of bread, you could do it quickly with a long hub (level 5) of the knife, or slowly with a short hub (level 1). Coagulation is of no importance in the case of bread, but in surgical practice swifter cutting implies less coagulation and vice versa.

Apart from the type of instrument used (sharp, blunt, pointed, flat), the operation of the instrument is of importance.

The desired effect of ultrasound energy on the tissue depends on the synergistically combined application of ultrasound energy and mechanical force (tension and/or pressure on the tissue). When the CS/LCS shears are used, the side of the selected instrument blade (sharp, blunt, flat) is pressed against the Teflon-coated tissue pad with a variable degree of force. In addition, variable tension on the tissue can be exerted overall with the closed instrument. The "strength" of the ultrasound energy is selected by choosing the amplitude of the axial vibration of the blade (i.e., choosing from levels 1 to 5), and the amount of applied ultrasound energy is determined by the "application time" factor.

> Editor's comment: Depending upon personal preference, the surgeon emphasizes control predominantly by varying the level setting, or predominantly by varying pressure and tension. There is more than one "truth" in ultrasonic cutting and coagulation.

Sharp blades, exertion of tension and/or pressure on the tissues, and high ultrasound amplitude (level 5) lead to rapid tissue dissection and/or transection (Fig. 2.**21**). Blunt blades and/or instrument tips, low tension and/or pressure in the tissues, and low amplitude (levels 1, 2, or 3) lead to coaptation, and also to coagulation depending on the time of effect of the energy.

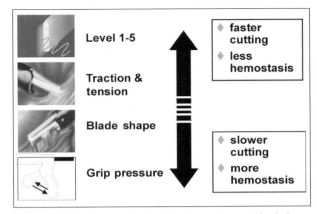

Fig. 2.**21** Practical use of the UltraCision shears. The balance between cutting and coagulation can be controlled by changing the level, applying more or less tension and traction, selecting a special blade or blade side, or applying more or less grip pressure.

Tissue Alterations with UltraCision and Electrosurgery

Local Tissue Temperature

In contrast to HF cautery, with UltraCision no electric current is passed through the patient. All of the risks associated with the application of electric current are thus avoided. The various effects of UltraCision in the tissues are achieved at temperatures of no more than 150 °C (Fig. 2.**22**). Coaptation leads to fragmentation of proteins and coagulation to denaturing of protein compounds. Cavitation occurs at body temperature, coaptation in the range between body temperature and below 100 °C, and coagulation at a temperature of up to 150 °C. In this way there is no burning, carbonization or smoke formation, as with cautery or the laser when temperatures of up to 400 °C may be reached.

Temperatures of over 150 °C, which cause burns and/or carbonization, do not occur when UltraCision is used. Conversely, to gain biological effects (e.g., hemostasis, tissue cutting) comparable to UltraCision using HF cautery or a laser can only be achieved at temperatures greatly in excess of 150 °C (Fig. 2.**23**).

Depth of Energy Penetration

When HF cautery is used, the maximum depth of penetration (Fig. 2.**24**) of the thermal electrical effect is reached soon after application of the HF current. When UltraCision is used, the depth of penetration of the flow of energy (measured in millimeters) has a linear correlation with time (measured in seconds). The possibility of deeper penetration of tissue can be controlled more precisely when using UltraCision by means of the "application time" factor.

After a five-second application time, which must not be exceeded during practical use of UltraCision, the

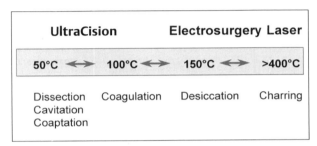

Fig. 2.**22** Local tissue temperature with UltraCision, electrosurgery, and laser.

Temp. (°C)	Visual Change	Biological Change
37-50	Swelling	Heating, retraction, reduced enzyme activity
50-65	Blanching	Coagulation
65-90	white/gray	Protein denaturation
90-100	Puckering	Drying of tissue
> 100	Drying	H_2O boils, Cell explosion
> 150	Charring	Carbonisation
300-400	Blackening	Smoke generation

Fig. 2.**23** Macroscopic and microscopic tissues changes with UltraCision, electrosurgery, and laser at various local tissue temperatures.

depth of penetration is less than half of an equal time of HF cautery. In practice, this means that with respect to coagulation achieving an effect equivalent to HF cautery will take longer with UltraCision, but the effect on tissues will be more readily controllable. Apart from the depth of penetration of the energy, the temperature in the tissues, and therefore the risk of unwanted thermal injury, is lower.

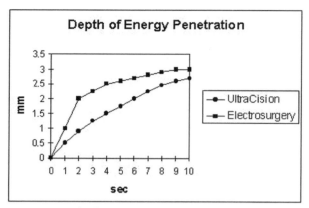

Fig. 2.**24** Depth of energy penetration (liver) using UltraCision or electrosurgery.

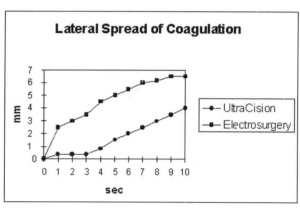

Fig. 2.**25** Lateral spread of energy (liver) using UltraCision or electrosurgery.

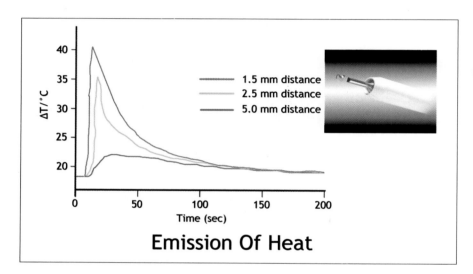

Fig. 2.**26** Emission of heat in relation to distance from the active blade. Heat alterations occur only in closest proximity to the active blade.

Lateral Energy Spread

Lateral spread of the energy flow, and the effect that can be achieved with it, reaches submaximum values after three seconds using HF cautery (Fig. 2.**25**). When UltraCision is used, there is a linear correlation between the time of application and the lateral spread of the effective energy flow.

The risk of distant tissue damage is lower with UltraCision than with HF cautery because of the lower lateral spread of the coagulation zone per se, and because of the effect that is controllable by the time factor.

Safe use of UltraCision allows low-risk dissection, even close to vulnerable structures (e.g., bowel, ureter, blood vessels) where use of the HF cautery carries a high potential for risk or is ruled out altogether.

Lateral Heat Emission

The lateral heat emission rate has been measured with temperature sensitive probes under various conditions (Fig. 2.**26**). Thus, it could be shown that temperature changes due to energy transformation occur only in close proximity to the active blade, whereas distant tissue is not (or at least very rarely) affected by heat alterations.

Conclusion

The application of ultrasonic energy to endoscopic surgery offers many advantages over the use of electromagnetic energy such as electrosurgery or laser surgery, without giving up the advantages of the latter energy forms. UltraCision allows tissue to be cut and coagulated with efficacy equal to that of electrosurgery. Unlike electrosurgery, however, there is no risk of stray electrical current injury, grounding pad failures, or electrical injury to the operator, since there is no electrical current in the surgical field. In addition, because of the lower heat generation, ultrasonic energy produces little smoke and minimal tissue charring or desiccation, leaving tissue planes and operative fields better visualized.

3 UltraCision Scalpel and Other Energy Modalities

W. Feil

Principles of High-Frequency Surgery

High-frequency electrical coagulation (HF cautery) in monopolar and bipolar form has been used in all branches of surgery for decades to deal with even the smallest sources of bleeding and to divide tissue (Fig. 3.1).

In HF surgery, high-frequency alternating current (500 to 1000 kHz; 100 to 20 000 V) is used on patients. The patient is thus connected directly to the electric circuit.

The principle of HF surgery is based upon an electrically-induced, localized development of heat that leads to denaturing of protein compounds, destruction of cells and tissues, and burning or carbonization.

When cutting with the HF cautery, the great heat at the tip of the instrument causes cells to burst from the release of water vapor. As a result of the extremely high temperature, there is immediate drying of the tissue, and burning and carbonization of the structures in the area affected by the instrument.

With the monopolar method (Figs. 3.2, 3.3a–c), which is the predominant method used, the electric current is sent directly through the patient. At the active instrument tip, the current density is bundled toward a large-surface, neutral electrode that is applied to the patient. The current density, which is high at the point, causes the liberation of heat energy and leads to coagulation and encrustation of the tissue.

With the bipolar method of HF surgery (Fig. 3.4), there is a flow of current between the limbs of a special forceps. In this case, the major part of the electrical current flows between the limbs of the instrument.

Disadvantages of HF Surgery

A fundamental disadvantage of HF cautery is the fact that electrical current is sent through the body of a (usually anesthetized) patient. As a result, all of the risks of using an electrical current are present (Table 3.1). The international literature reports numerous cases in open surgery of severe burns to patients due to leakage current, and even of explosions during the use of the HF cautery on the bowel.

In the event of the slightest damage to the surgical gloves, the surgeon's own hands may receive electrical shocks and burns when HF surgery is used.

Video-endoscopic operations are particularly burdened by complications associated with the use of electrosurgical methods (Table 3.2). Numerous cases

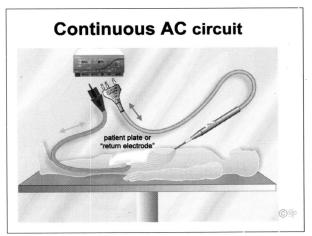

Fig. 3.**1** Flow of electrosurgical current in a complete monopolar unit. The current circuit is closed through the patient's body.

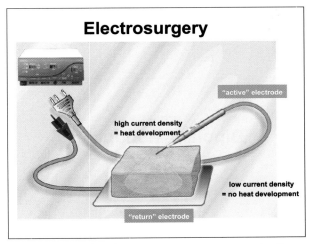

Fig. 3.**2** Monopolar electrosurgery: current passes to dispersive electrode. Current density focuses at tip of active electrode.

Table 3.**1** Disadvantages of HF surgery

Electrical current flows directly through the patient.
Electric shock and/or burns (on patient and/or surgeon).
Extensive, deep tissue damage (carbonization.)
Unnoticed distant tissue due to leakage current.

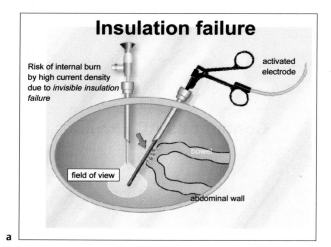

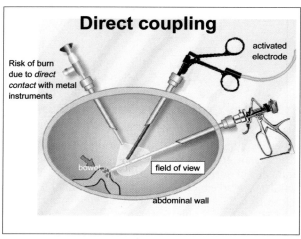

a

b

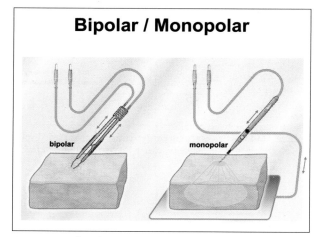

c

Fig. 3.**3 a, b, c** Monopolar electrosurgery: current passes through tissue to ground pad in videoscopic surgery. The current pathway follows the criteria of lowest electrical resistance.

---

have been reported in the literature in which tissue damage occurred distant from the actual operation area, resulting in very major postoperative complications. For laparoscopic cholecystectomy alone, there have been more than 30 different documented situations of electrosurgically-induced injuries.

Fig. 3.**4** Bipolar electrosurgery: most current is confined between two electrodes represented by the jaws of the bipolar forceps. When the conductivity of the sealed vessel is reduced (because it is dehydrated by local heat) the current pathway is guided through the adjacent structures, following Ohm's law.

Table 3.**2**   Causes of the complications of HF surgery

Unrecognized coagulation: direct thermal injury from an instrument tip that is briefly out of the surgeon's field of vision.

Absent or defective insulation of the instrument.

Direct contact, if an activated electrode is inadvertently brought into contact with the laparoscope or any other conductive instrument.

Contact with metal clips or other instruments.

Steel ports and/or hybrid ports.

Capacitive coupling, which is defined as the passage of current across the insulated part of a unipolar instrument electrode to an adjacent conductor (e.g., bowel loop).

Current flow through fluids and leakage currents.

In monopolar HF surgery, the electric current can arc to the tissue and cause injury far beyond the videoscopic field of vision and thus remain unnoticed by the surgeon. Such "current marks" in the intestinal tract can lead, after a delay of up to a week, to perforation and life-threatening peritonitis.

Rapid arcing of the electric current to the duodenum can occur during mobilization of adhesions between the duodenum and gallbladder with the HF cautery hook (Fig. 3.**5 a**). Even after a mere quarter-second contact time, there was an injury to the duodenum in the case illustrated that remained without sequelae.

Unnoticed bilateral duodenal perforations are often reported in the literature. The mortality of duodenal perforation is about 50%, as the bilateral perforations are often diagnosed and treated adequately only long after discharge to home care, due to the short postoperative period in hospital after cholecystectomy.

Defective insulation occurs in conventional cautery hooks mainly because of repeated cleaning procedures with, for example, sharp instruments or with the Ti polisher, when attempts are made to remove burnt-on and carbonized tissue remnants from the instrument. Insulation defects also arise from scrubbing on sharp-edged steel ports.

Due to short circuiting, injuries occur outside the videoscopic field of vision in the hollow organs of the intestinal tract or in the common bile duct.

Complications induced by electrosurgery also occur frequently in open surgery, but usually this "collateral damage" is ignored. Skin burns are the most common type of distant electrosurgical injury (Fig. 3.**5 b**). It can only be speculated about the frequency of complications induced by electrosurgical injury to inner organs, e.g., bowel wall at the site of an anastomosis.

Modern HF cautery often includes a so-called "cutting aid." With this, a peak current is applied immediately after pressing the foot pedal. This uncontrollable high energy leads rapidly to injuries of the gallbladder when the hook is used (Fig. 3.**6**). Leakage of bile makes the further course of the operation difficult, involves a possible risk of contamination, and causes the awkward and time-consuming loss of the stone in the abdomen.

A systemic problem with the HF hook is the absence of an adhesive effect. When hemostasis is attempted, burnt tissue often remains stuck to the forceps after coagulation is complete, and tears open small vessels again when the instrument is removed. This phenomenon also occurs in laparoscopic surgery (e.g., hemostasis in the liver bed) and is highly disagreeable. The cause is that the electrical conductivity of the desiccated, scorched tissue is reduced to zero.

Leakage currents due to uncontrolled and unpredictable conduction of the electric current in liquids are particularly dangerous. With video-endoscopic surgery, when bleeding occurs it is seldom possible to stop the injury adequately and to coagulate it because of the limited number of instruments, which in turn is due to the limited number of available ports.

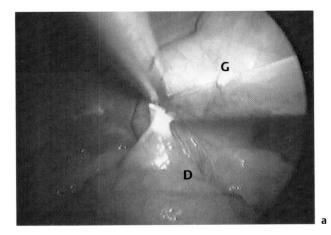

a

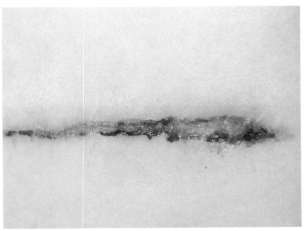

b

Fig. 3.**5 a** Adhesion between gallbladder (*G*) and duodenum (*D*) transected with monopolar electrosurgery: thermal lesion in the duodenal wall. This burn mark may cause perforation in up to a few days postoperatively. **b** Alternate site burn on the skin due to aberrant current conduction following open surgery with a monopolar electrocautery device.

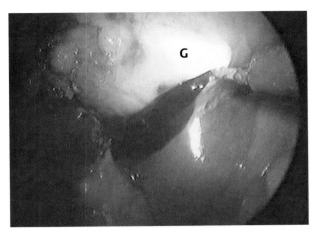

Fig. 3.**6** Thermal lesion of the gallbladder (*G*) and consecutive bile extravasation caused by electrosurgical hook dissector when a cautery device with "cutting aid" is used.

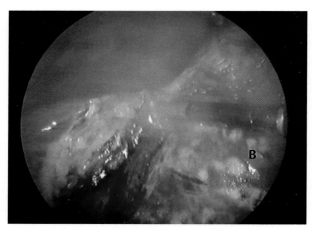

Fig. 3.**7** Laparoscopic cholecystectomy. Burn marks (*B*) in the liver produced by the proximal parts of the coagulating shears. Mostly unnoticed during surgery, since the surgeon is understandably focused on the "region of interest" at the resection site.

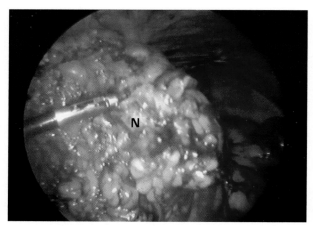

Fig. 3.**8** Extensive tissue necrosis (*N*) and consequent formation of smoke following electrosurgical coagulation in greater omentum.

Table 3.**3** Technological advantages of the UltraCision scalpel

No electrical current flows through the patient
No burns harm the patient
No distant tissue damage due to unnoticed leakage currents
No carbonization of tissue
No smoke formation
No depth effect, minimal lateral propagation of the energy flow
No neuromuscular stimulation
No neutral electrode
No electric shocks and/or burns harm the surgeon

The surgeon's focus is usually maintained at the point of direct action; for example, in laparoscopic cholecystectomy with the cautery shears, the interest is at the branches of the instrument. Thus, it may remain unrecognized that proximal parts of the instrument at the joints have had contact with tissue and have caused burn marks (Fig. 3.**7**).

Besides the development of extensive tissue necrosis, a particularly troublesome disadvantage of HF cautery in laparoscopic surgery is the often considerable smoke production (Fig. 3.**8**). The impairment of vision by the smoke often makes repeated deflation of the pneumoperitoneum necessary, causing considerable delays.

> Editor's comment: UltraCision produces not smoke, but "fog." These small water drops can be eliminated easily by suction or by leaving one port valve slightly open.

The recognized hazards of mainly monopolar HF surgery (Figs. 3.**3**, 3.**4**) have led to some suggested precautions. It is recommended to use the bipolar technique whenever possible. By passing from one jaw to another, the current does not spread to surrounding tissue (Fig. 3.**4**). The bipolar technique does not generate capacitive coupling. In spite of its recognized advantages, bipolar electrosurgery has not been accepted by the surgical community in laparoscopic surgery. The American College of Surgeons stated that 86% of its surgeons prefer monopolar to bipolar surgery (the remaining 14% use bipolar or laser) and that the coagulation mode is preferred to the cut mode. Presumably, surgeons in Europe and elsewhere have similar preferences.

> Editor's tip: The development of the UltraCision scalpel eliminated the disadvantages of HF current technology for video-endoscopic surgery and establishes a new technology for tissue dissection, tissue division, and hemostasis.

Technological Advantages of the UltraCision Scalpel

In video-endoscopic surgery, nearly all of the risks and complications associated with HF surgery can be avoided by the use of the UltraCision Scalpel (Table 3.**3**). This applies especially (corresponding to the frequency of occurrence) to injuries of the biliary tract and intestinal tract due to cautery hooks, problems with insulation, local short circuits through ports, or unnoticed leakage currents.

Dissection, cutting, and hemostasis are possible in a single procedure when using multifunction instruments in comparison to the use of HF cautery. The low depth of penetration and the minimal lateral spread of

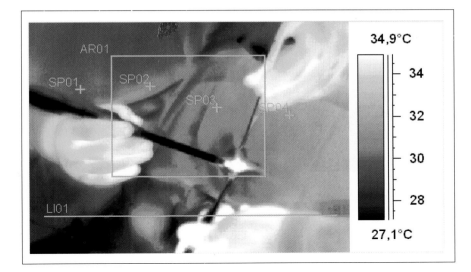

Fig. 3.**9** The ThermaCAM infrared video camera offers the opportunity to measure temperature to the nearest 0.1 °C. With the AGEMA Report software, spots (*SP01–05*), lines (*LI01*) or areas (*AR01*) can be selected for investigation.

energy reduce the risk of accidental tissue damage compared to HF cautery.

Infrared Thermography

The new technique of the ultrasonically activated scalpel posted a milestone in surgery. However, this technology had to withstand demanding comparisons to existing, widespread, and successful devices, mainly electrosurgery. In the attempt to prove the hypothesis that the ultrasonically activated scalpel provides a system that is able to extremely enhance tissue-friendly surgery without lateral damage, it became necessary to use infrared video-thermography for in-vivo and in-vitro research studies. In this way, absolute temperatures and the temperature changes at and around the activated blade and/or the tip of a cautery probe were investigated under various conditions.

A comparison was made between a conventional cautery device (Martin ME 400 Generator) and an UltraCision generator with a 5 mm HC blade and 5 mm LCS C5 shears. Thermography was performed with a ThermaCAM PM595 (FLIR Systems, Sweden) in vivo intraoperatively and ex vivo on human tissue. The ThermaCAM (focal plane array; uncooled microbolometer 320×240 pixels; spectral range 7.5 to 13 μm; measurement range 40 to 500 °C; validity ± 2 °C; sensitivity at 30 °C = 0.1 °C; standard bitmap output 8 bit) was connected to a SONY Vaio PCG X9 laptop computer (MESONIC, Austria) via an SCSI flashcard interface.

After calibration of the system, and fixing the expected temperature range, the object is taken with the ThermaCAM and bitmaps saved for further evaluation. Temperature can be measured at spots (SP01 to SP04), lines (LI01), or definable fields (AR01) (Fig. 3.**9**). For this investigation, spot measurement was used.

Data evaluation was performed with AGEMA Report 5.4 software. The camera automatically shows a visible picture (Fig. 3.**9**) by measuring the complete range of all temperatures in the total field of investigation. The digital data, which are recorded to an accuracy of 0.1 °C, cannot entirely be made graphically visible to the eye, even by using all possible differentiable colors to represent the data. To make the data presentable, the AGEMA software allows the user to pick out a temperature scale of interest and to modify the color scale for a defined range of temperature.

UltraCision (UC) Versus Electrosurgery (HF): Liver Ex Vivo

When both devices were investigated on the ex vivo human liver, the local temperature was 74.2 °C (HF) and 47.1 °C (UC) after one second (Fig. 3.**10**), 155.7 °C (HF) and 41.9 °C (UC) after three seconds at the instrument tip and 72.9 °C (HF) and 35.6 °C (UC) on the dissected tissue (Fig. 3.**11**). Four seconds later, the tissue had cooled down to 59.3 °C (HF) and 29.1 °C (UC) (Fig. 3.**12**).

The incision on the liver tissue clearly showed the difference between the cool cut of the ultrasonic scalpel and the extreme heat around the tip of the cautery probe. It also showed clearly that the temperature distribution in the tissue followed local (and thus predictable) rules of thermic bridging with the ultrasonic scalpel. With the electrocautery probe, however, tissue heating follows the rules of electrical conductance and current pathways. Accordingly, the extent and direction of tissue heating is unpredictable, because the electric conductivity cannot easily and reproducibly be assumed with the naked eye.

Besides the different temperature distribution, the cautery device produces significantly more heat for the same incision in the parenchyma.

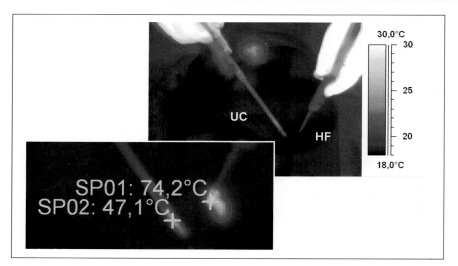

Fig. 3.**10** Human liver ex vivo: plain cut with a cautery probe (*HF*) and an UltraCision blade (*UC*). After one second, the temperature at the active blade tip is significantly higher at *SP01* (*HF*) than at *SP01* (*UC*).

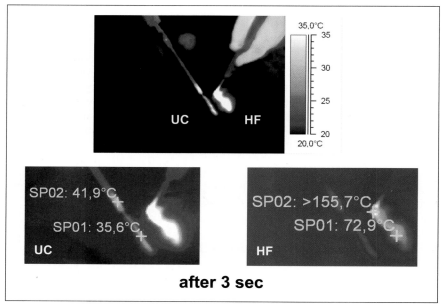

Fig. 3.**11** Human liver ex vivo: plain cut with a cautery probe (*HF*) and an UltraCision blade (*UC*). After three seconds, the temperature at the active blade tip and in the incision line is significantly lower with UltraCision (*UC*) as compared to electrocautery (*HF*).

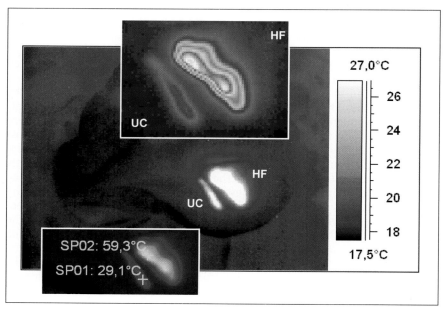

Fig. 3.**12** Human liver ex vivo: plain cut with a cautery probe (*HF*) and an UltraCision blade (*UC*). Four seconds later, the tissue is still hot after electrosurgery (SP02). Digital color correction with an alternate color scale (valid only for the upper insert) impressively shows the difference between UltraCision (*UC*) and electrocautery (*HF*). After electrosurgery, tissue remains significantly more heated and heat is confined to a larger area. After exposure to UltraCision (*UC*) for the same amount of time, tissue is cooler and temperature changes are confined solely to the cutting line.

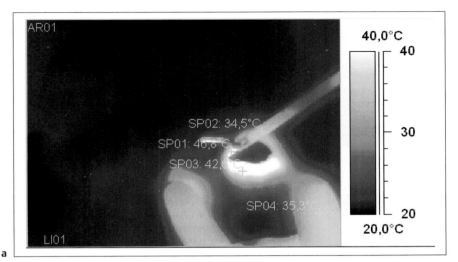

a

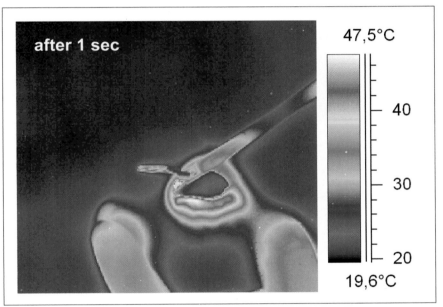

b

Fig. 3.**13 a:** UltraCision 5 mm CS shears in human mesentery ex vivo: after one second, local temperature around the blade is slightly elevated. *SP04* (note the surgeon's finger). **b:** UltraCision 5 mm CS shears in human mesentery ex vivo: color correction shows that after one second the temperature changes are confined to the blade and the tissue closest to the activated blade. The temperature changes in the distal parts of the shaft of the instrument are due to energy losses at the connection to the tip of the instrument.

UltraCision: Mesentery Ex Vivo

With the 5 mm CS shears in the mesentery, in vivo temperature was 42.6 °C (tissue) and 46.8 °C (blade) after one second (Fig. 3.**13 a, b**), after four seconds when the tissue was dissected 124.6 °C (blade) (Fig. 3.**14 a, b**), after five seconds 55.4 to 61.1 °C (tissue) and 66.9 °C (blade) (Fig. 3.**15**).

With UltraCision, temperature peaks of more than 100 °C are reached directly at the active blade. The blade cools down swiftly to an acceptable temperature that is not harmful for the tissue.

Editor's tip: Surgeons sometimes find that one can indeed burn one's own finger with the UltraCision blade, as 50 °C is felt as hot. Usually it is the left index finger that touches a blade tip that has not yet cooled down sufficiently.

Thermography clearly shows that within a 4- to 5-second period of coagulation and cutting in the mesentery (and this reflects the everyday situation in surgery), temperatures exceed 100 °C only at the blade itself. At a very short distance from the blade, the temperature cools rapidly to body temperature. The region of temperatures above 63 °C, which is the zone that may

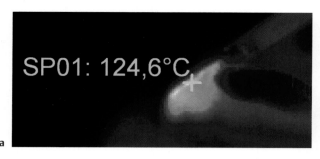

a

after 4 sec

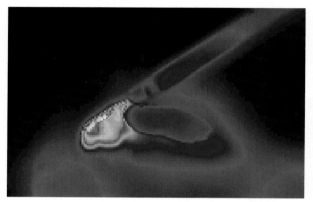

b

Fig. 3.**14a**   UltraCision 5 mm CS shears in human mesentery ex vivo: in the moment of tissue dissection, temperature at the blade is above 100 °C. **b** UltraCision 5 mm CS shears in human mesentery ex vivo: color correction shows that after four seconds, temperature changes are confined to the blade—only the blade and the tissue in the jaws of the instrument becomes hot.

Fig. 3.**15**   UltraCision 5 mm CS shears in human mesentery ex vivo: one second after tissue transection with the shears, the blade (*SP03*, *SP04*) and the tissue (*SP01*, *SP02*) have cooled down (the tip of the blade is still too hot to touch, however).

confine the tissue to irreversible protein denaturation, is limited to the closest vicinity of the blade. Thus one can state that the risk of lateral damage is minimized with the ultrasonic scalpel.

UltraCision and Electrocautery In Vivo

When the subcutaneous tissue was cut the temperature was 68.5 to 89.3 °C with HF and 39.8 to 46.7 °C with UltraCision. When the tissue was coagulated the temperature was 124.4 to 178.3 °C with electrocautery and 52.8 to 87.4 °C with UltraCision (Fig. 3.**16**).

Not unexpectedly, tissue cutting with a cautery device and with UltraCision reflected the same significant temperature differences as with the liver ex vivo. When bleeders were coagulated, this difference also presented impressively. With UltraCision, bleeders were stopped with coaptation (below 63 °C) or coagulation. Temperatures that regularly occur with cautery devices were never reached with UltraCision.

The data from infrared thermography definitively show the advantages of the ultrasonically activated scalpel. It is indeed possible to produce burn marks and tissue necrosis with the ultrasonically activated scalpel, but in practice, activation of the blade is usually confined to such a short period (no longer than five seconds) that the risk of lateral heat damage is minimized, as has been shown clearly not only by thermography but also by other studies.

UltraCision and Its Competitors

Ultrasonically activated cutting and coagulating systems are available as UltraCision (Ethicon Endo Surgery), AutoSonix (Tyco), and SonoSurg (Olympus). All systems have a power supply generator, a piezoelectric transducer that is housed in the hand piece, and a functional tip. The transducer consists of a stack of piezoelectric crystals sandwiched between two metal cylinders. It converts electrical energy into mechanical vibration at a frequency of 23 000 Hz (AutoSonix) or 55 500 Hz (UltraCision; SonoSurg). The amplitude of the vibration varies (depending on the selected level) between 25 and 100 μm (UltraCision) and 80 and 200 μm (AutoSonix).

The coagulation effect is determined by the local velocity of sound, which is a mathematical function of amplitude and frequency. Accordingly, the local velocity of sound is about equal for all available devices. The lower frequency of AutoSonix is compensated for by its higher maximal amplitude.

While the cutting/coagulation force is a function of frequency and amplitude, this force is unequally distributed along the instrument. Usually the tip of an instrument is an anti-node presenting a region of maximal amplitude. For example, toward the base of ul-

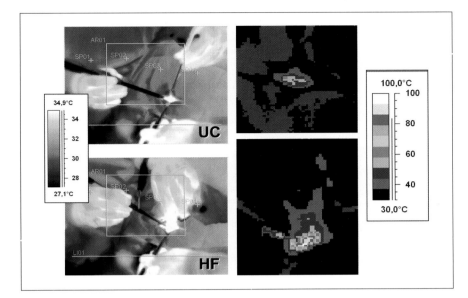

Fig. 3.**16** Coagulation of subcutaneous bleeders with UltraCision (*UC*) and electrocautery (*HF*) in vivo: the original frames from the camera with the automatic temperature distribution bar are shown at left. On the right, the color correction with respect to the local area of interest makes the differences in temperature and heat distribution clearly visible.

trasonically activated shears, the amplitude decreases by about 50% in UltraCision and by about 10% in Auto-Sonix (Fig. 3.**17**). The difference is caused by the different frequency of the generator. This effect is at least partially compensated by the fact that there is more pressure at the base of the shears.

In practice, it is found that, for example, the UltraCision CS/LCS shears cut at first from the tip of the instrument. This effect is compensated in the new generation of curved 5 mm shears by a blade whose tip is not exactly at an anti-node. This is impressively presented in the thermography of an activated shear (Fig. 3.**18**). Thus, the "tip-cuts-first effect" is significantly reduced.

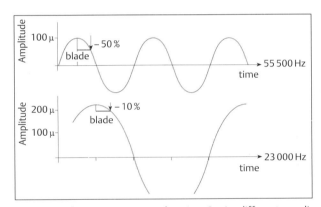

Fig. 3.**17** UltraCision compared to AutoSonix: different amplitude and different frequency. At comparable blade lengths, UltraCision has a decrease of amplitude from the tip to the base of the blade by 50%, and AutoSonix by 10%, when the tip of the blade is located at an anti-node.

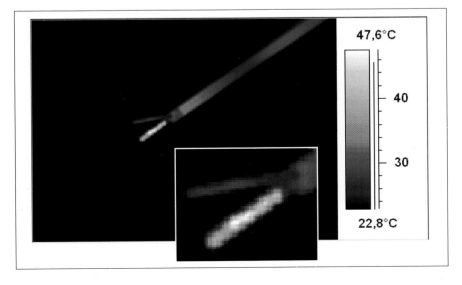

Fig. 3.**18** The activated blade of the new 5 mm curved tip shears shows the hot spot (the anti-node) in the middle of the blade that compensates for the decrease of amplitude along the blade. The shaft of the blade also demonstrates the effectiveness of nodes and anti-nodes in respect to temperature changes due to energy losses.

Suggested Reading

Amaral JF, Chrostek C. Experimental comparison of the ultrasonically activated scalpel to electrosurgery and laser surgery for laparoscopic use. Min Invas Ther & Allied Technol 1997; 6: 324–31.

Amaral JE. Laparoscopic cholecystectomy in 200 consecutive patients using an ultrasonic activated scalpel. Surg Laparosc Endosc 1995; 5: 255–62.

Cuschieri A, Shimi S, Banting S, VanderHelpen G. Endoscopic ultrasonic dissection for thoracoscopic and laparoscopic surgery. Surg Endosc 1993; 7: 197–99.

Farin G. Ultrasonic dissection in combination with HF surgery. End Surg All Tech 1994; 2: 211–13.

Fowler DL. Laparoscopic right hemicolectomy. In: Tooull J, Gossot D, Hunter JH, editors. Endosurgery. New York: Churchill Livingstone; 1996, pp. 665–73.

Fowler DL, White S. Laparoscopic sigmoid resection with the Harmonic Scalpel (Abstr).Surg Endosc 1994; 8: 503.

Geis WP, Kim HC, McAfee PC, Kang JG, Brennan EJ. Synergistic benefits of combined technologies in complex minimally invasive surgical procedures. Surg Endosc 1996; 10: 1025–28.

Gossot D, Fritsch S, Cälärier M. Laparoscopic splenectomy: optimal vascular control using the lateral approach and ultrasonic dissection. Surg Endosc 1999; 13: 21–25.

Gossot D, Buess B, Cuschieri A, et al. Ultrasonic dissection for endoscopic surgery. Surgl Endosc 1999; 13: 412–17.

Grosskinsky CM, Hulka JF. Unipolar electrosurgery in operative laparoscopy. Capacitance as a potential source of injury. J Reprod Med 1995; 40: 549–52.

Hambley R, Hebda PA, Abell E, Cohen B, Jegasothy BV. Wound healing of skin incisions produced by ultrasonically vibrating knife, scalpel, electrosurgery, and carbon dioxide laser. J Dermatol Surg Oncol 1988; 14: 11.

Laycock WS, Trus TL, Hunter JG. New technology for the division of short gastric vessels during laparoscopic Nissen fundoplication: a prospective randomized trial. Surg Endosc 1996; 10: 71–3.

Meijer DW, Bannenberg JJG. HF Electrosurgery for endoscopic surgery. In: Toouli J,Gossot D, Hunter J, editors. Endosurgery. New York: Churchill Llvingstone; 1996, pp. 97–102.

Nduka CC, Super PA, Monson JRT, Darzi AW. Cause and prevention of electrosurgical injuries in laparoscopy. J Am Coll Surg 1994; 179: 161–70.

Richards SR, Simpkins SS. Comparison of the harmonic scissors and endostapler in laparoscopic supracervical hysterectomy. J Am Assoc Gynecol Laparosc 1995; 3: 87–90.

Robbins ML, Ferland RJ. Laparoscopic-assisted vaginal hysterectomy using the laparosonic coagulating shears. J Am Assoc Gynecol Laparosc 1995; 2: 339–43.

Rothenberg SS. Laparoscopic splenectomy using the Harmonic Scalpel. J Laparoendosc Surg 1996; 6: 61–3.

Schwarz RO. Total laparoscopic hysterectomy with the Harmonic Scalpel. J Gynecol Surg 1994; 10: 33–4.

Spivak H, Richardson WS, Hunter JG. The use of cautery, laparosonic coagulating shears, and vascular clips for hemostasis of small and medium-sized vessels. Surg Endosc 1998; 12: 183–85.

Stringer NH. Laparoscopic myomectomy with the Harmonic Scalpel: a review of 25 cases. J Gynecol Surg 1994; 10: 241–45.

Suzuki K, Fujita K, Ushiyama T, Mugiya S, Kageyama S, Ishikawa A. Efficacy of an ultrasonic surgical system for laparoscopic adrenalectomy. J Urol 1995; 154: 484–86.

Swanstrom LL, Pennings JL. Laparoscopic control of short gastric vessels. J Am Coll Surg 1995; 181: 347–51.

Tucker RD. Laparoscopic electrosurgical injuries: survey results and their implications. Surg Laparosc Endosc 1995; 5: 311–17.

Wetter LA, Payne JH, Kirshenbaum G, Podoll EF, Bachinsky T, Way LW. The ultrasonic dissector facilitates laparoscopic cholecystectomy. Arch Surg 1992; 127: 1195–98.

4 Education, Training, and Personal Experience

W. Feil

UltraCision in Practical Use

The use of UltraCision means a considerable change in surgical technique for the surgeon who is used to high-frequency (HF) electrosurgery. A basic requirement for the successful use of UltraCision is a precise knowledge and understanding of the technical basis and characteristics of the UltraCision scalpel.

The initial learning phase is limited to the first two weeks, when the basic functions of UltraCision are experienced stepwise in practical use and are converted for one's own area of use. This learning phase can be shortened by attending appropriate theoretical and practical courses.

Although UltraCision was developed primarily for use in laparoscopic surgery, it is a good idea for the novice to initially use the UltraCision scalpel only in open surgery in selected operations.

The usual initial (and logistically understandable) attempt to use the hand piece with a blade, like the handle of the cautery, gives poor results. Putting into practice the theoretical knowledge of the significance of tension and pressure and of the need for a counter-pressure for hemostasis leads rapidly to acceptance of the functions of UltraCision.

After practical experience in open surgery, use of the dissecting blades for laparoscopic surgery can proceed without problems. Lysis of adhesions, cholecystectomy, and hernia repair are recommended operations for getting started. The absence of obscuring smoke and the possibility of risk-free dissection close to hilar structures (as compared to cautery) are obvious advantages in laparoscopic cholecystectomy.

After a habituation period of two to four weeks, the surgeon will have implemented the advantages of the new technology in his individual surgical technique. UltraCision can be used in all elective open and laparoscopic operations in the habituation phase. After one month, it is thus possible to reduce gradually the intellectual preoccupation with technical matters in order to concentrate entirely on the progress of the operation.

Editor's tip: When I tried the short blade for the first time in my own pioneer period, my first impression was that UltraCision did not work properly and that cutting was extremely slow. My mistake was that I tried to use it like a cautery device. At that time I had no basic theoretical information, because it is always the same with us surgeons: we get a new toy and play with it! Today, with the implementation of theoretical and practical courses, this misapprehension is easily avoided.

After a few weeks of accommodation, UltraCision can be used in all open and laparoscopic (elective and acute) operations. The HF cautery is replaced completely by UltraCision, and attachment of a neutral electrode (for safety) is omitted.

Editor's tip: It is also possible to change from a cautery device to UltraCision at a moment's notice if necessary, as indeed I have done. Everything that can be done with a cautery device can be done with UltraCision, and even more. It is unnecessary to have the cautery device on the table "just to be sure," except for psychological reasons.

Implementation of UltraCision

The first UltraCision system was implemented in the Department of General Surgery (96 beds and ICU) of the Donauspital (total 1000 beds) in Vienna, Austria during September 1996. My personal series of more than 1500 operations (two-thirds open and one-third laparoscopic) commenced at that time, when I stopped using electrocautery from one day to the next. The consequence of my growing expertise was the implementation of the system not only by surgeons in my own department but also those in other departments as well.

Today our surgical department uses three generators. Theoretical and practical two-day courses in UltraCision are held regularly, not only for general surgeons but also for all other surgical disciplines. UltraCision systems are available and regularly used also in the hospital's Departments of Gynecology and Obstetrics, Orthopedic Surgery, Urology, Pediatric Surgery, and Otorhinolaryngology.

Beside the fact that the main task of any surgical department is to serve the local population for all types of general surgery, the formation of special interests and necessities reflects various regions of special competence: esophageal, gastrointestinal, colorectal, hepatobiliary, thyroid surgery; all types of visceral tumor surgery; and the full range of laparoscopic and thoracoscopic indications.

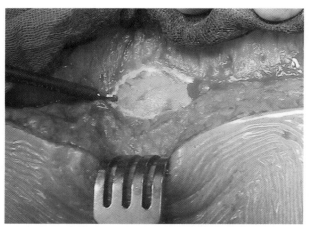

Fig. 4.**1**   Cutting of the abdominal fascia with a 5 mm SH sharp blade. Cutting speed is controlled by tension resulting from prestretching the tissue.

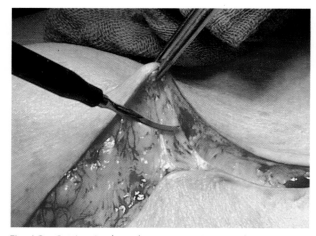

Fig. 4.**2**   Cutting in the subcutaneous tissue with a 5 mm HF blade. This blade allows swift cutting with the sharp lateral sides of the blade. The blunt, convex side is used for coagulation with pressure to the underlying tissue; the concave side is used for loading tissue and coagulation under direct visual control.

Practical Experience and Development of New Instruments in Open Surgery

Starting in 1996, the practicality of UltraCision as a substitute for HF cautery, and as a dissecting instrument in daily routine work, was tested in an open prospective study.

The HS2 blade, which was the only short blade available at that time, was used, for example, to open the abdomen, for dissecting and resecting the thyroid and the cervical esophagus, in the perineal phase of abdominoperineal resection, and in the parenchymatous phase (liver, kidney). All intra-abdominal dissec-

tion stages, division of tissue, and initial hemostasis were performed with the CS shears (pistol grip) and optionally with the longer LCS shears. Ligatures and/or transfixions were only required for the large vessels.

The reusable, sickle-shaped HS2 blade was succeeded by the disposable 5 mm blade, which always provides a sharp and pointed instrument.

> Editor's tip: It was clear to the surgical community that curved blades and curved shears would be better, but it was a very difficult task for the materials scientists to fashion a substance that could withstand the force of the vibration in a curved blade without shattering.

The first curved blade was the HC blade used for harvesting of the internal mammary vessels in heart surgery. When this shape proved itself the HC was succeeded by the sharper HF blade, which does a perfect job in cutting and also in coagulation when a local counterpart for obtaining pressure is present.

> Editor's tip: In my opinion, the sickle-shaped blade will disappear in time, since a sickle is truly not the typical surgical instrument!

Laparotomy

Laparotomy is the perfect procedure to make the first contact with this ultrasonic cutting and coagulating device.

After incising the skin with the scalpel, all further steps of the laparotomy up to complete opening of the abdominal cavity can be undertaken with a blade. When a sickle-shaped blade is used, the blunt convex side of the dissecting blade proves itself in the subcutaneous tissue. For hemostasis in the subcutaneous tissue, it has proved to be beneficial to grasp the skin with a gauze pledget between the thumb and index finger, to evert it and so provide the necessary counterpressure for coaptation.

Incision of the fascia (Fig. 4.**1**) of the linea alba with the sharp, concave side of the dissecting blade demands markedly more force (tension) than during incision using cautery, and also takes somewhat longer. The additional time is offset by the fact that the usual change of instruments (forceps, cautery) is avoided in the further course of the laparotomy.

Hemostasis in the preperitoneal adipose tissue is best obtained with the broad cheek of the blade, which then only has to be turned through 90° for further incision. Larger vessels are isolated with the cavitation technique, under-run, coapted with the broad cheek, and then cut after a 90° turn. Following laparotomy, lysis of adhesions is likewise possible in the regions that are accessible with the hand piece. Changeover to the CS shears usually ensues following laparotomy.

The introduction of the new HF blade (Fig. 4.**2**) made all these procedures easier because the handling of this blade is more ergonomic and the blade is extremely sharp.

> Editor's tip: From the economic point of view, it is questionable if it indeed makes sense to use a disposable blade in major surgery only for opening of the abdominal cavity.

All steps of dissection following skin incision, however, can also be performed with (preferably) the 5 mm shears when the jaws are left open and the blade is activated downwards with pressure to cut the tissue. Small bleeders can be grasped in the same way as with a bipolar forceps and coagulated. This technique avoids the search for a local counterpart as is the case when a blade is used.

> Editor's tip: When the 5 mm C14 shears are used for opening the abdomen following skin incision with the activated blade down, it is recommended to leave the jaws open in order to have full control over the activated blade and have no energy losses to the Teflon pad. In certain cases, it can make sense to perform the incision of the fascia with a steel scalpel in order to save time. With the shears, all connective and subcutaneous tissues are incised—and muscle transection done—absolutely bloodlessly.

Thyroid Surgery

Thyroid surgery is another appropriate field in which to gain experience with the ultrasonic cutting and dissecting technique. It is possible to do most of the preparation and resection with a blade. With an HC blade, the tissue can be loaded on the blade (Fig. 4.**3**) and coagulated under direct vision (Fig. 4.**4**). The coapted/coagulated tissue can be cut easily when the blade is rotated to the sharper lateral side (Fig. 4.**5**).

If resection of the thyroid gland is performed closest to the capsule, it may be possible to transect the vessels after coagulation with the blade. However, it is recommended to dissect the pole vessels between clamps to play it safe.

> Editor's tip: Thyroid surgery with the 10 mm shears was unsatisfactory because the instrument is too clumsy for the delicate structures in the neck region. The implementation of the 5 mm curved shears (CS14C) gave us a perfect tool for this type of surgery.

With the 5 mm curved-tip shears, preparation and dissection in thyroid surgery has become easy. All vascular structures that could not be controlled with the blade can now be coagulated and transected safely with the shears.

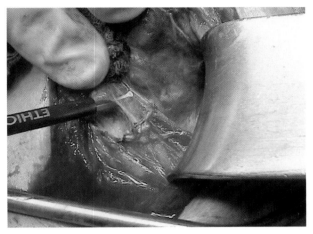

Fig. 4.**3** Thyroid surgery. The tissue is loaded on the concave side of a HC blade.

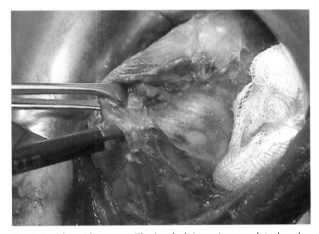

Fig. 4.**4** Thyroid surgery. The loaded tissue is coagulated under direct visual control.

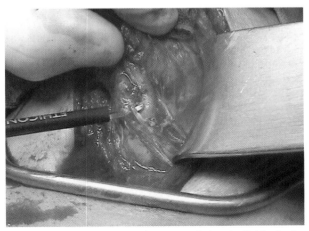

Fig. 4.**5** Thyroid surgery. When coagulation is finished, the blade is twisted to the sharp side and tissue is cut easily.

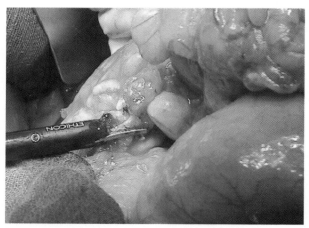

Fig. 4.**6**   Total gastrectomy. Transection of the gastroduodenal artery with the UltraCision CS shears.

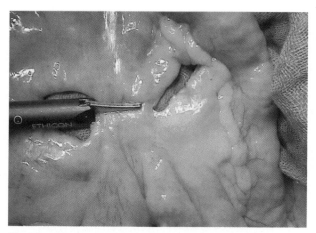

Fig. 4.**7**   Preparation of a Y-Roux sling. Dissection of the mesentery with the UltraCision CS shears.

Esophageal Myotomy

Myotomy following resection of a Zenker's diverticulum and distal myotomy in achalasia are perfect indications to show the benefit of UltraCision.

The cervical incision and the entire dissection, including complete exposure of the diverticulum, can be carried out with a blade or the 14 cm shears. The diverticulum is removed using a T35 stapler.

The subsequent cervical esophagomyotomy is performed with a blade or with the shears. During the myotomy, typical venous vessels, sometimes tending to bleed awkwardly, are found in the plane between mucosa and muscle. Hemostasis in this situation is always problematic, and the use of cautery is extremely dangerous. Local application of hemostyptics (e.g., POR8) was often the only possibility. With UltraCision, the myotomy could be performed without risk.

Cervical myotomy in the context of removal of a Zenker's diverticulum is equivalent in technical terms to distal esophageal myotomy for achalasia. Laparo-

scopic myotomy for achalasia with the 5 mm curved shears is a 30 minutes operation without any bleeding, with perfect visualization, and with excellent results for patients.

Esophageal Resection

In transthoracic esophagectomy, thoracotomy and all dissection in the chest cavity can be performed with the UltraCision shears. Dissection of the tumor-bearing esophagus from the endangered and vulnerable structures (azygos vein, aorta, trachea, vagus nerve, and phrenic nerve) is performed easily and without risk using UltraCision.

Using the UltraCision shears, it is possible to coapt and divide in one step the thin-walled and vulnerable large-diameter vessels in the adherent layer between stomach and spleen in such a way that the vascularization of the stomach, which is absolutely necessary when the stomach is to be pulled up, is not jeopardized and no injury is caused to the spleen. The use of UltraCision reduces instrument changing during the operation to a minimum.

All stages of transhiatal esophageal resection and esophageal replacement by stomach interposition in the abdomen, dissection in the mediastinum and the neck can be carried out with UltraCision.

Gastrectomy

UltraCision has been used in a series of gastric resections. In gastric resection, all stages of dissection were undertaken with the UltraCision shears. It is particularly advantageous to be able to perform a Kocher mobilization of the duodenum and the entire dissection of the gastrocolic ligament and the division of the splenic hilum with UltraCision. The conventional technique with frequent instrument changes (clamp, clamp, scissors, ligature, scissors, ligature, scissors, adjusting position, scissors, clamp, …) can be completely omitted (Fig. 4.**6**).

It is possible to perform the entire dissection promptly, in one operation, without changing instruments while maintaining the position. The constant direction of gaze and permanent maintenance of ocular focus reduces fatigue and contributes to preserving the surgeon's full concentration on the surgical procedure.

In stomach resection, clamps and ligatures or transfixions need only be used for the large central vessels. Oncologically correct lymphadenectomy along the large vessels was also performed without risk using UltraCision.

Opening the proximally stapled stomach after resection to construct a partial inferior proximal gastrojejunostomy was performed with the sharp blade of the CS shears after initial hemostasis within the wall of the stomach.

Preparation of a Y-Roux sling (Figs. 4.**7**–4.**9**) is easily done with the UltraCision shears. Transfixions are

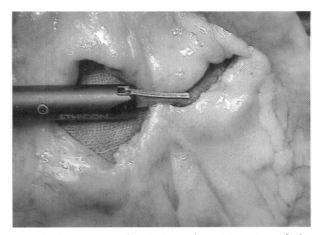

Fig. 4.**8** Preparation of a Y-Roux sling. Dissection of the mesentery with the UltraCision CS shears. No transfixation means optimal length of the sling.

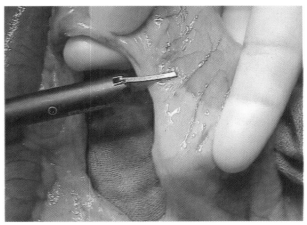

Fig. 4.**9** Preparation of a Y-Roux sling. Dissection close to the bowel wall without injury of the small bowel.

omitted; thus the optimal length of the sling is guaranteed.

Under certain conditions it is also feasible to dissect larger vessels like a splenic vein with the UltraCision CS shears (Fig. 4.**10**). This procedure is recommended for the new 5 mm curved tip shears, as cutting may be done too quickly and the coagulation zone to the lateral side may be too narrow otherwise.

Colon and Rectum

UltraCision was used in the following colorectal operations: ileocaecal resection; right and left hemi-colectomy; transverse colectomy; sigmoid colectomy; (deep) anterior resection; abdominoperineal (intersphincteric) resection of the rectum with coloanal anastomosis; intestinal reconstruction. In all of these operations, following laparotomy the UltraCision shears were used (Fig. 4.**11**). Clamps with ligatures or transfixions were necessary only for the few large central vessels.

With UltraCision it is possible to undertake the entire dissection of the rectum down to the floor of the pelvis in one step without altering the visual direction or ocular focus, thereby, maintaining full concentration at all times on the progress of the operation.

> Editor's tip: The new curved tip is the best choice for visceral surgery. In most cases the 14 cm-long shears are a fine choice. In certain cases of low rectum resection and transhiatal esophageal resection, or in obese patients, the 23 cm-long shears are preferable.

It is particularly advantageous to be able to perform an oncologically correct dissection of the entire colon area in one stage without having to make adjustments and instrument changes. This fact is especially apparent in

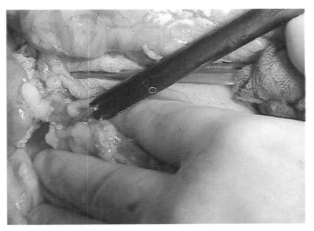

Fig. 4.**10** Total gastrectomy. Dissection of a splenic vein with the UltraCision CS shears.

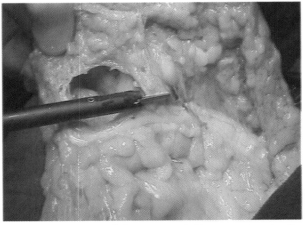

Fig. 4.**11** Dissection of the gastrocolic ligament close to the colon wall with the UltraCision CS shears. No ligatures are needed; there is no damage to the colon wall.

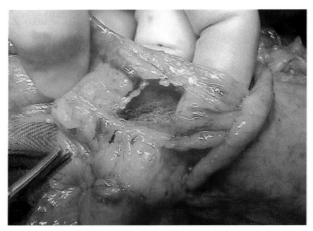

Fig. 4.**12** After transection of the gastrocolic ligament, a thicker vein is perfectly sealed. The lateral zone of tissue necrosis is extremely small when compared to electrosurgical burn marks or tissue included in ligatures.

mobilization of the splenic flexure, which is considerably easier with UltraCision. Even under difficult conditions (poor vision, obese patient, inexperienced assistance), it was possible to control the adjustment of the operative field with the left hand, and perform the entire mobilization in one go with the shears in the right hand.

Oncologically correct and precise anatomical mobilization and lymphadenectomy along the aorta, at the lower border of the pancreas and along the gonadal vessels and the ureter were also possible with the UltraCision shears and there was no oozing to impair vision.

> Editor's tip: Dissection with the UltraCision shears means a clear cut and a very narrow zone of lateral damage with perfect sealing of vessels (Fig. 4.**12**).

Use of the UltraCision shears in the pelvis for resection of the rectum with total *en bloc* resection of the mesorectum has proved to be particularly advantageous. Experience in rectal surgery has shown that the constant changing of the position of instruments and lights detracts from the progress of the operation and from the surgeon's concentration.

> Editor's tip: With UltraCision, colorectal surgery takes place in a de facto bloodless field. Using the UltraCision CS shears, one must bear in mind that the shears cut first at the tip of the instrument (Fig. 4.**13 a–c**).

A further advantage in rectal surgery is that the overall view in the pelvis is considerably better due to the use of the UltraCision shears. The assistant is occupied with retracting the abdominal wall, the pelvic inlet, and holding back loops of bowel; while the surgeon holds the rectum him/herself in the various phases with one hand and guides the instrument with the other hand. The absence of other hands for positioning, suction, removing clamps, guiding a forceps, or using the cautery improves the view in the pelvis significantly.

a

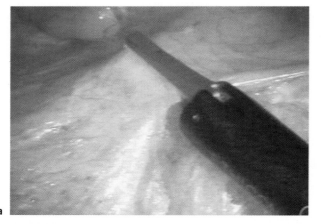

b

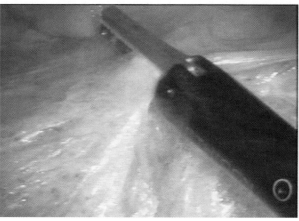

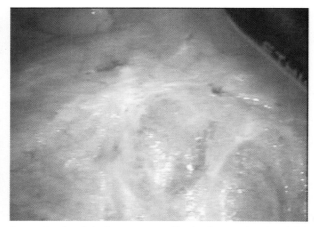

c

Fig. 4.**13 a** Coagulation of a vessel-bearing structure with the UltraCision CS shears. **b** The UltraCision CS/LCS shears start cutting at the tip of the instrument. **c** Cutting is completed and the vessel stumps remain sealed properly.

Liver Resection

All of the stages of dissection in liver resection as far as the parenchymal phase were performed with UltraCision. During the parenchymal phase itself, the use of UltraCision did not offer any technical advantage compared to the conventional operative method (digital fracture and transfixion), but caused delay when the liver had been clamped. The UltraCision scalpel was subsequently used again for hemostasis.

UltraCision, however, is very suitable for taking wedge-shaped tissue samples from the liver; hemostasis and cutting occur at the same time and the quality of the tissue for histological examination does not suffer from the applied heat, as compared to removal with cautery (Fig. 4.**14 a, b**).

UltraCision cannot be unequivocally recommended for use during the parenchymal phase of major liver resections after establishing warm ischemia of the organ with a Pringle's maneuver. The clear distinction from other ultrasound techniques, which are geared particularly to the parenchymal phase, seems necessary so as not to awaken false expectations.

Any preparation ahead of the parenchyma resection can easily be performed with the UltraCision shears, especially the preparation in the hilus, and along the inferior vena cava with all its annoying small vessels that have to be transected at the back side of the liver before the liver veins are completely isolated.

Pancreas Resection

All dissecting stages can be performed with the UltraCision shears. Division of the pancreas with the CS shears is problem-free and without bleeding in most cases. The pancreatic duct itself can be left sealed in a left-sided resection. In a Whipple's procedure, the pancreas can also be transected with the shears, but it may occur in cases with a very soft parenchyma that a narrow pancreatic duct is so closely sealed that it may not be found for drainage or anastomosis.

> Editor's tip: In practice it is recommended to transect the pancreatic parenchyma in very small gaps so that the duct is sealed and hence difficult to be found for anastomosis and/or drainage.

In partial duodenopancreatectomy, the entire dissection can be performed with the UltraCision shears. The ultrasound dissection technique has proven to be particularly advantageous in dissecting the pancreas off the portal vein.

> Editor's tip: The new curved-tip shears (14 and 23 cm lengths) will replace the 10 mm shears in visceral surgery. The additional use of a blade is unnecessary, as the shears can be used with the jaws open and the blade down like a scalpel.

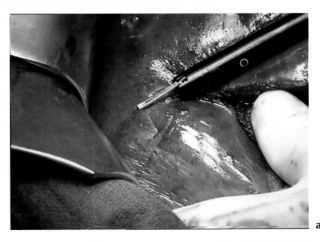
a

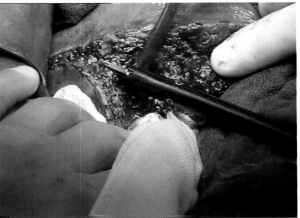
b

Fig. 4.**14 a, b** Anterolateral bisegmentectomy of the liver with the UltraCision CS shears.

Practical Experience and Development of New Instruments in Laparoscopic Surgery

UltraCision was primarily constructed for laparoscopic surgery. Laparoscopic cholecystectomy was the first domain for this new technology. The implementation of this new technique to other endosurgical indications was initially limited by the fact that a local counterpart to obtain pressure for adequate hemostasis with the blade was not always available. Thus, a local counterpart had to be provided permanently close to the activated blade—the Teflon pad of the shears. The development of the shears meant a huge step forward toward new endosurgical indications.

Laparoscopic Cholecystectomy

In an open prospective study, the practicability of UltraCision was tested as a substitute for HF cautery and as a dissecting instrument in routine laparoscopic procedures. All intra-abdominal stages of dissection, initial

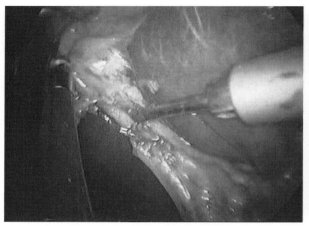

Fig. 4.**15** Laparoscopic cholecystectomy. Preparation of the cystic duct with a 10 mm reusable SH blade.

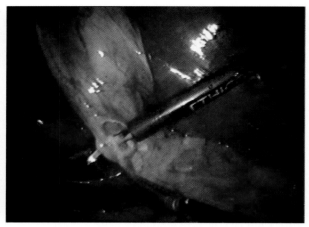

Fig. 4.**16** Laparoscopic cholecystectomy. The peritoneum is incised with a 5 mm HC blade.

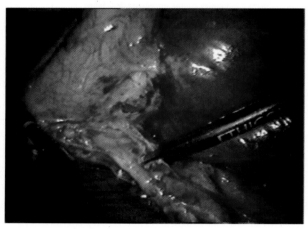

Fig. 4.**17** Laparoscopic cholecystectomy. The cystic duct and artery are dissected with a 5 mm HC blade.

hemostasis, and tissue division were performed with the sharp or blunt 10 mm or 5 mm dissecting blade and/ or the 10 mm LCS shears. Meanwhile, most cholecystectomies are performed with the 5 mm CS shears.

Four ports (511, 512, and 355 twice) were placed for laparoscopic cholecystectomy and the 30° optic was used. The dissecting blade or the curved blade was used initially for dissection of the structures in Calot's triangle. A common practice in laparoscopic cholecystectomy is the encircling of the cystic artery and cystic duct and adequate axial exposure of these structures before dividing them (Fig. 4.**15**).

With the curved blade, the inner surface of which is sharp and ends in a point and is open at an angle of only 40°, the danger of vessel injury appears higher for the inexperienced surgeon than when the blunt blade is used. The blunt blade has a rounded tip and a more favorable 60° opening angle.

With the relatively blunt HC blade the dissection of the peritoneal covering is easily performed (Fig. 4.**16**). The risk of accidental vessel injury seems less with the blunt blade (Fig. 4.**17**).

Altogether, it is possible to perform the dissection of the cystic artery and duct much more exactly and under vision with UltraCision as compared to HF surgery. Especially when there are considerable acute or chronic inflammatory changes in the hilar region, the superiority of UltraCision is apparent; there is no danger of distant thermal tissue injury under normal conditions, and fine dissection is possible even under difficult local conditions.

The cystic duct is always treated with clips, the cystic artery only when a blade is used. In a few cases of slight oozing, subsequent safe coagulation with UltraCision was possible and was successful in the immediate vicinity of the metal clips. When the 5 mm shears are used, the only structure to be transected between clips is the cystic duct.

Retrograde removal of the gallbladder from the liver bed was performed either with the dissecting blade (Fig. 4.**18**) or with the shears (Fig. 4.**19**). The decision on

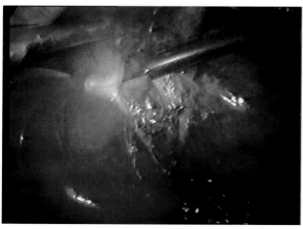

Fig. 4.**18** Laparoscopic cholecystectomy. The gallbladder is peeled out with a 5 mm HC blade.

using the shears is made after assessing the local situation: if it is a "bland" cholecystectomy, it is dissected out with the dissecting blade. Preliminary hemostasis is achieved using the cavitation effect with the blunt outer curve or the flat cheek of the instrument; removal of the organ itself is performed with a technique that is comparable to use of the conventional cautery hook.

When there are extensive, acute, or chronic alterations of the gallbladder, the shears are used. In certain cases a "dome down" cholecystectomy (Fig. 4.**20**) is necessary. It is apparent that dissecting out from the liver bed under these more difficult conditions was markedly easier, less bloody, and better visualized than with HF surgery. Accidental hemorrhage from the liver bed can always be stopped with the flat side of the blade or with the shears.

> Editor's tip: Use of UltraCision for laparoscopic cholecystectomy leads overall to a shortening of operating time and brings the conversion rate close to zero, even in difficult cases.

Independently of whether the shears were used or dissection was performed with the dissecting blade, there was no accidental perforation of the gallbladder in laparoscopic cholecystectomy; though this is a recognized occurrence with HF surgery.

> Editor's tip: In laparoscopic cholecystectomy, it is recommended to choose the UltraCision instrument after having a look at the operative field: if it is a "simple" procedure with a clearly visible triangle of Calot and no inflammation, the (less expensive) HC blade is fine. If instead there are many adhesions, or if there is severe inflammation, or if the anatomy in the triangle of Calot is not clear at the first view, the 5 mm curved-tip shears are the best choice from the beginning of the operation. To start with a blade and then switch to shears if bleeding occurs is too risky and expensive.

When using the shears, the instrument remains in the right plane "automatically" when the organ is exposed, due to the initial cavitation. As a result, slipping from the optimal plane of dissection into the parenchyma of the liver or into the lumen of the gallbladder (which often occurs when the cautery hook is used under difficult operative conditions) does not occur.

When UltraCision is used, there is release of water vapor that can briefly impair vision. This "fog" condenses rapidly, depending upon the size of the drops, and vision becomes clear again after one or two seconds. The time-consuming partial removal of smoke from the pneumoperitoneum, familiar from HF surgery, is no longer necessary with UltraCision.

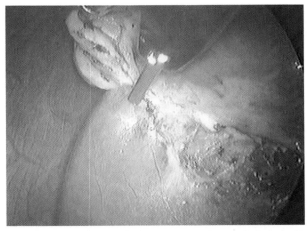

Fig. 4.**19** Laparoscopic cholecystectomy. Removal of the gallbladder with the LCS shears.

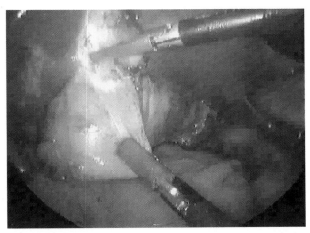

Fig. 4.**20** Laparoscopic cholecystectomy. "Dome down" cholecystectomy with the straight 5 mm shears.

Laparoscopic Reflux Surgery

Open Nissen fundoplication was the surgical gold standard for gastro-esophageal reflux disease (GERD) prior to the implementation of H2-blockers and proton-pump blockers. Conservative therapy with these drugs achieves rapid relief from symptoms due to acid reduction, but does not eliminate biliary reflux, which itself may lead to Barrett's esophagus and/or cancer. Symptoms re-establish when conservative therapy is canceled and motility disorders of the esophagus may present after a longer history of recurrent inflammation in the distal esophagus. These arguments, combined with the option to perform the Nissen fundoplication laparoscopically, have led to a renaissance of this surgical procedure.

The indication for laparoscopic Nissen fundoplication in patients with hiatal hernia and/or GERD is evidence-based on preoperative examinations, of which

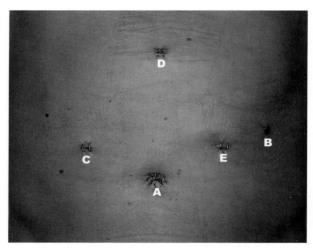

Fig. 4.**21**   Position and placement of the ports for laparoscopic reflux surgery. *A* 511 camera port, *B* 355 port for Endo-Babcock, *C* 355 port for Endo-dissect, *D* 355 port for 5 mm probe, *E* 512 port for UltraCision and sutures.

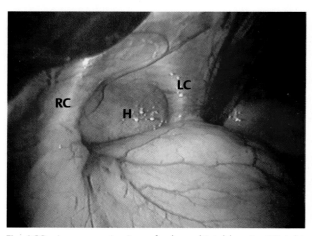

Fig. 4.**22**   Laparoscopic view of a large hiatal hernia. *RC* right crus, *LC* left crus, *H* hiatal hernia sack.

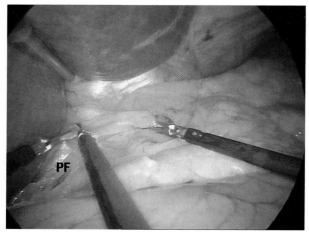

Fig. 4.**23**   Incision of the pars flaccida (*PF*) of the lesser omentum to gain access to the right crus of the diaphragm with the 5 mm CS shears.

the following are mandatory: X-ray examination, endoscopy (± biopsy) and manometry and facultatively 24 h-pH-metry.

Patients with motility disorders should be treated with a Toupet procedure instead of a Nissen. Patients with Barrett's esophagus undergo additional treatment (e. g., laser ablation of metaplastic epithelium) or even resection, when high-grade dysplasia or cancer is present.

For the laparoscopic Nissen procedure, patients are positioned in a modified Lloyd-Davies position.

> Editor's tip: It is helpful to move the patient into a somewhat half-sitting anti-Trendelenburg position, in order to emphasize the surgical approach to the abdominal esophagus even in obese patients with huge herniations.

After establishing a pneumoperitoneum, the ports are placed (Fig. 4.**21**), the camera is inserted via the umbilical port, and a 5 mm steel-probe is introduced via the sub-xyphoidal port in order to elevate the left liver (Table 4.**1**). The position of the trocars depends upon the individual anatomy of the patient—mainly the distance between umbilicus and xyphoid. In tall patients, the camera port should be positioned at an adequate distance above the umbilicus. Before introducing the "working port" for the UltraCision scalpel and for the grasping tools, it is useful to measure the distance up to the hiatus to ensure that the esophagus could be reached with the appropriate instruments.

> Editor's tip: For retraction of the liver, in most cases the 5 mm steel probe is sufficient to elevate the left liver lobe. The probe is handled by an assistant or alternatively is fixed to a holding-system. Otherwise a robotic device is fixed to the OR-table, in order to reduce personnel for this procedure. In very obese patients the use of a liver retractor can be helpful.

The indication is confirmed by observing a large hiatal hernia (Fig. 4.**22**). The preparation is started with the sharp and/or blunt side of the UC 10 mm LCS shears or with the 5 mm curved-tip shears. The peritoneum of the pars flaccida of the lesser omentum is incised close to the right crus, preserving the hepatic branches of the vagal nerve (Fig. 4.**23**). The right crus is prepared

Table 4.**1**   The following choice of instruments is recommended

- One 511, 10 mm port (camera)
- One 512, 10 mm port
- Three 355, 5 mm ports
- UltraCision 5 mm CS (preferable) or10 mm LCS shears
- Two 5 mm grasping instruments (pref. Endo-grasp, Endo-dissect)
- One probe (5 mm)
- Two needle-holders (pref. SRNH1)
- 2/0 unresorbable sutures (pref. Ethibond)
- Knot pusher (pref. ESS), or SW 100 automatic suturing system

downward to finally expose the reunification with the left crus. Thereafter, the incision of the peritoneum is continued over the abdominal esophagus (sparing the left vagal nerve) and the left crus is carefully prepared (Fig. 4.**24**).

Using the 10 mm LCS shears in this situation may result in an impaired view to the tip of the instrument under certain conditions (Fig. 4.**25**).

Special care during the initial preparation is taken to preserve an additional left hepatic artery in the upper part of the pars flaccida in about 15% of cases. More frequently, thicker veins leading from the left side of the diaphragm and crossing over the abdominal esophagus penetrate the left triangle ligament of the liver. These structures may be sacrificed and easily transected with the blunt side of the blade.

On the left side of the inferior and dorsal part of the crus, in most cases a small network of veins and a smaller artery are found and transected carefully with UltraCision. Otherwise, if dissected only bluntly, these vessels cause irresistible oozing, since the stump of the little artery retracts unreachably behind the left crus. It is reported that bleeding from this side is a major cause of conversion to an open procedure.

> Editor's tip: During preparation, the UltraCision shears can also be used as a grasping, holding, and dissecting instrument, in order to avoid frequent instrument changes and to enhance fluent progress of the intervention.

The right vagal nerve is bluntly separated from the esophagus; minor vessels between the epineurium and the esophagus are transected with the UltraCision scalpel. If possible, a small retroesophageal window is created at this time.

> Editor's tip: Preparation close to the delicate vagal nerve is an excellent argument for the use of the UltraCision Scalpel. As there is no electric current and tissue temperature does not increase too much, the risk of injury to the nerve is minimized.

In most cases with significant herniation, the abdominal esophagus is too short, dorsal fixation of the mesogastrium (left gastrics) is too extensive, and the anatomy is not distinctly clear due to herniation and chronic inflammation. In these cases the window can be prepared later on when the greater curvature and the (if existing) angle of His are exposed with the spleen out of the field of operation.

Mobilization is continued at the greater curvature of the stomach. The incision of the peritoneum starts in the oral part of the upper-third of the stomach (Fig. 4.**26**), above the unification of the right and left gastroepiploic artery with anastomotic branches. Access is gained into the lesser sac with UltraCision and the greater curvature is skeletized up toward the spleen.

With the UltraCision 5 mm shears, the dissection of the stomach can be performed close to the gastric wall

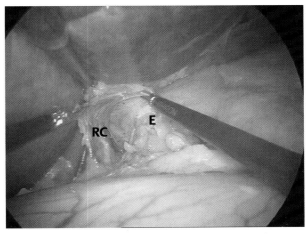

Fig. 4.**24** Completion of the peritoneal incision along the anterior side of the esophagus (*E*); preparation of the right crus of the diaphragm (*RC*) with the 5 mm CS shears.

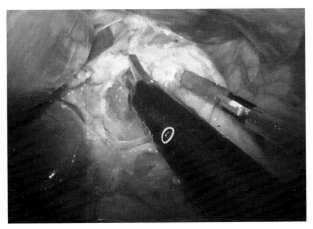

Fig. 4.**25** Preparation of the crura and of the anterior wall of the esophagus with the 10 mm LCS shears.

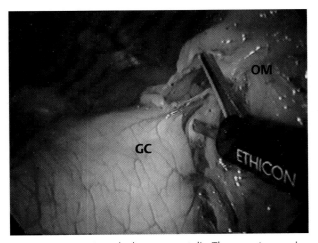

Fig. 4.**26** Access into the bursa omentalis. The omentum majus (*OM*) is dissected from the greater curvature (*GC*). Stomach and omentum are held with Endo-grasps, the peritoneum is punctured with the blade of the 10 mm LCS shears (jaws opened, level 5). The vessel is grasped, coapted, and transected.

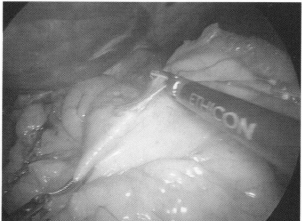

Fig. 4.**27** Access into the bursa omentalis with the 5 mm CS shears.

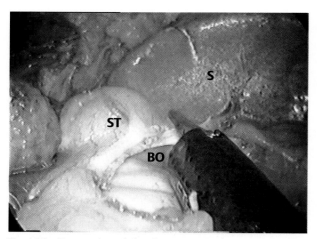

Fig. 4.**28** Transection of the short gastrics close to the spleen with the flat side of the 10 mm LCS shears. *S* spleen, *ST* stomach, *BO* bursa omentalis.

(Fig. 4.**27**). In the vicinity of the spleen it is necessary to work carefully. When the 10 mm shears are used it is recommended to switch to the flat side in order to reduce the risk of parenchymal injury with the edge of the blade (Fig. 4.**28**). UltraCision allows dissection of the stomach even in those situations where the gastric wall is closely attached to the spleen and no distinct plane of dissection can be identified.

After completing the gastric dissection, it is feasible also in difficult cases to clearly identify both crura down to their reunification, to separate the vagal nerve, and to create the retroesophageal window (Fig. 4.**29**). The crura are reunified with three stitches of non-resorbable 2/0 material (Ehibond or Prolene). The vagal nerve is positioned between the crura under the first suture (Fig. 4.**30**).

> Editor's tip: In patients with endobrachyesophagus and with a short abdominal esophagus due to chronic inflammation, it can be difficult to guide a straight instrument through the retroesophageal window. In such cases a flexible instrument can resolve the problem. It could also be helpful to place a holding suture on the greater curvature and pull the plication through the window by grasping this suture.

The plication is guided through the retroesophageal window after insertion of a gastric tube as a placeholder. After the plication has been guided through the window, the plication should remain in position and not slip back after withdrawal of the pulling instrument. This technique, and an adequately thick gastric tube, ensures that the plication is not too tight. The plication is fixed with three sutures of 2/0 non-resorbable material, with or without stitching the esophagus. The gastric tube is removed, and (when the esophagus has not been stitched before) an additional suture is placed

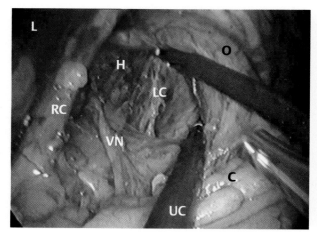

Fig. 4.**29** The retroesophageal windows are created. *L* liver, *RC* right crus, *LC* left crus; *H* hiatal hernia, *VN* nervus vagus, *C* cardia, *E* esophagus. The esophagus is gently elevated with a 5 mm Endo-grasp and the window created by blunt dissection. Remnant membranes are cut with the 10 mm LCS shears (*UC*).

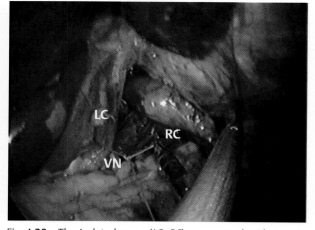

Fig. 4.**30** The isolated crura (*LC*, *RC*) are sutured with two or three Ethibond sutures (2/0) using the ESS knot pusher (*ESS*). The vagal nerve (*VN*) is positioned at the lowest point of the inferior reunification of the crura.

between the plication and the lesser curvature of the stomach to prevent slipping of the plication (Fig. 4.**31**).

> Editor's tip: The plication can be fixed by stitching the esophageal wall. This technique could cause laceration of the esophageal wall or cause damage of the anterior vagal nerve. Another method to prevent the plication from slipping is to place an additional suture between the lesser curvature and the plication to avoid the telescope phenomenon.

If there are no endoshears on the table, it is possible to use UltraCision to cut the sutures intracorporeally.

In a personal series of 150 cases with laparoscopic Nissen or Toupet operations following the described procedure, no conversions were necessary. All patients underwent preoperative manometry, X-ray examination, and endoscopy with biopsy. Mean OR time was 60 minutes (range 50 to 85 minutes). UltraCision was used solely in all cases; electrocautery and/or clips were never used. The suction device was used in three cases (45 ml), when bleeding occurred from adhesions or from a chronically inflamed tissue around the esophagus. There were no major postoperative complications.

Because of a severe motility problem with pathological manometry three months after a Nissen procedure, two patients had to be reoperated. Endoscopy did not show any sign of stenosis; relaparoscopy showed a regular plication. The Nissen was opened and a Toupet plication performed. The patients are now symptom-free. Two other patients' Nissen had to be dilated endoscopically after a Nissen procedure two and three times, respectively, to remain symptom-free thereafter.

The 10 mm LCS shears with the needle-holder handgrip, and later the 5 mm CS curved-tip shears, were the standard instruments in this series. These instruments provide all advantages of a multifunction instrument. The needle-holder handgrip of the 10 mm shears offers a more ergonomic approach when compared to the classic pistol-grip. The choice of the grip depends upon the surgeon's personal preference and on the shape of the other instruments used, in order to achieve an ergonomic position of the surgeon's shoulder girdle. For the 5 mm curved-tip shears, the pistol-grip is not such a disadvantage because this instrument can be brought into an adequate position and the whole shaft can be rotated. The lack of this function is a clear disadvantage of the 10 mm shears.

> Editor's tip: As in most surgical procedures using UltraCision, the tissue effect of the locally applied ultrasound energy can be controlled by varying blade shape, switching between level 1 and 5, and modifying grip pressure and tissue tension. Thus a synergy between the cutting and coagulation can be obtained in order to achieve the appropriate result.

The risks of electrosurgery are avoided by the use of UltraCision. In laparoscopic reflux surgery, all steps of the

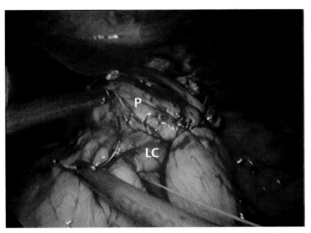

Fig. 4.**31** The fundoplication is fixed with three 2/0 Ethibond sutures. An additional suture is placed between the lesser curvature (*LC*) and the plication (*P*) to prevent the telescope phenomenon by slipping of the plication.

preparation can be made precisely without any loss of blood under perfect vision. The synergistic use of coaptation, coagulation, and cutting means that the entire dissection can be performed easily with a single instrument. The fact that the shears can also be used for grasping facilitates the operation significantly and reduces OR-time, since the usual, frequent instrument changes are avoided. Due to the fact that no electric current is present when UltraCision is used, the risk of electric or thermal injury to delicate structures (esophagus, vagal nerve) is also avoided. Hence the esophagus can be mobilized under difficult circumstances without any risk of damage that could lead to intraoperative or postoperative perforation. The fine vessels can be prepared, coapted, and transected in one step without instrument changes and without application of clips or the electric current that would otherwise char delicate tissue structures.

The results from the personal series and from the recent literature show that laparoscopic Nissen fundoplication using UltraCision gives excellent results. Surgical complications that might lead to intraoperative conversion or major postoperative complications can be completely avoided. OR-times are reduced and the use of additional costly instruments is minimized.

Laparoscopic Hernia Operation (TAPP Repair)

In the transabdominal preperitoneal (TAPP) procedure, a 511 port is used umbilically with the 30° optic, plus a 355 and a 512 port. Dissection of the peritoneal fold was performed, preferably with the sharp 40° curved blade, or also with the blunt 60° dissecting blade or with a 5 mm HC blade.

Editor's tip: For TAPP repair, a blade is fine for preparation. In cases of recurrent hernia with lots of adhesions or impacted hernia, the shears may be a better choice.

Anatomical exposure of the structures (epigastric vessels, spermatic cord structures, nerves) was achieved from the technical surgical aspect in a manner comparable in its results to the former practices (endoshears and HF cautery).

UltraCision, however, allows an even more precise exposure of the structures than HF surgery, without the risk of thermally induced injuries to vessels, nerves, and the spermatic cord.

After insertion of the Prolene mesh and fixation with the EMS stapler, the peritoneal fold was closed with a continuous 2/0 JB PDS suture with Lapra-Ty clips. The suture end was cut with the blade of the UltraCision scalpel.

Laparoscopic Colon Surgery

A perfect step into laparoscopic colon surgery is the construction of a Hartmann's fecal diversion in patients with inoperable rectal carcinoma, severe perineal fistulation in Crohn's disease, or severe radiation injury in the pelvis with proctitis and recurrent hemorrhage and/or stenosis.

After placement of the ports (511 umbilical; 355 exactly at the site of the planned stoma; 355 in the right mid-abdomen; 512 in the right lower abdomen for the stapler), the sigmoid colon is mobilized with the LCS shears. Transection of the mesentery was performed close to the bowel wall while dividing the marginal arcade. The bowel lumen was divided with the endo-linercutter EZ45 (blue). This was followed by proximal dissection of the sigmoid colon with the shears, and finally delivery of it through the port on the patient's left side.

Placement of clips, insertion of sutures or suture loops, or the insertion of further rows of staples is unnecessary. The entire dissection, hemostasis, and division of tissue structures were performed with UltraCision.

In laparoscopic colon surgery, port placement depends upon the patient's anatomy and on the site of resection. Using the 5 mm curved tip shears means that the main instrument can be used over all 5 mm ports when necessary. The 312 port is placed at the appropriate site for the insertion of the linear cutter.

Advantages of UltraCision

The advantage of UltraCision, which is apparent the first time it is used, lies in the principal difference between the ultrasound technology and conventional HF cautery: there is no electric current through the patient. All of the risks of using electric current are avoided.

A new era of surgical dissection technology has been introduced with UltraCision. This extremely clean and uncompromisingly bloodless dissection technique, usable even in inaccessible locations and very close to sensitive tissue structures in oncological surgery, ultimately means crucial benefits for the patient.

The introduction of UltraCision signifies a milestone in the further development of surgery. Video-endoscopic operations are becoming significantly safer due to the new ultrasound technology, and the range of indications can be gradually broadened because of the improved technical surgical possibilities for hemostasis and tissue division.

Costs

Implementation of UltraCision means a considerable primary investment. Subsequent costs arise through the use of disposable items. On the other hand, there is a saving on other disposable items in video-endoscopic surgery (tissue forceps, shears, clips, staplers) (Table 4.2).

There is also a significant reduction in blood units, because surgery with UltraCision is quite miserly with blood.

When shears are used, the otherwise necessary repeated instrument changes are avoided according to the various application modalities. This allows shortened operating times. The staffing requirements in the operating theater can also be reduced.

Table 4.2   UltraCision shears versus clips in laparoscopic fundoplication

Variable	Clips	LCS	p value
Patients	$n=10$	$n=10$	
Time for transection of short gastric vessels	37.4 ± 5.7 min	23.7 ± 6.1 min	$p<0.05$
Blood loss	20.1 ± 18.1 ml	14.2 ± 13.1 ml	n.s.
Costs (USD)	$925\pm185	$734\pm62.3	$p<0.05$

From: Surg Endos 1996: 10: 71–73.

Suggested Reading

Ata AA, Bellemore TJ, Meisel JA, Arambulo SM. Distal thermal injury from monopolar electrosurgery. Surg Laparosc Endosc 1993; 3: 323.

Amaral JF. Laparoscopic application of an ultrasonically activated scalpel. Gastrointestinal Endoscopy Clinics of North America 1993; 3: 381.

Amaral JF. Ultrasonic energy in laparoscopic surgery. Surg Technol Int III: 155.

Amaral JF. The experimental development of an ultrasonically activated scalpel for laparoscopic use. Surg Laparosc Endosc 1994; 4: 92.

Amaral JF. Tissue injury with ultrasonic energy and electrosurgery in the porcine stomach. Second Asian Pacific Congress for Endoscopic Surgery, Hong Kong 1995.

Amaral JF. Laparoscopic cholcystectomy in 200 consecutive patients using an ultrasonically activated scalpel. Surg Laparosc Endosc 1995; 5: 255.

Amaral JF. Depth of thermal injury: ultrasonically activated scalpel vs. electrosurgery. Surg Endosc 1995; 9: 226.

Amaral JF, Fowler DL. Laparoscopic esophagomyotomy and seromyotomy using an ultrasonically activated scalpel. Society for Minimally Invasive Therapy, Orlando, 1993.

Berry SM, Ose KJ, Bell RH, Fink AS. Thermal injury of the posterior duodenum during laparoscopic cholecystectomy. Surg Endosc 1994; 8: 197.

Bell RCW. Can doing more be faster? An ultrasonic scalpel and speed of fundoplication. Surg Endoscopy 1996; 10: 223.

Feil W. Schilddrüsenresektion mit UltraCision. Acta Chirurgica Austriaca 1997; Suppl. 130: 23.

Feil W. Sphinktererhaltende Rektumresektionen mit UltraCision. Acta Chirurgica Austriaca 1997; Suppl. 130: 80.

Feil W. UltraCision: Erste Erfahrungen in der offenen Chirurgie. Acta Chirurgica Austriaca 1997; Suppl. 130: 128.

Feil W. UltraCision: Erste Erfahrungen in der laparoskopischen Chirurgie. Acta Chirurgica Austriaca 1997; Suppl. 130: 130.

Fowler DL. Mesenteric dissection without clips or staples. American College of Surgeons, Chicago, 1994.

Fowler DL. Use of ultrasonically activated scalpel and shears in endoscopic surgery. Third International Congress on New Technology and Advanced Techniques in Surgery, Luxembourg, 1995.

Fowler DL, White ShA. Laparoscopic gastrectomy: five cases. Surg Laprosc Endosc 1996; 6: 98.

Geis WP, McAfee PC, Kim HC. The combined use of head-mounted display, robotic enhancement and Harmonic Scalpel technologies in complex minimal invasive surgical procedures. The Society for Minimally Invasive Therapy, Seventh International Meeting, Portland, Oregon, 1995.

Geis WP, Kim HC, McAfee PC, Kang JG, Brennan EJ. Synergistic benefits of combined technologies in complex, minimally invasive surgical procedures. Surg Endosc 1996; 10: 1025.

Lange V, Millott M, Dahsan H, Eilers D. Das Ultraschallskalpell: erste Erfahrungen beim Einsatz in der laparoskopischen Chirurgie. Chirurg 1996; 67: 387.

Laycock WS, Trus TL, Hunter JG. New technology for the division of short gastric vessels during laparoscopic Nissen fundoplication. Surg Endosc 1996; 10: 71.

Luciano AA, Soderstrom RM. Essential principles of electrosurgery in operative laparoscopy. J Am Assoc Gynec Lap 1994; 1: 189.

Markowicz S, Chrostek CA, Amaral JF. Surgical laparoscopic energy and lateral thermal damage. The Society for Minimally Invasive Therapy, Berlin, 1994.

Meltzer RC, Hoenig DM, Chrostek CA, Amaral JF. The ultrasonically activated scalpel vs. electrosurgery for seromyotomy: acute and chronic studies in the pig. Society of the American Gastrointestinal Endoscopic Surgeons, Nashville, 1994.

Moossa AR, Easter DW, Sonnenberg E, Casola G, Agostino H. Laparoscopic injuries to the bile duct. Ann Surg 1992; 215: 203.

Nduka CC, Super PA, Monson JRT, Darzi AW. Cause and prevention of electrosurgical injuries in laparoscopy. J Am Coll Surg 1994; 179: 161.

Ohgami M, Otani Y, Kumai K, Kitajima M. Laparoscopic curative surgery for early gastric cancer. Third International Congress on New Technology and Advanced Techniques in Surgery, Luxembourg, 1995.

Ott D. Smoke production and smoke reduction in endoscopic surgery: preliminary report. End Surg 1993; 1: 230.

Rothenberg SS. Laparoscopic splenectomy using the Harmonic Scalpel. J Laparoendoscopic Surgery 1996; 6: S61.

Saye WB, Miller WM, Hertzmann P. Electrosurgical thermal injury. Surg Laparosc Endosc 1991; 1: 223.

Swanstrom LL, Pennings JL. Laparoscopic control of short gastric vessels. J American College of Surgeons 1995; 181: 347.

Tucker RD. Laparoscopic electrosurgical injuries: survey results and their implications. Surg Laparosc Endosc 1995; 5: 311.

Tucker RD, Voyles CR. Laparoscopic electrosurgical complications and their prevention. AORN J 1995; 62: 51.

Voyles CR, Tucker RD. Unrecognized hazards of surgical electrodes passed through metal suction-irrigation devices. Surg Endosc 1994; 8: 185.

Voyles CR, Meena AL, Petro AB, Haick AJ. Electrocautery is superior to laser for laparoscopic cholecystectomy. Am J Surg 1990; 160: 457.

5 Esophageal Resection With the UltraCision Blade and Shears

B. Walther

In spite of the time-consuming and technically demanding nature of esophageal resection, and its dismal prognosis (it is associated with probably the highest mortality rate of any elective operation), surgical correction of esophageal cancer is still considered the mainstay of treatment (3, 13, 15).

The importance of the surgical approach for postoperative comfort is evident in minor procedures after introduction of laparoscopic bile and antireflux surgery. The approach is of little consequence for postoperative morbidity, mortality, and long-time survival in major esophageal surgery for malignant disease with extensive mediastinal dissection close to the airways and the heart, where clearance of the abdominal and thoracic aorta from fat and lymph nodes in often respiratory (tobacco use) and immunologically (alcohol use) compromised patients is required (5, 11, 14). Hard evidence for an increased rate of wound metastases following laparo/thoracoscopic cancer surgery has accumulated and further diminished the enthusiasm for removing the esophagus by minimal invasive approaches (7, 8, 12). This, and the failure to show lesser postoperative morbidity, mortality, and better long-time survival with minimal invasive methods, are the reasons for the present unanimous recommendation that open surgery should remain the standard of esophagectomy (11, 14).

> Editor's tip: By now, minimally invasive esophagectomy is technically feasible, but open surgery should remain the standard until future studies conclusively demonstrate the advantages of minimally invasive approaches.

Esophagectomy through an upper-midline incision and a right thoracotomy approach was described in 1946 by Ivor Lewis. This is still the most popular method, followed by the transhiatal method, described experimentally in 1913 and successfully performed clinically in 1924 and again in 1933 (4, 6, 17). Throughout the years, the majority of surgeons have used the stomach as their premier choice of conduit for reconstruction, with the colon as the second choice (13).

In distal pancreatectomy, the incidence of pancreatic fistula is significantly reduced with the ultrasonic dissector compared to conventional techniques, as found in a randomized clinical trial (16). In another randomized trial, the operation time was significantly reduced in thyroidectomies with the use of the ultrasonic shears (18). These arguments, and the convincing results with the ultrasonic shears in laparoscopic mo-

bilization of the gastric fundus in antireflux procedures, led me to venture to use this instrument in major open procedures as well.

Indication and Preoperative Management

At the Department of Surgery at Lund University, Lund, Sweden, the indication for esophageal resection is cancer of the esophagus 90% of the time (half of which is adenocarcinoma and the other half squamous cell carcinoma), and benign esophageal disease 10% of the time. The preoperative preparation consists of (besides a careful clinical evaluation) fibre-endoscopy of the esophagus, where the level of the tumor is recorded. In patients with a tumor that allows the endoscope to pass, the stomach, the substitute of choice in the majority of patients, is also assessed. In other patients, radiological evaluation of the projected conduit is performed. When chest X-rays and ultrasounds of the liver reveal no signs of metastases, we explore the patient.

Operation

The following instruments are recommended:
- For skin incision: scalpel
- For subcutaneous tissue, chest wall muscles, intercostal muscles, pleura and linea alba: UltraCision 10 cm with 5 mm blade (DH 105)
- For mediastinal and intraabdominal dissection: UltraCision 23 cm with 5 mm curved shears for open surgery (CS-23C)
- For the azygos vein: doubly secured with suture ligation and ligation (4.0 Prolene and 2.0 Prolene, respectively)
- For the inferior phrenic veins: suture ligation with 4.0 Vicryl in connection with the phrenotomy
- For the left gastric artery: doubly ligated with 2.0 Vicryl
- For phrenotomy: bipolar PowerStar

> Editor's tip: Development of robots with multidirectional specific instruments, including ultrasound instruments, might be the future of esophageal resection.

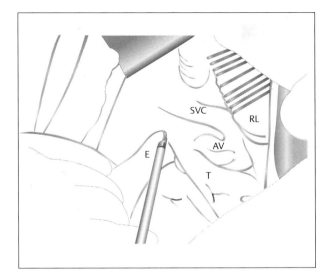

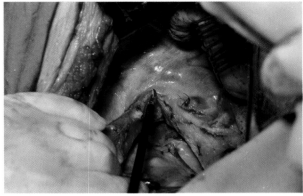

Fig. 5.**1**   The mediastinum is dissected, using the 23 cm long UltraCision curved shears (CS-23C), from the diaphragm to the apex of the chest, with the inactive blade towards sensible structures. *SVC* superior vena cava, *RL* right lung, *AV* ligated azygos vein, *E* esophagus, *T* trachea.

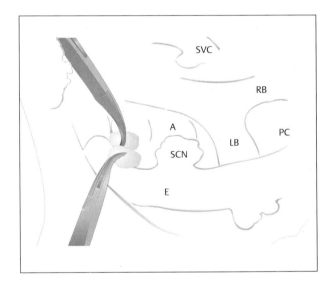

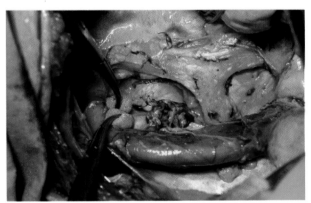

Fig. 5.**2**   For complete hemostasis, the UltraCision shears (CS-23C) were used throughout the procedure except for ligation of the azygos vein. *A* aortic arch, *E* esophagus with subcarinal nodes (*SCN*), *LB* left main brochus, *T* trachea, *PC* pericardium, *SVC* superior vena cava.

Anastomosis in the Neck

In patients who require neck anastomoses, the operation is started with a right posterolateral thoracotomy performed with the 10 cm UltraCision with a 5 mm blade (DH 105) in the fifth interspace. Using the 23 cm long curved shears (CS-23C), the mediastinum is dissected, from the diaphragm to the apex of the chest, along the aorta, left pleura, and pericardium, and upward along the superior vena cava and trachea, with removal of fat, nodes, esophagus, azygos vein and the thoracic duct en bloc (Fig. 5.**1**). The subcarinal nodes and the aortopulmonary window are included in the dissection (Fig. 5.**2**). The thorax is drained and closed and the patient placed in the supine position.

The abdomen is explored through a midline incision with the same blade as used for the thoracotomy. After division of all left gastroepiploic arteries ("the short gastrics"), the omentum is resected outside of the right gastroepiploic arcade with the shears, using the edges of the laparotomy incision as the touch spot and the 23 cm long shears as a lever for easy adjustment of tension in the tissue (Fig. 5.**3 a, b**).

Fat and nodes along the upper part of the abdominal aorta and along the celiac trunk are dissected in the same way (Fig. 5.**4**). The left gastric artery is doubly ligated with 2.0 absorbable material (Fig. 5.**5**).

The duodenum and head of pancreas are mobilized to allow the pylorus to reach the hiatus. Pyloroplasty is performed only when deemed necessary, and the

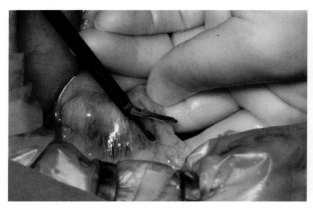
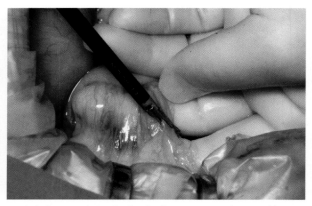

Fig. 5.**3 a** With open jaws, and the shears activated, a small hemostatic hole is made in the fat. **b** The most expedient and hemostatic division is achieved by using only the foremost two-thirds of the shears.

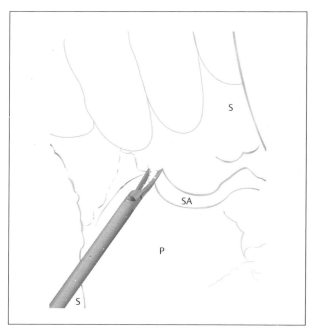
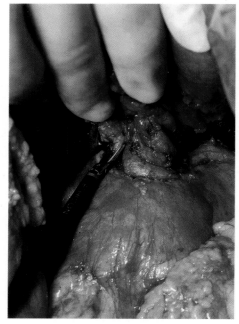

Fig. 5.**4** With the inactive blade toward the vessels, the splenic artery and the hepatic artery are dissected. *P* pancreas, *SA* splenic artery, *S* stomach.

spleen is not removed. A gastric tube is created (Fig. 5.**6**; Fig. 5.**7 a**).

The right gastric and the right gastro-epiploic arteries provide the vascular supply of the tube. To prevent subsequent vascular compromise of the substitute, an anterior phrenotomy of the hiatus is done. Here, we use a pair of scissors due to the hard fibrotic strands, which are impossible for the shears to cope with.

A cervical incision is made parallel to the medial part of the left sternocleidomastoid muscle. The prepared gastric tube is gently pushed from below through the mediastinum and delivered to the neck. After adjustment of the length, the gastric tube and the esophagus are divided and the anastomosis sutured. (Fig. 5.**7 b**)

Anastomosis in the Chest

In patients with tumors in the distal third of the esophagus, a stapled intrathoracic anastomosis is performed (Fig. 5.**7 c**). The operation is started with the gastric mobilization and finished with the anastomosis in

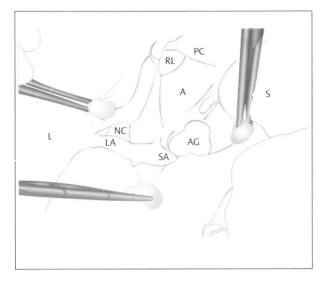

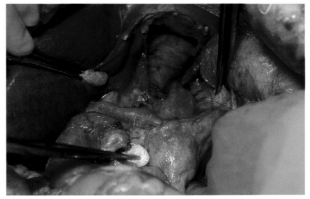

Fig. 5.**5**   The abdominal dissection is finished. The left gastric artery and the inferior phrenic veins are the only structures ligated. *A* aorta, *PC* pericardium, *RL* right lung, *C* crus (a cuff of diaphragm resected), *S* stomach, *L* liver, *AG* left adrenal gland, *LA* liver artery, *SA* splenic artery.

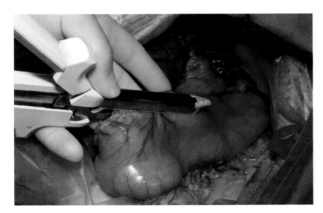

Fig. 5.**6**   The gastric tube is created by serial applications of a linear cutting stapling device, TLC75 (Ethicon Endosurgery) parallel to and at a distance of 6 cm from the greater curvature. *S* stomach; *TLC* a 75 mm linear cutter.

Fig. 5.**7**   (*A*) Approximately 8 cm proximal to the pylorus at the Crow's foot the gastric tube is created by serial applications of a linear cutting stapling device, TLC75. (*B*) The anastomosis in the neck is done with a running, single-layer, end-to-end technique with 4.0 polydioxanone (PDS II) through all layers. (*C*) The thoracic esophagogastrostomy is performed end-to-greater curvature, by insertion of a circular stapling device through the subsequently resected lesser curvature.
▽

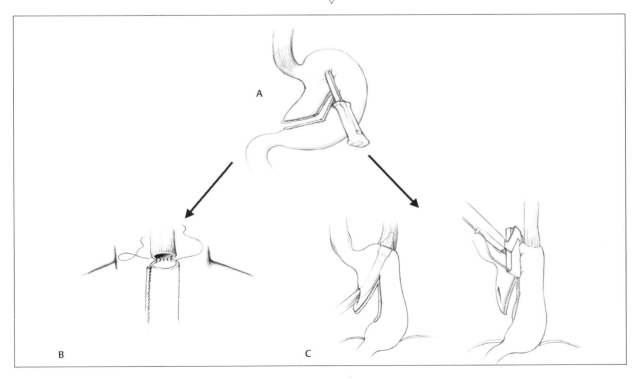

the right chest. The dissection and the handling of the stomach and the esophagus are consistent with that of the neck group. Circular stapling devices (cartridge sizes 25, 28, 29, or 31 mm) have been used to construct the esophagogastric anastomosis in the right apex of the chest. The stomach is resected with a linear stapling device, not nearer than 2 cm to the circular anastomosis (Fig. 5.7c). The two "doughnuts" from the circular stapler are checked for completeness. With the anastomosis under saline, its integrity is checked by inflating air through the nasogastric tube. If a leak is present, or an anastomotic ring is incomplete, the defect is sewn over with an absorbable 4.0 suture.

Irrespective of approach, all gastric tubes are placed in the posterior mediastinum. The pleura are drained with two chest-tubes. No drain is left in the abdomen or neck.

> Editor's tip: Our experience in open and thoracoscopic approaches suggests that the fluid outflow from chest drainage is lowered when using UltraCision. Randomized trials have never been conducted in this area, however.

Summary of the Esophagectomy Procedure

Whether a neck or a chest anastomosis is performed, the mediastinum is dissected exclusively with the 23 cm long curved shears (CS-23C) from the diaphragm to the right apex of the chest through a right thoracotomy, done with the dissecting hook (DH 105).

The gastric mobilization is achieved with the curved shears (CS-23C). The decussating, hard, tendinous strands, which form the anterior part of the hiatus divided in connection with the phrenotomy, is the only part of the abdominal procedure that the ultrasonic shears cannot cope with. Here, we use a diathermic pair of scissors (the bipolar PowerStar) for division.

The duodenum and head of pancreas are mobilized to allow the pylorus to reach the hiatus. Pyloroplasty is performed only when deemed necessary, and the spleen is not removed. The gastric tube, substituting for the esophagus, is created by serial applications of a linear cutting stapling device (a TLC 55 from Ethicon, Stockholm, Sweden) parallel to and at a distance of 6 cm from the greater curvature, starting approximately 8 cm proximal to the pylorus at the Crow's foot.

When a patient needs an esophagogastrostomy in the neck, a running, single-layer end-to-end technique with 4.0 Polydioxanone (PDS II, Ethicon) is used through all the layers. In the chest, the esophagogastrostomy is constructed end-to-greater curvature, by insertion of a circular stapling device (a TLH 90 or TL 60, Ethicon) through the subsequently resected lesser curvature. In the two techniques, everting staple lines in the proximal part of the substitute are at hand and the circulation in the most critical part easily evaluated.

 Hints and Pitfalls

To avoid annoying tears in the splenic capsule, two precautionary measures should be carried out. First, no abdominal exploration or dissection is started without gauze behind the spleen. Second, the gastric mobilization starts with the most difficult part, i.e., the separation of the stomach from the spleen. This is best achieved by dissection along the left crus (level 5) downward entering the lesser sack from above. With the left index finger behind the gastro-splenic ligament, the short gastric vessels are readily divided one at a time without tension with the 23 cm shears (level 2) to the unification of the left and right gastroepiploic arteries. This is in contrast to what is done laparoscopically, where the fundic mobilization is more convenient from below towards the spleen.

The long-shafted curved shears (CS-23C) can be used as a lever with the edge of the laparotomy incision as a touch spot and pressure and tension accordingly adjusted during the abdominal dissection. In the thorax, the ribs function as touch spots.

To avoid mechanical injuries in dissection along the celiac axis to the hepatic and splenic arteries, the azygos vein, and the inferior pulmonary veins, the inactive blade is turned toward the vessels. This is also true for the dissection along the membranous part of the trachea and the pericardium.

The shears may also be used to cut the ends of the few necessary sutures, two in the abdomen (for the left gastric artery and the inferior diaphragmatic vein), and one in the thorax (for the azygos vein).

Rotating the shears results in more surface of the tissue against the active blade of the instrument. This speeds up the division but still retains the reliable hemostatic function. Consequently, by practicing this we increasingly have substituted level 2 with level 5.

 Personal Experience

In a prospective series, we included 310 open esophagectomies from May 1990 through April 2002. The postoperative mortality was 0.97 % (3 of 310). The latest 60 have been performed with the straight and curved UltraCision shears for open surgery without hospital mortality or reoperation. The median hospital stay was 14 days (range 8 to 83 days).

The 5 mm thick, 23 cm curved UltraCision shears with needle-holder handgrip (CS-23C) were our usual preference. In the beginning of the series, we used the 10 mm shears with a straight and rotating active blade, and frequently used all three sides of the blade. Admittedly, we gradually stopped rotating the blade, instead using only the blunt side. We have now substituted the straight instrument for a curved instrument with a fixed blade (CS-23C), whose characteristics correspond to the blunt side of the straight and rotating blade.

The reliable and durable hemostatic function of UltraCision was obvious, even with the first patient. There was now no need for the regular turn with the diathermy forceps around the wound edges for complete hemostasis before closing the abdominal and thoracic incisions. This, and the fact that none of the 60 patients was reoperated because of postoperative hemorrhage, led us to the conclusion that the UltraCision shears are a reliable hemostatic-dissecting instrument.

 ## Discussion

Hemostatic dissecting instruments have been available for decades. The bipolar diathermy PowerStar scissors arrived in the 1990s, with excellent dissecting and coagulating qualities. The entry of UltraCision, however, resulted in an instrument which avoided all the risks of electricity.

The advantage of an instrument capable of atraumatic surgical dissection and division of vessels up to 3 mm with reliable hemostasis is very great. In a short report from Laycock, the advantage of division of the short gastrics with the UltraCision scalpel in laparoscopic Nissen fundoplication was evident (10). Mobilizing the stomach from the spleen in open esophagectomies is even more demanding, especially in large distal esophageal tumors growing close to or into the left diaphragm. Here the UltraCision shears (CS-23C) allow separation of the stomach and the spleen without damage to any of the organs (level 2) even if there is no distinct plane for dissection. The lateral spread of thermal injury of only 1 mm at five seconds of activation of the instrument is especially appreciated around this area of the stomach, since this part, where the circulation is most compromised, will subsequently constitute the anastomosis to the esophagus (1, 2, 9).

In long operations, like en bloc esophagectomies with extensive dissection in the upper-abdomen and mediastinum, the durability of the instrument is tested. In 10 out of the 60 esophagectomies performed with the shears, we had to use two instruments to finish the operation. In all ten cases the reason was breakdown of the closing mechanism. When we avoided tar at the base of the two blades by grasping tissue only with the foremost two-thirds of the jaws, and replaced the shears with the blade through the abdominal and thoracic wall, we have completed the procedures using only a single UltraCision shears.

Here are two hints to achieve a clean and well-functioning instrument throughout long procedures: use only the foremost two-thirds of the shears; and have the instrument activated a couple of seconds after withdrawal from the tissue. In fact, a clean instrument after hours of operation testifies to satisfying experience with the ultrasonic technique.

The efficiency of ultrasonic instruments, measured by operation time and blood loss, can be illustrated by a comparison to the era of ligation, clips, and diathermy. This has been done in randomized studies for left pancreatectomies and thyroidectomies; these studies demonstrate the superiority of the ultrasonic technique (16, 18). After the introduction of UltraCision instruments, we have found that the abdominal part of the esophagectomy procedure has been shortened from four to three hours, and the blood loss (quantified as number of gauze) has diminished from 30 to 20. As for the thoracic part, however, no time reduction has been noticed, presumably because operation time in the thorax is more dependent upon tumor size and location than upon the specific dissecting instruments used.

> Editor's tip: Several alternatives for esophageal resection and replacement with laparoscopic, thoracoscopic, video-assisted, or completely endoscopic techniques have been reported. All of these alternatives have advantages and disadvantages according to the indications, instrumental requirements, cost, and feasibility. In these operations, ultrasound energy based instruments are very helpful, avoiding the need for multiple changes of instruments.

 ## References

1. Amaral JF. The experimental development of an ultrasonically activated scalpel for laparoscopic use. Surg Laparoscop Endoscop 1994; 4:92–9.
2. Amaral JF. Ultrasonic dissection. Endosc Surg Allied Technol 1994; 2:181–85.
3. Birkmeyer JD, Siewers AE, Finlayson EVA, et al. Hospital volume and surgical mortality in the United States. N Engl J Med 2002; 346:1128–1137.
4. Clairmont P. Zur Radikaloperation des Ösophaguskarzinoms. Zbl Chir 1924; 51:42–6.
5. Collard JM. Role of videoassisted surgery in the treatment of oesophageal cancer. Ann Chirurg, Gynaecol 1995; 84:209–14.
6. Denk W. Zur Radikaloperation des Ösophaguskarzinoms. Zentralbl Chir 1913; 40:1065–68.
7. Dixit AS, Martin CJ, Flynn P. Port-site recurrence after thoracoscopic resection of oesophageal carcinoma. Aust N Z J Surg 1997; 67:148–49.
8. Downey RJ, McCormack P, Lo Cicero J III. Dissemination of malignant tumours after video-assisted thoracic surgery: a report of twenty-one cases. The Video-Assisted Thoracic Surgery Study Group. J Thorac Cardiovasc Surg 1996; 111:954–60.
9. Hoenig DM, Chrostek CA, Amaral JF. Laparosonic coagulating shears: alternative method of hemostatic control of unsupported tissue. J Endourol 1996; 10:431–33.
10. Laycock WS, Trus TL, Hunter JG. New technology for the division of short gastric vessels during laparoscopic Nissen fundoplication: a prospective randomized trial. Surg Endosc 1996; 10:71–3.
11. Luketich JD, Schauer PR, Christie NA, et al. Minimally invasive esophagectomy. Ann Thorac Surg 2000; 70:906–12.
12. Neuhaus SJ, Texler M, Hewett PJ, Watson Dl. Port-site metastases following laparoscopic surgery. Br J Surg 1998; 85:735–41.
13. Reed CE. Surgical management of esophageal carcinoma. Oncologist 1999; 4:95–105.

14. Smithers BM, Gotley DC, McEwan D, Martin I, Bessell J, Doyle L. Thoracoscopic mobilization of the esophagus. Surg Endosc 2001; 15:176–82.
15. Sugimachi K. Advances in the surgical treatment of oesophageal cancer. Br J Surg 1998; 85:289–90.
16. Suzuki Y, Fujino Y, Tanioka Y, et al. Randomized clinical trial of ultrasonic dissector or conventional division in distal pancreatectomy for non-fibrotic pancreas. Br J Surg 1999; 86:608–11.
17. Turner GG. Excision of the thoracic oesophagus for carcinoma with construction of an extrathoracic gullet. Lancet 1933; 2:1315–16.
18. Voutilainen PE, Haglund CH. Ultrasonically activated shears in thyroidectomies. A randomized trial. Ann Surg 2000; 231:322–28.

6 Reflux Surgery (Nissen and Toupet)

O. J. McAnena

The vast majority of patients with gastroesophageal reflux disease (GERD) are managed adequately with simple lifestyle modifications and proton-pump inhibitors. A significant minority with severe symptoms of reflux, however, is refractory to medical management, or they relapse quickly when treatment is discontinued.

Open Nissen fundoplication was the surgical "gold standard" for GERD prior to the introduction of H2-receptor antagonists and proton-pump inhibitors. When surgical and medical treatments of complicated GERD were compared in a prospective, randomized trial, surgically-treated patients fared better (16). Because open antireflux surgery was performed with a long incision, however, by either a laparotomy or thoracotomy with its attendant morbidity, most patients chose to avoid surgery unless it was a last resort.

The development in the early 1990s of minimally invasive techniques for performing antireflux surgery dramatically changed the paradigm for the surgical management of GERD and hiatus hernia (8, 11).

Laparoscopic Nissen fundoplication has become the established treatment modality in refractory gastroesophageal reflux disease (3, 4, 6, 7, 12, 13, 15, 37). Partial fundoplications are generally reserved for patients with poor esophageal motility associated with gastroesophageal reflux. The Toupet fundoplication has been the main alternative in those situations (21, 28, 29).

Indication and Preoperative Management

Indications for antireflux surgery include complications of GERD that may be resistant to medical therapy, complications associated with paraesophageal hiatal hernia, relapses once medical therapy has been discontinued in a young patient, or with a patient who does not want lifelong medical therapy.

Objective evidence of reflux disease is mandatory before contemplating antireflux surgery (38). The minimal diagnostic evaluation is esophagogastroduodenoscopy to assess the gastroesophageal mucosa for evidence of esophagitis and to screen for evidence of Barrett's esophagus (10, 32).

Endoscopic evidence of reflux esophagitis is a minimal requirement in a patient with typical symptoms. If Barrett's esophagus with severe dysplasia is discovered on biopsy, the patient should probably undergo esophageal resection rather than antireflux surgery as there is a high incidence of adenocarcinoma in this group.

Twenty-four-hour pH monitoring is the "gold standard" test to confirm the presence of gastroesophageal reflux. It also correlates subjective symptoms with reflux events and differentiates between upright and supine reflux (10, 32).

Contrast radiological studies may be helpful to gauge the size of a hiatal hernia, to localize precisely the gastroesophageal junction in relation to the esophageal hiatus (and therefore infer the presence or absence of esophageal shortening), and to qualitatively assess the adequacy of peristalsis and speed of gastric emptying.

Esophageal manometry should be performed in all patients considered for antireflux surgery. Manometry assesses the length, location, and pressure of the lower esophageal sphincter and its ability to relax during swallowing. Furthermore, both the amplitude and efficacy of swallowing-induced peristalsis of the esophageal body is assessed. Manometry, therefore, identifies the rare individual with a primary motility disorder (achalasia, scleroderma) with symptoms of GERD. A partial fundoplication such as Toupet's procedure is less likely to result in dysphagia or gas bloat syndrome in these individuals.

Where symptoms include significant nausea and vomiting—and in those individuals with severe insulin-dependent diabetes—a scintigraphic gastric emptying test should be performed to help exclude a gastric emptying abnormality. If a marked delay in gastric emptying is identified, a pyloroplasty or pyloromyotomy may be performed at the time of surgery.

Lifestyle modifications, which are among the hallmarks of medical therapy, should also be implemented. Weight reduction in overweight individuals combined with abstinence from alcohol, chocolate, coffee, and cigarette smoking, which all affect the LOS, are to be recommended.

> Editor's tip: There are a number of patients who present with typical symptoms of GERD without evidence of endoscopic esophagitis. These patients must undergo a complete assessment of the foregut to analyze the origin of the symptoms.
> We recommend barium upper GI series in all patients. Twenty-four-hour pH monitoring is used in a selective manner: atypical or extraesophageal symptoms; absence of response to a well-conducted PPI therapy; no endoscopic signs of esophagitis.

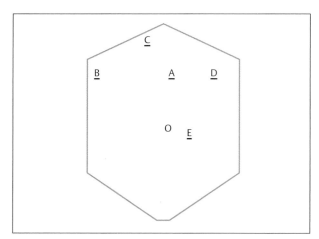

Fig. 6.1 Drawing showing the port positions for laparoscopic Nissen fundoplication. (*A*) 10 mm port for the 30° telescope placed midway between umbilicus and xiphisternum. (*B*) 10 mm port below right costal margin for liver retractor. (*C*) 5 mm port that penetrates the falciform ligament from right to left, for De-Bakey forceps access. (*D*) 10 mm port below left costal margin for access with LSC shears. (*E*) 10 mm port below and to left of the umbilicus for retraction of stomach using blunt-ended Bab-cock forceps.

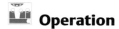 **Operation**

Laparoscopic Nissen Fundoplication

Several different techniques have been described for performing laparoscopic antireflux surgery. The description given here will outline our current approach (25). The patient is placed in a modified Lloyd-Davies position, the hips being placed in a neutral position. The surgeon stands between the patient's legs, with an assistant on either side. Two video monitors are positioned at either side of the head of the table to allow easy viewing by the surgeon and assistants. The table is maintained in a steep, head-up position—gravity displaces the abdominal viscera from the subdiaphragmatic area.

The following choice of instruments is recommended:

- Four 10 mm ports (camera, LCS shears, liver retractor, and Babcock retractor)
- One 5 mm port (DeBakey tissue forceps)
- UltraCision 10 mm LCS shears
- Two needle holders
- 2/0 unresorbable sutures (preferably silk nurolon or Ethibond)
- 30° angled telescope

The following instruments may be used additionally or alternatively:

- UltraCision 5 mm LCS shears
- Instrument holder or robotic device
- 2/0 Prolene sutures

Laparoscopic access is via four 10 mm ports and one 5 mm port. The camera port is placed midway between the xiphisternum and the umbilicus. The 10 mm ports are sited in the right and left subcostal areas for liver retraction and LCS shears access, respectively. A 10 mm port is positioned below the umbilicus to the patient's left to facilitate access for a Babcock retractor on the stomach. The final 5 mm port is sited in the right of the epigastrium to facilitate access with a DeBakey tissue forceps. This last port traverses the falciform ligament from right to left, and reduces the risk of "crossing swords" with the LCS shears and/or telescope (Fig. 6.**1**).

> Editor's tip: The availability of 5 mm LCS shears permits one to use four 5 mm ports, since there is no need for clips or other 10 mm instruments, and only one 10 mm port for the laparoscope. Placement of trocars is somewhat different, however (Fig. 6.**1**).

The operating assistant on the patient's right side holds the liver retractor to elevate the left lobe and also functions as cameraman. The stomach is placed under tension, using a Babcock tissue forceps inserted via the infraumbilical port on the patient's left side and held in position by the second operating assistant. The lesser omentum is divided, beginning just above the hepatic branch of the vagus nerve to the level of the right sling of the right crus of the diaphragm, with the LCS shears. The phrenoesophageal membrane is then divided in a transverse direction, with care being taken to divide only the most anterior portion, thus avoiding injury to the underlying esophagus. The gastric fundus is then pulled inferiorly and to the right. The proximal gastrophrenic ligament is divided to mobilize the proximal gastric cardia. A meticulous dissection is then taken around the esophageal hiatus. The LCS is used to dissect both hiatal slings of the right crus and to create a posterior esophageal window. The mediastinum is entered posterior to the esophagus and the posterior vagus nerve is identified and preserved. The initial mediastinal dissection is complete and the esophagus is free from the pleura, the aorta, and the right crural slings (Fig. 6.**2**).

> Editor's tip: The intramediastinal dissection must be extended to permit 2 to 3 cm of the lower esophagus to stay without traction in the abdomen, below the diaphragm. If this is not obtained, one should consider the possibility of a shortened esophagus and apply adequate techniques (Collis gastroplasty).

The gastric fundus is then mobilized. The greater curve of the stomach is mobilized from the angle of His to the spleen, with division of a variable number of short gastric vessels high on the greater curvature. This may be performed from spleen to angle of His or vice versa, depending on the anatomy encountered.

Vessel division occurs by grasping between the flat aspect of the LCS instrument's active limb and passive arm, applying gentle pressure, and then activating the device using the footswitch. The vessels are thus divided without blood loss (Fig. 6.**3**).

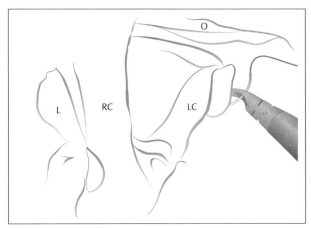

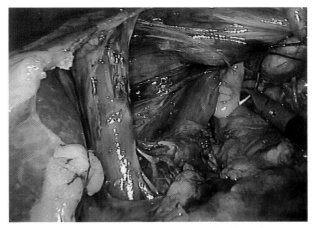

Fig. 6.2 Right and left slings of right crus dissected with scalpel and retroesophageal window created. *L* liver, *RC* right limb of right crus, *LC* left limb of right crus, *E* esophagus. The esophagus is gently elevated and the window created by blunt dissection. Remnant membranes are cut with the 10 mm shears.

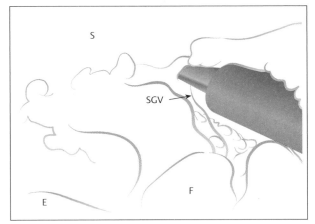

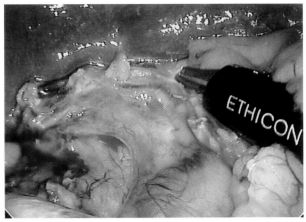

Fig. 6.3 Short gastric vessel division with the LCS shears. *S* spleen, *F* fundus, *E* esophagus, *SGV* short gastric vessel. Vessel division occurs by grasping between the flat aspect of the LCS instrument's active limb and passive arm, applying gentle pressure, and then activating the device using the footswitch.

Editor's tip: The LCS 5 mm shears can be used as a grasping, holding, and dissecting instrument. Even cutting the sutures can be done with the LCS, avoiding the need for other instruments and thus reducing total costs.

When dividing the short gastric vessels, the surgeon must slightly release the traction on the tissues in order to give time for the LCS to ensure coagulation. In this fashion, power level 5 can be used during the entire procedure; level 3 being reserved for possible local bleeding control.

The superior aspect of the bare area of the posterior stomach is mobilized and congenital adhesions between the left sling of the right crus and greater curvature taken down. Excision of the fat pad found at the angle of His aids formation of a mobile wrap, although this step is not always necessary. Grasping forceps are then used to bring the floppy gastric wrap thus created through the posterior esophageal window to lie, without tension, on the right side of the esophagus (Fig. 6.4).

The 360° stomach wrap is secured loosely around the esophagus with two silk sutures, one incorporating the esophagus to maintain the intra-abdominal esophageal segment and prevent wrap slippage. Two silk sutures are also placed to approximate the right crural sling, taking care to avoid the underlying aorta (Fig. 6.5). Bouginage of the esophagus is not routinely used.

Editor's tip: There are two main floppy 360° fundoplications. One is constructed with the upper part of the mobilized fundus that is passed on the right side of the esophagus. Both anterior and posterior walls of the fundus are passed, and the valve is created with the anterior wall of the fundus at the left side of the esophagus and the junction of the posterior and anterior walls at the right side.

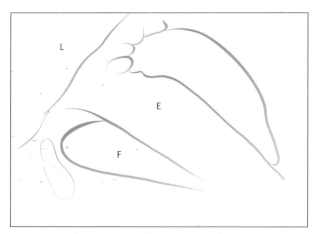
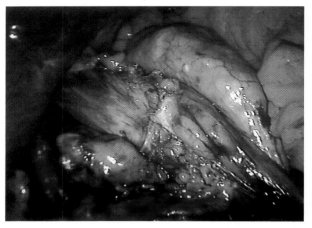

Fig. 6.**4** Fundic wrap rotated to the back of the esophagus without tension, prior to suturing in position. *E* esophagus, *F* leading edge of wrapped fundus, *L* liver.

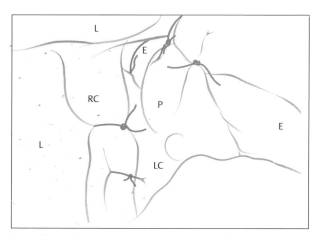
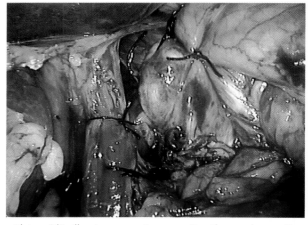

Fig. 6.**5** Fundoplication complete and right crural sling opposed. *E* esophagus, *L* liver, *P* plication, *RC* and *LC* right and left limbs of right crural sling opposed. The 360° wrap is secured with two 2/0 silk sutures, one incorporating the esophagus. Two silk sutures are also used to oppose the right crural sling and prevent further herniation.

The "DeMeester's" valve is different: the posterior wall of the mobilized fundus is passed to the right side of the esophagus and is attached to the anterior wall from the left side of the esophagus, thus incorporating the esophagus in a fold of the gastric fundus. Both valves must be very short—less than 2 cm.

We no longer use silk, which seems not to be as unabsorbable as we had thought (no sutures are found in reoperated patients). We use a mersilène suture, 00.

Crural repair must be performed in all patients and adapted to the size of the hiatal orifice: at the end of the repair, the esophagus must be lying without compression in the repaired orifice.

At the end of the procedure, a bupivacaine irrigation (of 10 ml of a 0.5 % solution in 500 ml of 0.9 % saline) onto the diaphragm is used to reduce shoulder tip pain (5).

Summary of the Nissen fundoplication:
- Division of the pars condensa of the lesser omentum (gastrohepatic ligament),
- Division of the phrenoesophageal membrane and gastrophrenic ligament,
- Mobilization of the distal esophagus from the mediastinum and crura. Reduction of the hiatus hernia,
- Creation of a posterior esophageal window,
- Mobilization of the gastric fundus by division of appropriate short gastric vessels,
- Closure of the crura,
- Creation of a tension-free fundoplication and prevention of slippage.

Toupet Fundoplication

Partial fundoplications are generally reserved for patients with poor esophageal motility associated with GERD, although some centers employ a partial fundoplication routinely (17, 26, 27). The Toupet fundoplication incorporating a 200° to 270° wrap has been the main alternative in these situations (36).

The general approach and initial dissection for laparoscopic partial fundoplications are identical to

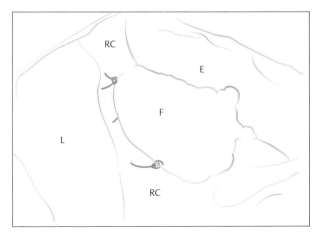

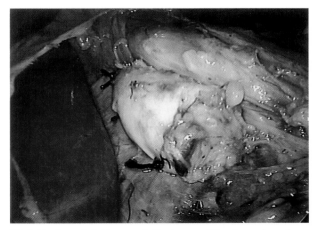

Fig. 6.**6** Posterior aspect of gastric fundus wrap secured to right crural slings using three interrupted 2/0 silk sutures. *L* liver,

RC right sling of right crus of diaphragm, *F* leading edge of gastric fundus to right of esophagus, *E* esophagus.

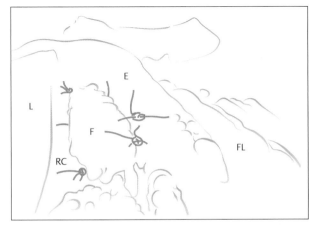

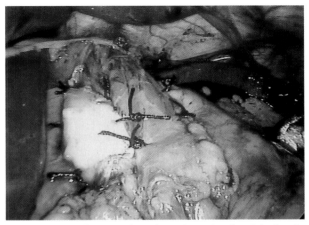

Fig. 6.**7** Completed Toupet fundoplication. *L* liver, *RC* right crus of diaphragm, *F* fundoplication leading edge, *E* esophagus, *FL* fundus to left of esophagus. Three interrupted 2/0 silk sutures are

placed between the anterolateral esophageal wall and the fundic wrap on either side at the 11 o'clock and 1 o'clock positions. The wrap is also secured to the right crus to prevent slippage.

those for the Nissen fundoplication. The gastrohepatic omentum, phrenoesophageal membrane, and gastrophrenic ligaments are divided. The esophagus is dissected away from the mediastinal structures and crura, and the vagus nerves are identified and preserved. Although it may be possible to perform a partial fundoplication without fundic mobilization and division of the short gastric vessels, our policy has been to perform short gastric division routinely. The mobile fundus is pulled left to right behind the esophagus and the crura are re-approximated as before.

The precise technical details of the Toupet fundoplication vary considerably among surgeons. Some authorities describe fixation of the fundoplication to the crura, whereas others omit this step. Most individuals use multiple interrupted, non-absorbable sutures to fix the fundoplication between 200° and 270° around the esophagus.

The wrapped fundus is pulled well to the patient's left to expose the posterior aspect of the fundus and the crura. Several sutures are placed between both the posterior left aspect of the wrapped fundus and the

left sling of the right crus, and between the posterior right aspect of the fundus and the right sling of the right crus (Fig. 6.**6**). These sutures are intended to stabilize the fundus and prevent any tendency for the wrap to de-rotate and to migrate. Several interrupted sutures are placed between the anterior esophageal wall and the fundic wrap on either side at the 11 o'clock and 1 o'clock positions. A dilator is probably unnecessary, but may help by making the esophagus assume a more tubular structure. We generally place three sutures between the right anterolateral aspect of the esophagus (at the 11 o'clock position on the esophageal wall) and the leading edge of the wrapped portion of fundus. The sutures in the esophageal wall should be fairly deep but not full thickness. The medial fundus to the left of the esophagus is then grasped and pulled towards the left anterolateral aspect of the esophagus. Three interrupted sutures are then placed between the fundus to the left of the esophagus and the left anterolateral aspect of the esophagus at the 1 o'clock position (Fig. 6.**7**). The area is examined for hemostasis.

Postoperative care of patients who have undergone laparoscopic partial fundoplication is identical to that for Nissen's. A nasogastric tube is not routinely placed and the patient is allowed clear fluids the evening of the operation and a soft diet the following morning. Rapid resumption of normal activities is encouraged, although activities requiring the Valsalva maneuver (such as lifting heavy objects) and contact sports are to be avoided for six weeks.

⚠ Hints and Pitfalls

- Smaller ports may be used for liver retraction, LCS shears, and Babcock retraction.
- Technical aspects common to all fundoplications include the need to dissect away from the esophagus to avoid injury to the esophageal wall. The esophagus must never be grasped directly or manipulated with the tip of a pointed instrument.
- Vessel division occurs by grasping between the flat aspect of the instrument's active limb and passive arm, applying gentle pressure, and then activating the device using the footswitch. The vessels are thus divided without blood loss.
- When the thoracic angle is very narrow in asthenic patients, the relatively thick shaft of the 10 mm shears can compromise the vision of the surgical field at the hiatus. In such cases the 5 mm LCS shears are an appropriate alternative.
- At the end of the procedure, a bupivacaine irrigation (of 10 ml of a 0.5 % solution in 500 ml of 0.9 % saline) onto the diaphragm may reduce shoulder tip pain (5).

Editor's tip:
- The complete dissection (esophagus, SGV) can be done safely with the 5 mm LCS. There is no need for other dissecting, cutting, or coagulating instruments.
- A vascular lacet placed around the cardia helps in preventing any instrumental injury when manipulating the esophagus and gives good traction and exposure during the different reconstructive steps.
- Floppiness of the valve is obtained when there is no tendency for the right limb of the valve to go back to the spleen after the retroesophageal passage of the fundus. Care must be taken to avoid twisting of the fundus during this passage.
- Postoperative left-shoulder pain is due to the crural repair, is common, and can last up to two weeks.

Personal Experience

One hundred and ten consecutive patients who underwent laparoscopic Nissen's fundoplication as described above have been analyzed (25). Exclusive use was made of the LCS shears. Patients were referred who suffered persistent reflux symptoms despite medical treatment, or who relapsed as soon as medication was discontinued. Seventy-one patients had intractable GERD or relapsing GERD after discontinuation of medical treatment, while 14 declined lifelong medical therapy. Twenty-four younger patients were offered surgery, following pH studies that confirmed severe reflux. All underwent preoperative manometry, pH studies, and endoscopy. They had been on either omeprazole or lansoprazole for 3 to 84 months preoperatively. The mean age was 41.2 years (range 12–69). There were 66 male and 44 female patients. Mean preoperative DeMeester symptom score was 4 (Table 6.**1**).

The mean anesthetic time was 89.6 minutes (range 45–185 minutes). Three patients required conversions to an open procedure; one due to camera failure and two for bleeding related to short gastric vessel division. The two cases of bleeding occurred early during the series. There was one inadvertent esophageal perforation in a patient with marked adhesions around the esophagus, secondary to transmural esophagitis. This was sutured laparoscopically without sequelae. Two patients with a foreshortened esophagus and severe inflammatory reaction around the esophagus had a Toupet fundoplication.

A mild degree of dysphagia was very common postoperatively (64%) but had resolved in all but seven patients at the one-month follow-up. Six patients required endoscopy within the first month for assessment of dysphagia; four required dilatation. Of the six, all but two were symptomatic at six months. The other two had dysphagia that failed to settle with dilation and the wrap was taken down at two and six weeks postoperatively, respectively. At the six-month follow-up, these patients' symptoms were unchanged from preoperatively. Early satiety was noted postoperatively in most patients, but had settled by six weeks in all. No patient had a splenectomy.

The mean postoperative hospital stay was 2.1 days (range 1–8). Of the 110 patients selected for laparoscopic fundoplication, 107 (97.6 % of the total) had their operation completed laparoscopically. Of these 107,

Table 6.**1** DeMeester symptomatic scoring system

Score	Heartburn	Regurgitation	Dysphagia
0	None	None	None
1	Minimal	Minimal	Minimal
2	Moderate	Moderate	Moderate
3	Incapacitated	Incapacitated	Incapacitated

103 had a successful result, with a dramatic resolution of symptoms with a mean DeMeester symptom score of 1.4 postoperatively at six months.

The 10 mm LCS was the standard instrument employed in this series. The LCS provides all the advantages of a multifunction instrument, and was used exclusively for surgical cutting, coagulation, and dissection of tissues. Scissors and diathermy were not used in any case.

> **Editor's tip:**
> - Postoperative dysphagia is common in all patients and lasts for four weeks.
> - Shortened esophagus should be approached with lengthening techniques.
> - In more than 400 fundoplications performed with the help of the LCS, we had no conversion, no postoperative bleeding, no splenic trauma.
> - The new 5 mm LCS with curved blades allows more precise, rapid, and safe dissection.

Discussion

Antireflux surgery is a qualitative operation designed to improve quality of life safely. In early series of laparoscopic antireflux surgery, where electrocautery was used almost exclusively, numerous severe complications were frequently reported (24). Intraoperative bleeding, esophageal perforation with conversion, postoperative bleeding, and peritonitis due to esophageal or gastric wall necrosis were largely attributed to the use of electrocautery.

The use of an ultrasonic activated dissector, the LCS, offers significant advantages in the performance of laparoscopic fundoplication. Because the LCS relies on mechanical energy as a mechanism for cutting and diathermy, the risk of injury from electrical current arc or dissipation is minimized. Safe and reliable blood vessel division, including division of short gastric vessels, can be achieved with minimal lateral thermal damage, because the temperature generated by the LCS is only a quarter of that generated by other modalities of coagulation. The operating field is blood-free and smokeless. Furthermore, a single disposable instrument can replace clips, scissors, and diathermy, resulting in reduced operating times and case-related operating costs. Several prospective randomized trials have shown the LCS to perform division of the short gastric vessels more rapidly and more cheaply than clipping and sharp division (19, 34).

Technically, we feel that division of the short gastric vessels from the angle of His to the spleen, freeing the fundus, and mobilizing the superior aspect of the retroperitoneal bare area of the stomach are essential steps in the creation of a floppy wrap.

Partial fundoplications, predominantly the Toupet, have been used because of concerns that the complete fundoplication may be hypercontinent, resulting in the well-described complications of the Nissen fundoplication, such as dysphagia, inability to belch, and the gas bloat syndrome. From our series, these complaints have been very few. Concerns that the long-term reliability of such repairs is not as good as the Nissen fundoplication remain controversial (17, 22, 23, 31). To keep the outcomes of laparoscopic antireflux surgery in perspective, they should be compared with those of open antireflux operations. One prospective randomized trial comparing the two has revealed similar symptomatic outcomes with a reduced hospital stay in the laparoscopic group (18). Long-term follow-up for open Nissen fundoplication has shown control of reflux symptoms in more than 90 % of patients.

Early results of LARS have been encouraging (2, 12, 13, 15, 30, 41, 42). Perioperative rates of mortality and splenic injury are both near zero and conversion rates in most series are less than 5 %. Dysphagia is a common problem soon after operation, especially following a complete fundoplication, but diminishes over time so that later only 5 to 10 % of all patients will experience occasional mild dysphagia (35, 39). Recurrent reflux symptoms are present in up to 5 % of patients, and wrap disruption or migration either into the chest or down onto the stomach occurs in up to 7 % of patients (14). This is minimized by closure of the crural slings and fixation of the wrap to the esophagus.

The long-term outcome after Toupet fundoplication does not appear to be as good as following a Nissen fundoplication, although this remains controversial and data are scarce. Patti and colleagues using partial fundoplications selectively for patients with "dysfunction of esophageal peristalsis" showed improvement in esophageal peristalsis with an equivalent improvement in postoperative pH testing (28, 29). However, Jobe and colleagues showed worse outcomes using Toupet fundoplication than with Nissen in an unselected group of patients (17). Bell and colleagues, in a series of 143 Toupet partial fundoplications, showed that the presence of complicated esophagitis and a defective lower esophageal sphincter were associated with a three-year failure rate of up to 50 %. They suggested that Toupet should be reserved for milder cases of GERD as assessed by manometry and endoscopy (1).

The results from our personal series and from the recent literature show that the advent of laparoscopic Nissen's and Toupet's fundoplication has significant implications for the surgical management of gastroesophageal reflux disease. The reliability, safety, and versatility of the LCS make it an essential addition to the armamentarium of laparoscopic surgeons performing this operation.

References

1. Bell RWC, Hanna P, Mills MR, Bowry D. Patterns of success and failure with laparoscopic Toupet fundoplication. Surg Endosc 1999; 13: 1189–94.
2. Collet D, Cadiere GB. Conversion and complications of laparoscopic treatment of gastro-oesophageal reflux disease. Am J Surg 1995; 169: 622–26.
3. Coster DD, Bower WH, Wilson VT, Brebrick RT, Richardson GL. Laparoscopic partial fundoplication vs. laparoscopic Nissen-Rissetti fundoplication. Short term results of 231 cases. Surg Endosc 1997; 11: 625–31.
4. Coster DD, Bower WH, Wilson VT, Butler DA, Locker SC, Brebrick RT. Laparoscopic Nissen fundoplication: a curative, safe, and cost-effective procedure for complicated gastroesophageal reflux disease. Surg Laparosc Endosc 1995; 5: 111–17.
5. Cunniffe MG, McAnena OJ, Dar M. Randomised trial of intraoperative bupivacaine irrigation for management of shoulder tip pain for laparoscopy. Am J Surg (in press).
6. Cushieiri A, Shimi S, Nathanson LK. Laparoscopic reduction, crural repair, and fundoplication of large hiatal hernia. Am J Surg 1992; 163: 425–30.
7. Dallemagne B, Taziaux P, Weerts J, Jehaes C, Markiewicz S. Chirurgie laparoscopique du reflux gastro-oesophagien. Ann Chir 1995; 49: 30–6.
8. Dallemagne B, Weerts JM, Jehaes C, et al. Laparoscopic Nissen fundoplication: preliminary report. Surg Laparosc Endosc 1991; 1: 138–43.
9. DeMeester TR, Bonavina L, Albertucci M. Nissen fundoplication for gastro-oesophageal reflux disease: evaluation of primary repair in 100 consecutive patients. Ann Surg 1986; 204: 9–20.
10. DeMeester TR, Wang CI, Wernly JA, et al. Technique, indications and clinical use of 24-hour oesophageal pH monitoring. J Thorac Cardiocasc Surg 1980; 79: 656–70.
11. Geagea T. Laparoscopic Nissen's fundoplication: preliminary report on ten cases. Surg Endosc 1991; 5: 170–73.
12. Gotley DC, Smithers BM, Rhodes M, Menzies B, Branicki FJ, Nathanson L. Laparoscopic Nissen fundoplication—200 consecutive cases. Gut 1996; 38: 487–91. Spechler SJ and the Department of Veterans Affairs Gastroesophageal Reflux Disease Study Group. Comparison of medical and surgical therapy for complicated gastroesophageal reflux disease in veterans. N Engl J Med 1992; 326: 786–91.
13. Hinder RA, Filipi CJ, Wetscher G, Neary P, Demeester TR, Perdikis G. Laparoscopic Nissen fundoplication is an effective treatment for gastroesophageal reflux disease. Ann Surg 1994; 220: 472–83.
14. Hunter JG, Swanstrom L, Waring P. Dysphagia after laparoscopic antireflux surgery. Ann Surg 1996; 224: 51–7.
15. Hunter JG, Trus TL, Branum GD, Waring JP, Wood WC. A physiological approach to laparoscopic fundoplication for gastroesophageal reflux disease. Ann Surg 1996; 223: 673–87.
16. Isolauri J, Luostarinen M, Isolauri E, et al. Natural course of gastroesophageal reflux disease: 17 to 22-year follow-up of 60 patients. Am J Gastroenterol 1997; 92: 37–41.
17. Jobe B, Wallace J, Hansen PD, Swanstrom L. Evaluation of laparoscopic Toupet fundoplication as a primary repair for all patients with medically resistant gastroesophageal reflux. Surg Endosc 1997; 11: 1080–83.
18. Laine S, Rantala A, Gullichsen R, Ovaska J. Laparoscopic vs. conventional Nissen fundoplication. Surg Endosc 1997; 11: 441–44.
19. Laycock WS, Trus TL, Hunter JG. New technology for the division of short gastric vessels during laparoscopic Nissen fundoplication. Surg Endosc 1996; 10: 71–73.
20. Lefebvre JC, Belva P, Takieddine M, Vaneukem P. Laparoscopic Toupet fundoplication: prospective study of 100 cases. Results at one year and literature review. Acta Chirurgica Belgica 1998; 98: 1–4.
21. Lund RJ, Wetcher GJ, Raiser F, et al. Laparoscopic Toupet fundoplication for gastro-oesophageal reflux disease with poor oesophageal body motility. J Gastrointestinal Surg 1997; 1: 301–08.
22. Lundell L, Abrahamsson H, Ruth M, Rydberg L, Lonroth H, Olbe L. Long term results of a prospective randomised comparison of total fundic wrap (Nissen-Rossetti) or semifundiplication (Toupet) for gastro-oesophageal reflux. Br J Surg 1996; 83: 830–35.
23. Mayr J, Sauer H, Huber A, Pilhatsch A, Ratschet M. Modified Toupet wrap for gastroesophageal reflux in childhood. Eu J Paediat Surg 1998: 8: 75–80.
24. McAnena OJ, Wilson P. Diathermy in laparoscopic surgery. Br J Surg 1993; 80: 1094–96.
25. McLaughlin R, McAnena OJ. Laparoscopic Nissen's fundoplication using an ultrasonic dissector. Min Invas Ther and Allied Technol 1999; 8: 49–54.
26. Mosnier H, Leport J, Aubert A, Kianmanesh R, Sbai Idrissi MS, Guivarc'h M. A 270 degree laparoscopic posterior fundoplasty in the treatment of gastroesophageal reflux. J Am Coll Surg 1995; 181: 220–24.
27. O'Reilly MJ, Mullins SG, Saye WB, Pinto SE, Falkner PT. Laparoscopic partial fundoplication: analysis of 100 consecutive cases. J Laparoendosc Surg 1996; 6: 141–50.
28. Patti MG, De Bellis M, De Pinto M, et al. Partial fundoplication for gastro-oesophageal reflux. Surg Endosc 1997; 11: 445–48.
29. Patti MG, De Pinto M, De Bellis M, et al. Comparison of laparoscopic total and partial fundoplication for gastro-oesophageal reflux. J Gastrointestinal Surg 1997; 1: 309–15.
30. Peters JH, DeMeester TR, Eubanks S, et al. The treatment of gastro-oesophageal reflux disease with laparoscopic Nissen fundoplication. Ann Surg 1998; 228: 40–50.
31. Rydberg L, Ruth M, Abrahamsson H, Lundell L. Tailoring antireflux surgery: A randomised clinical trial. World J Surg 1999: 23: 612–18.
32. Schindleback NE, Ippisch H, Klauser A, Muller-Lissner S. Which pH threshold is best in esophageal pH monitoring? Am J Gastroenterol 1991; 86: 1138–45.
33. Spechler SJ and the Department of Veterans Affairs Gastro-oesophageal Reflux Disease Study Group. Comparison of medical and surgical therapy for complicated gastro-oesophageal reflux disease in veterans. N Engl J Med 1992; 326: 786–91.
34. Swanstrom LL, Pennings JL. Laparoscopic control of short gastric vessels. J Am Coll Surg 1995; 181: 347–51.
35. Swanstrom LL, Wayne R. Spectrum of gastrointestinal symptoms after laparoscopic fundoplication. Am J Surg 1994; 167: 538–41.
36. Toupet A. Technique d'oesophago-gastroplastie avec phreno-gastropexie appliquee dans la cure radicale des hernies hiatales et comme complement de l'operation de Heller dans les cardiospasmes. Acad Chirurg 1963; 27: 394–99.
37. Trus TL, Laycock WS, Branum G, Waring JP, Mauren S, Hunter JG. Intermediate follow up of laparoscopic antireflux surgery. Am J Surg 1996; 171: 32–35.
38. Waring JP, Hunter JG, Oddsdottir M, et al. The preoperative evaluation of patients considered for laparoscopic antireflux surgery. Am J Surg 1995; 90: 35–38.
39. Watson DI, Chan A, Myers JC, Jamieson GG. Illness behaviour influences the outcome of laparoscopic antireflux surgery. J Am Coll Surg 1997; 184: 44–48.
40. Watson DI, Jamieson GG. Antireflux surgery in the laparoscopic era. Br J Surg 1998; 85: 1173–84.
41. Watson DI, Jamieson GG, Devitt PG, et al. Changing strategies in the performance of laparoscopic Nissen fundoplication as a result of experience with 230 operations. Surg Endosc 1995; 9: 961–66.
42. Weerts JM, Dallemagne B, Hamoir E, et al. Laparoscopic Nissen fundoplication: detailed analysis of 132 patients. Surg Endosc 1993; 3: 359–64.

7 Esophageal Myotomy for Achalasia

O. J. McAnena, C. Power, D. Maguire

Achalasia is a motor disorder of the esophagus. It is characterized by impaired swallowing-induced relaxation of the lower esophageal sphincter (LES) and absent esophageal peristalsis that affects 0.03–1.1/105/ patient per year (24). It may present at any age, from childhood onwards, but symptoms have typically been present for years at examination (13, 33). A history of dysphagia felt at the upper sternum is usually volunteered. Initially, this is often intermittent and occurs either for solids or liquids, but ultimately it progresses to both. Other symptoms include regurgitation of undigested food (typically nocturnal), halitosis, aspiration, and nocturnal cough. Approximately 50% of patients complain of retrosternal pain.

Indication and Preoperative Management

Accurate patient evaluation is necessary in order to manage patients effectively. Endoscopy is essential for excluding a secondary cause, since malignancy-induced achalasia (typically caused by tumors of the distal esophagus/cardia) mimics both the clinical and manometric manifestations of achalasia (32). While plain radiology is of limited use, chest films may be required to evaluate pulmonary complications (aspiration or abscess) prior to surgery. Esophageal contrast studies classically have shown decreased esophageal peristalsis with failure of LES relaxation (10, 21, 28). Early in the course of the disease, however, only a breakdown of peristalsis with failure to clear barium may be observed. Careful examination of the distal esophagus/cardia is mandatory to rule out secondary achalasia, but there is still a significant risk of missing an early neoplasm due to the distortion produced by retained secretions and food debris.

Patients with suspected achalasia should undergo esophageal manometry. Manometric features include: (a) impaired peristalsis of the esophageal body; (b) elevated LES pressure (average >50 mmHg in achalasia, while normal is 15 to 30 mmHg); and (c) impaired LES relaxation on swallowing (40% as opposed to >90% in

normal patients) (6). Esophageal contractions are low in amplitude (20–40 mmHg) and simultaneous, but earlier in the course of the illness high amplitude simultaneous contractions may be seen.

Operation

Laparoscopic Technique

The patient is placed in a modified Lloyd-Davies position, with the hips in a neutral position. The surgeon stands between the patient's legs, with an assistant on either side. The table is maintained in a steep, head-up position.

The following choice of instruments is recommended:

- Four 10 mm ports (camera, LCS shears, liver retractor, and Babcock retractor)
- One 5 mm port (DeBakey tissue forceps)
- UltraCision 5 or 10 mm LCS shears
- Two needle holders
- 30° angled telescope

After establishing a pneumoperitoneum, the camera port (10 mm) is placed midway between the xiphisternum and the umbilicus. A 30° viewing lens is used, since this facilitates visualization of the cardia. Two further 10 mm ports are then placed in the right (for liver retractor) and left (UltraCision dissector) subcostal areas. A 5 mm port is placed to the right of the midline in the epigastrium (for DeBakey forceps) and traverses the falciform ligament. Finally, a 5 or 10 mm port is placed to the left of and slightly below the umbilicus for insertion of Babcock forceps (used to retract the stomach caudally) (Fig. 7.1).

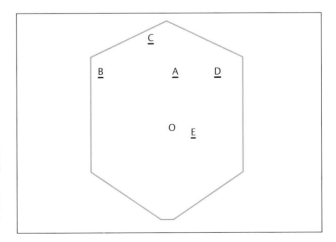

Fig. 7.1 Placement of trocars for esophageal myotomy. (*A*) 10 mm port for the 30° telescope placed midway between umbilicus and xiphisternum. (*B*) 10 mm port below right costal margin for liver retractor. (*C*) 5 mm port that penetrates the falciform ligament from right to left, for DeBakey forceps access. (*D*) 10 mm port below left costal margin for access with LSC shears. (*E*) 10 mm port below and to left of the umbilicus for retraction of stomach using blunt-ended Babcock forceps.

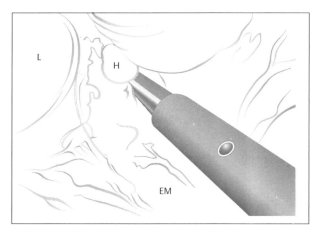
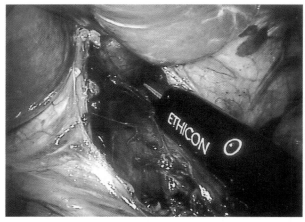

Fig. 7.**2**   UltraCision shears dissecting the phrenicoesophageal membrane. *L* liver, *H* hiatus, *EM* esophageal mucosa.

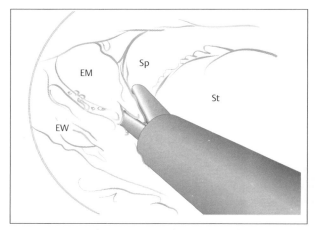
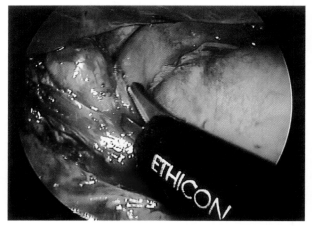

Fig. 7.**3**   Starting the myotomy at the esophageal side of the cardia. *EM* esophageal mucosa, *EW* esophageal muscle wall, *Sp*, spleen, *St* stomach.

Editor's tip: Usually placement of trocars for myotomy is similar to Nissen fundoplication. Thirty-degree lenses are recommended to facilitate visualization of the cardia and lower esophagus through the hiatus.

After placement of the trocars, the liver retractor (left port) is used to elevate the left liver lobe. The right hiatal sling is identified by division of the phrenicoesophageal membrane and connective tissue, and the plane between the anterior, anteromedial, and anterolateral esophagus and the hiatal sling is clarified using the UltraCision shears (Fig. 7.2). The distal 7 to 10 cm of the esophagus within the mediastinum is displayed on its anterior surface.

Editor's tip: The initial part of the dissection is similar to the fundoplication technique: the pars condensa of the lesser omentum is incised above the hepatic branches of the vagal nerve, giving access to

the right crus, which is the first important landmark. It is recommended to avoid complete mobilization of the entire circumference of the esophagus and cardia in order to maintain the antireflux attachments of the cardia.

Traction on the fat pad at the lower cardia helps in the exposure of the cardia and the lower esophagus. This is the key element in acquiring accessible esophageal length.

The LCS is used to dissect and display the lower esophagus and cardia and to divide the small veins crossing the cardia and the superior part of the fat pad, in order to expose properly the entire length of the cardia. The anterior vagus nerve must be identified and dissected in order to be kept away from the myotomy site.

The anterior myotomy is commenced by dividing/separating the longitudinal and circular muscle fibers until the mucosa is reached (Fig. 7.3). The myotomy is established in the middle of the anterior surface of the

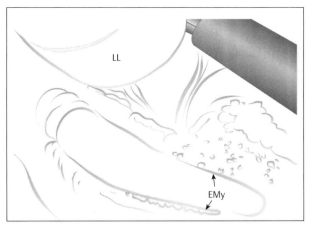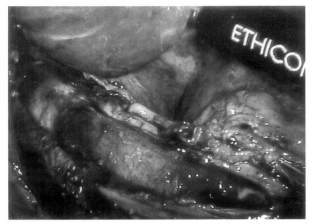

Fig. 7.**4** Endoscopic control of the myotomy, demonstrating some persisting transverse fibers at the gastric side of the cardia. *LL* left lobe of liver, *EM* esophageal mucosa, *EMy* esophageal myotomy.

esophagus. UltraCision facilitates this, because it allows the surgeon to separate the tissues using a single instrument for precise muscle separation and vessel division under direct vision, thereby decreasing the risk of mucosal damage.

> Editor's tip: The best point to start with this step is the esophageal side of the cardia. The plane between the muscular layers and the mucosa is easily entered. UltraCision facilitates this because it allows the surgeon to separate the tissues without bleeding and to identify clearly this plane. But the surgeon must place the LCS in a proper position with the inactive blade toward the mucosa to avoid injury.
>
> In patients with multiple previous endoscopic dilatation sessions, it is recommended to start 4–5 cm above the gastroesophageal junction, where the plane is more accessible because it is less fibrotic.

When the mucosa is reached, the development of the tissue plane between it and the circular muscle is facilitated.

> Editor's tip: This is usually done by blunt dissection with the inactivated LCS, or the suction-irrigation device that helps clear the view of this plane. Hemostasis is usually unnecessary since bleeding stops spontaneously.

Once this has been developed, the myotomy is then completed. Electrocautery can be used for this with a hook-like instrument, but one must be concerned for the potential for a diathermy-induced mucosal injury. The LCS is used for this as collateral tissue injury is less of a problem and instrument interchange is also limited.

In order to check the extent of myotomy, simultaneous endoscopy may be used (Fig. 7.**4**) to ensure that the length of myotomy is appropriate.

The myotomy has to be completed by extending the section of the muscular fibers down the cardia at a 1 or 2 cm distance (Fig. 7.**5**).

> Editor's tip: One should keep in mind that there have been reports of postoperative mucosal necrosis with the LCS. If it is used, proper control of the placement of the active/inactive blades is mandatory. We use conventional scissors without cautery. The myotomy is extended for 6 cm on the lower esophagus and 2 cm back on the gastric side of the cardia when transverse fibers can be observed with the endoscope in place. This part can be done with the LCS with the same care. The total length of the myotomy is usually 8 cm.
>
> Next, the myotomy bed is checked for perforations by submerging the esophagus in an irrigation fluid and insufflating it with the endoscope or nasogastric tube. Small mucosal holes can be safely repaired with absorbable sutures.
>
> We perform systematically an antireflux repair with an anterior fundoplication (Dor technique) that is fixed on both edges of the myotomy and both crura (Fig. 7.**6**).

Thoracoscopic Technique

The patient is placed in the right lateral position; under general anesthesia with a double lumen endotracheal tube. The left lung is collapsed. A 10 mm port is placed posteriorly in the sixth or seventh intercostal space for the telescope. The second and third ports are placed in the sixth interspace in the anterior axillary line and in the seventh interspace in the mid-axillary line. The inferior pulmonary ligament is divided, while retracting the lung upward using a retractor. The esophagus is grasped by Babcock forceps and the overlying parietal pleura divided. The vagal trunks are identified and the myotomy begun with the LCS or hook. First the longitudinal and then the circular muscle fibers are divided

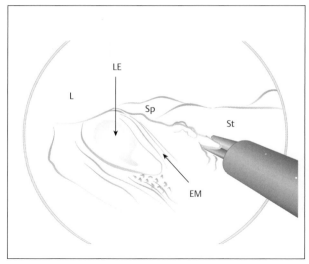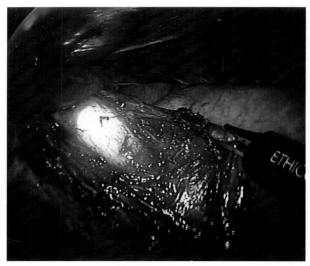

Fig. 7.**5**   The completed myotomy division of the LOS (the light of the endoscope is used to confirm the completeness of the myotomy). *L* liver, *LE* light from endoscope, *Sp* spleen, *St* stomach, *EM* esophageal mucosa.

with the activated instrument. The completeness of the myotomy is assessed by simultaneous endoscopy, which facilitates clear assessment of the depth of the myotomy. The myotomy is extended distally to the stomach with minimal dissection of the crura and is carried proximally about 8 cm above the gastroesophageal junction. With the thoracoscopic approach, the procedure is made more difficult by the cardiac and diaphragmatic movements.

> Editor's tip: The same care must be taken when performing the myotomy with the LCS in terms of control of the placements of the blades.

One of the claimed advantages of the thoracoscopic approach is the avoidance of an added antireflux repair, since all the attachments of the cardioesophageal junction are kept intact.

Summary of the Laparoscopic Myotomy

- Exposure of the anterior surface of the cardia and lower esophagus (6–8 cm).
- No division of the posterior and lateral attachments of the cardia.
- The myotomy is established in the middle of the anterior surface of the esophagus and cardia.
- The length of the myotomy is usually 6 cm on the esophagus and 2 cm on the stomach.
- Definition of the distal end point is best aided by intraoperative esophagogastroscopy.
- An anterior antireflux repair (Dor technique) is recommended.
- UltraCision facilitates the dissection and the performing of myotomy because:

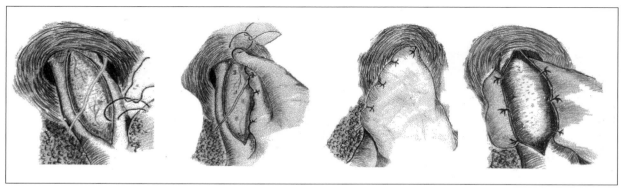

Fig. 7.**6**   *From the left:* A Dor wrap is performed by initially recreating the angle of His with a single suture between the fundus and the cut edge of the myotomy. Two further sutures are then placed so as to attach the fundus to the diaphragm. The fundus is then rolled over the myotomy and sutured in place (bougi- nage of the esophagus may help to keep the wrap suitably loose). In contrast, a Toupet wrap is performed by bringing the fundus behind the esophagus and then attaching the fundus to the cut edge of the myotomy.

Table 7.**1**   Publications on laparoscopic esophageal myotomy (*H*), some of which included Dor (*D*) or Toupet (*T*) fundoplication

Reference	Year	Procedure	Number	% Satisfied	% Dysphagia	% Reflux
1	1995	H+D	17	94	6	0
26	1995	H+D	25	96	4	
8	1996	H+D	12		16	
15	1997	H+D or T	40		10	5
22	1998	H+T	30	90	0	10
34	1998	H	27	89	11	14
29	1999	H+T	63		10	11

1. Collateral visceral damage is less likely,
2. Instrument interchange is reduced,
3. Hemostatic division of the musculature reduces the likelihood of mucosal perforation.

 ## Hints and Pitfalls

- Ensure absolute hemostasis.
- Dissect at least 1 cm onto anterior gastric surface.
- Beware of mucosal injury.
- Perform an "I maneuver" with the endoscope in the stomach at the end of the procedure to look at the esophagogastric junction.

 ## Discussion

No present therapy for achalasia reverses the underlying neuropathology or the associated esophageal aperistalsis and impaired LES relaxation. The target of therapy is to reduce the LES pressure allowing gravity to facilitate emptying. The most satisfactory means of treating achalasia are those that disrupt the distal esophageal musculature (forced balloon dilatation or myotomy). While dilatation has produced symptomatic relief in 65–80% of patients, esophageal perforation rates may be as high as 14% (mean 3–4%) (3, 20, 27). There is now a growing body of literature, however, that suggests surgical myotomy is superior to balloon dilatation (4, 7, 23).

Cardiomyotomy was first described in 1914 by Ernest Heller. This operation consisted of two myotomies on opposite sides of the esophagus via a laparotomy. The technique was modified in 1923 by a Dutch surgeon, who performed only a single myotomy. Throughout continental Europe and in South America, cardiomyotomy was historically performed via laparotomy, while in the United States, Canada, and Great Britain it was performed via the left chest (5, 12, 16, 19); excellent results being obtained with both approaches.

While previously the morbidity associated with open surgery (17) was believed by many to limit its application to those patients who had failed pneumatic dilatation therapy, the development of minimally invasive surgical technology has justifiably led to a renewed interest in surgery as the first-line treatment for achalasia. Reports have convincingly shown that minimally invasive approaches result in less morbidity, a shorter hospital stay, and an earlier return to normal activity than comparative open surgery (1, 22, 29). As minimally invasive procedures have evolved, there has been a marked shift toward laparoscopic as opposed to thoracoscopic approaches (18).

There are many years of follow-up on large numbers of patients who have undergone surgical myotomy, though our experience with the laparoscopic approach is much shorter. As seen from Table 7.**1**, our short-term results have been reasonable, but we will have to wait for longer-term follow-up.

Without an antireflux component, 14% of patients have symptomatic reflux while 28% have abnormal 24-hour-pH studies (2, 7). Reflux complications including esophagitis, Barrett's esophagus, and peptic esophageal stricture may occur (18). DeMeester and Stein have demonstrated that an antireflux procedure, done at the time of myotomy, decreased reflux in their series from 12 to 4% (9). The "ideal" antireflux procedure needs to be effective but non-obstructive to prevent dysphagia (due to the intrinsic esophageal body dysmotility) (11). The antireflux procedures used include anterior partial Dor fundoplication, posterior partial Toupet fundoplication, and 360° Nissen fundoplication. Most agree that a Nissen fundoplication is not the procedure of choice, since a relatively high incidence of long-term dysphagia has been associated with the complete Nissen wrap (31); the Dor or Toupet procedures are superior. When performing a wrap, the surgical technique described above is modified slightly (Fig. 7.**2**). The hiatal slings are fully defined, and division of the proximal short gastric vessels with UltraCision facilitates the loose wrap that is essential. For the Toupet procedure, a window must be developed behind the esophagus, taking care not to damage the posterior vagus. There is debate as to the best antireflux procedure, with varied results between reports (5, 25, 30). Some authors now suggest a more tailored approach using a Toupet procedure except for elderly patients and those with megaesophagus >7 cm when a Dor procedure is recommended (the Toupet may increase outflow obstruction by excessively angling the esophagus anteriorly) (14).

References

1. Ancona A, Anselimino M, Zanitto G, et al. Esophageal achalasia: Laparoscopic versus open Heller-Dor operation. Am J Surg 1995; 170: 265–70.
2. Andrello NA, Earlam RJ. Heller's myotomy for achalasia: Is an added anti-reflux procedure necessary? Br J Surg 1987; 74; 765–69.
3. Anselmino M, Perdikis G, Hinder RA, et al. Heller myotomy is superior to dilatation for the treatment of achalasia. Arch Surg 1997; 132: 233–40.
4. Black J, Vorbach AN, Collis JL. Results of Heller's operation for achalasia of the oesophagus. The importance of hiatal repair. Br J Surg 1986; 63: 949–53.
5. Bonavana L, Nosadini A, Bardini R et al. A. Primary treatment of esophageal achalasia: Long-term results of myotomy and Dor fundoplication. Arch Surg 192; 127: 222–27.
6. Cohen S, Lipshutz W. Lower esophageal sphincter dysfunction in achalasia. Gastroenterology 1971; 61: 814.
7. Csendes A, Braghetto I, Henriquez A, et al. Late results of a prospective randomized study comparing forceful dilation and oesophagomyotomy in patients with achalasia. Gut 1989; 30: 299–304.
8. Delgado F, Bolufer JM, Martinez-Abad M et al. Laparoscopic treatment of esophageal achalasia. Surg Laparosc Endosc 1996; 6: 83–90.
9. DeMeester TR, Stein HJ. Surgery for oesophageal motor disorders. In: Castell DO, editor, The Oesophagus. Boston: Little, Brown; 1992. p. 424.
10. Dodds WJ. Esophagus and esophagogastric region. In: Margulis AR, Burhenne HJ, editors, Alimentary Tract Radiology. St Louis: C.V. Mosby; 1983. p. 542.
11. Donahue PE, Schlesinger PK, Sluss KF et al. Esophagocardiomyotomy: floppy Nissen fundoplication effectively treats achalasia without causing oesophageal obstruction. Surgery 1994; 116: 719–25.
12. Ellis FH Jr. Oesophagomyotomy for achalasia: a 22-year experience. Br J Surg 1993; 80: 882–5.
13. Fellows IW, Ogilive AL. Atkinson M. Pneumatic dilation in achalasia. Gut 1983; 24: 1020.
14. Hunter JG, Richardson WS. Surgical management of achalasia. Surg Clin N Am 1997; 77: 993–1015.
15. Hunter JC, Trus TL, Branum et al. Laparoscopic Heller myotomy and fundoplication for achalasia. Ann Surg 1997; 225: 655–64.
16. Jara FM, Toledo-Pereyra LH, Lewis JW et al. Long-term results of esophagomyotomy for achalasia of esophagus. Arch Surg 1979; 114: 935–36.
17. Malthaner R, Todd T, Miller L, et al. Long-term results in surgically managed esophageal achalasia. Ann Thorac Surg 1994; 58: 1343–47.
18. Mattioli S, Di Simone MP, Bassi F et al. Surgery for oesophageal achalasia: longterm results with three different techniques. Hepatogastroenterology 1996; 43: 492–500.
19. Menzies-Gow N, Gummer JWP, Edwards DAW. Results of Heller's operation for achalasia of the cardia. Br J Surg 1978; 65: 483–85.
20. Okike N, Payne WS, Neufield DM et al. Esophagomyotomy versus forceful dilation for achalasia of the oesophagus: Results of 899 patients. Ann Thorac Surg 1979; 28: 119–25.
21. Ott OJ, Richter JE, Chen YM et al. Esophageal radiography and manometry: Correlation in 172 patients with dysphagia. Am J Roentgenol 1987; 149: 307.
22. Patti MG, Arcerito M, DePinto M, et al. Comparison of thoracoscopic and laparoscopic Heller myotomy for achalasia. J Gastrointest Surg 1998; 2: 561–66.
23. Pinotti HW, Felix VN, Zilberstein B, et al. Surgical complications of Chagas' disease: Megaoesophagus and achalasia of the pylorus and cholelithiasis. World J Surg 1991; 15: 198–204.
24. Podas T, Eaden J, Mayberry M, et al. Achalasia: A critical review of epidemiological studies. Am J Gastroenterol 1998; 93: 2345–47.
25. Raiser F, Perdikis G, Hinder RA et al. Heller myotomy via minimal access surgery. Arch Surg 1996; 131: 593–98.
26. Rosati R, Fumagilli U Bonavina et al. Laparoscopic approaches to esophageal achalasia. Am J Surg 1995; 169: 424.
27. Sauer L, Pellegrini CA, Way LW. The treatment of achalasia. Arch Surg 1989; 124: 929–31.
28. Stewart ET. Radiographic evaluation of the oesophagus and its motor disorders. Med Clin N Am 1981; 65: 1173.
29. Stewart KC, Finley RJ, Clifton JC, et al. Thoracoscopic versus laparoscopic modified Heller myotomy for achalasia: Efficacy and safety in 87 patients. J Am Coll Surg 1999; 189: 164–69.
30. Swanstrom LL, Pennings J. Laparoscopic esophagomyotomy for achalasia. Surg Endosc 1995; 9: 286–92.
31. Topart P, Deschamps C, Taillfer R, et al. Long-term effects of total fundoplication on the myotomized esophagus. Ann Thorac Surg 1992; 54: 1046–52.
32. Tucker HJ, Snape WJ, Cohen S. Achalasia secondary to carcinoma: Manometric and clinical features. Ann Intern Med 1978; 89: 315.
33. Vantrappen G, Hellemans J, Deloof W et al. Treatment of achalasia with pneumatic dilation. Gut 1971; 12: 268.
34. Wang P, Sharp KW, Holzman MD et al. The outcome of laparoscopic Heller myotomy without antireflux procedure in patients with achalasia. Am Surg. 1998; 64: 515–20.

8 Total Radical Gastrectomy

E. C. Tsimoyiannis

Gastrectomy, whether total or subtotal and when followed by extended lymphadenectomy or D2 dissection, markedly improves the long-term survival of patients with stage II and IIIA gastric cancer (6, 8). In several prospective randomized studies, D2 dissection was associated with increased post-surgical morbidity and mortality rates (2, 3). A significant part of this morbidity is due to the prolonged postoperative retention of intra-abdominal fluid (lymphorrhea) (5). The lymphatic dissection itself may have an adverse effect on the prognosis because of local tumor spillage from the many divided lymphatic vessels (7).

UltraCision shears have been shown to be a safe alternative to electrosurgery (1, 4, 15). This device mechanically denatures protein by disruption of hydrogen bonds within the protein structure. This disorganized protein forms a sticky coagulum that coapts the vessel walls, not only of the blood vessels, but also of narrow bile vessels (15). This finding led us to the hypothesis that with UltraCision shears it would be possible to coapt and obstruct the lymphatic vessels, thus avoiding lymphorrhea and tumor spillage (16).

Indication and Preoperative Management

Surgery provides the only possibility of a cure. Preoperative proof of the diagnosis (using gastroscopy and biopsies) and staging should be carried out using CT scans with double contrast and echoendoscopy.

In our department, all patients with advanced gastric cancer are treated preoperatively by total parenteral nutrition (TPN) infusion for six days and correction of anemia when necessary. In cases of pyloric stenosis, a nasogastric tube is placed during the TPN infusion; otherwise, the nasogastric tube is placed the day before surgery.

Operative staging by laparotomy or laparoscopy should be seen as an essential prerequisite to rational decisions regarding resectability. This staging demands an assessment of the extent of the tumor, the depth of invasion, the extent of lymph node involvement, the presence and extent of peritoneal deposits, and the presence of hepatic metastases. Laparoscopic assessment may be the best way to determine operability and staging. Ultrasonography of the liver can be performed laparoscopically at this staging procedure. By such a laparoscopic assessment, some unnecessary laparotomies (in cases of unresectable tumors) can be avoided.

After appropriate staging, an elective total or subtotal gastrectomy with D2 dissection is indicated in patients with gastric cancer stage II or IIIA.

Operation

Since the stomach is not vital to a relatively lengthy life span, the surgeon can consider anything up to and including: a total gastrectomy, removal of the omentum, removal of the spleen, removal of the distal portion of the esophagus, removal of the proximal portion of the duodenum, and even simultaneous removal of a portion of the transverse colon. Lesser resections of the stomach are anatomically, surgically, and oncologically possible, and the extent of resection can be determined partly according to the extent of the lesion, and partly by knowledge of its usual pathways of extension (9).

Curative resection should be attempted only on tumors of the stomach and neighboring lymph nodes, although the presence of attachments to surrounding structures does not preclude a resection, if those structures can be removed en bloc with the primary tumor. The aim of curative surgery in gastric cancer is the complete removal of all tumor bulk, both macroscopically and microscopically: (R0) resection.

The operative strategy should consider the location of the tumor, its histological character (Lauren classification), and the stage of disease according to the TNM classification (9).

A subtotal gastrectomy is performed in pT1–2 carcinomas located in the distal third of the stomach. In all other patients, a total gastrectomy is performed. The spleen is resected in carcinomas of the cardia, fundus, and upper part of the corpus, while the pancreas is resected only when directly involved by the tumor (11). An en bloc resection of the stomach with lymph node dissection of compartments I and II (D2 dissection) is the procedure of choice in all cases of stage II or IIIA and in young patients with stage IIIB or IV. In stage I, the lymph node dissection of compartment I is recommended (10, 11). Compartment I comprises all lymph nodes along the major and minor curvature of the stomach and especially the lymph node stations 1 through 6 (11) in those undergoing a total gastrectomy, and lymph node stations 3 through 6 (11) in those undergoing a subtotal gastrectomy. Compartment II comprises lymph node stations 7 to 12 (11, 12).

The UltraCision shears must be used in all steps of the dissection (Fig. 8.1), and only blood vessels more than 3 mm in diameter (left gastric vessels, splenic vessels) must be clipped or ligated. The dissection is begun by dividing the omentum from the transverse colon. The origin of the right gastric artery at the common hepatic artery is divided with UltraCision shears. Lymphatic-bearing tissues are swept toward the gastric side.

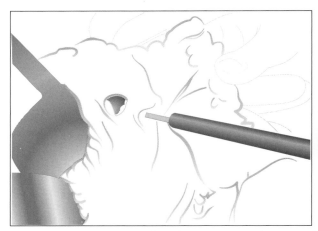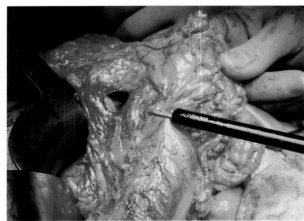

Fig. 8.**1**   Perioperative view of D2 dissection using UltraCision shears. Division of the gastrocolic ligament.

The right gastroepiploic artery is divided with UltraCision shears to its origin at the gastroduodenal artery. The left gastric artery and vein are ligated and divided. Ligation is applied to the splenic vessels in the cases of a splenectomy. In cases without a splenectomy, the short gastric vessels are divided using the UltraCision shears. All the steps of a lymphadenectomy—the division of the esophagus (in total gastrectomy) and the stomach (in subtotal gastrectomy)—are performed using the UltraCision shears. The duodenum is divided using a TA-55 stapler. For better control of hemostasis we use lower power (level 3) and the blunt surface of the UltraCision shears to cut the vessels, while we use higher power (level 5) and the sharper blade to divide lymphatic and small blood vessels. Sometimes, in obese patients, we use the laparoscopic UltraCision shears (they are longer) in the perisplenic and periesophageal areas.

In all D2 dissections, a subhepatic closed drainage must be left until intra-abdominal fluid outflow stops. In cases of splenectomy, a second closed drainage is left in the splenic bed. In cases of total gastrectomy, a feeding needle jejunostomy is performed for the infusion of commercial liquid foods between the first to eighth postoperative days to protect the esophagojejunal anastomosis from early oral feeding.

During the procedure, the blood transfusion is applied only in cases with massive blood loss. In cases of mild blood loss, the resultant anemia is treated postoperatively by epoetin A plus intravenous iron administration.

Hints and Pitfalls

- In specialized centers, extended lymph node dissection does not increase the mortality or morbidity rate of resection for gastric cancer, but does markedly improve the long-term survival of patients with stage II or IIIA tumors.

- Lymphadenectomy is beneficial not only in patients with frank lymph node metastases, but also in patients in whom no lymph node metastases can be detected by standard histopathological assessment. The benefit of radical removal of apparently uninvolved lymph nodes can be explained by the phenomenon of lymph node micro-involvement or micro-metastases (minute tumor islands with stromal reaction), which are usually not detected by standard histopathological assessment (12).
- The UltraCision shears can be used in all steps of a D2 gastric resection for advanced gastric cancer. By using this instrument the dissection is easier, occurs without bleeding, and requires only a few ligations or hemoclips.
- The better hemostasis when using the UltraCision shears leads to decreased blood loss and to decreased need of blood transfusion.
- The complete coaptation of the lymphatic vessel walls cut by the UltraCision shears leads to a decreased amount of postoperative lymphorrhea.
- The advantages of the application of UltraCision shears in D2 gastric resection are so pronounced that the disadvantage of the cost is completely eliminated.

 Personal Experience

During the past three years we have used the UltraCision shears in most lymph node dissections involving gastric cancer, colon cancer, pancreatic cancer, breast cancer, and thyroid cancer. In all these procedures the advantages are similar: faster procedure (because we do not spend time changing instruments and placing ligations or clips), better hemostasis, decreased lymphorrhea, and decreased blood transfusion (because of decreased blood loss).

Recently, we have completed a prospective randomized study comparing the effectiveness of the Ul-

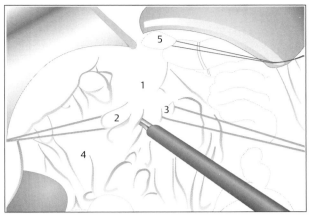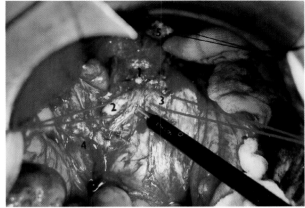

Fig. 8.**2**   Perioperative view of D2 dissection using UltraCision shears. Lymphatic dissection around the branches of the celiac axis. *1* left gastric artery, *2* common hepatic artery, *3* splenic artery, *4* duodenal stump, *5* esophagus.

traCision shears versus monopolar electrocautery in D2 gastric resections for stage II and IIIA gastric cancer (16). In the patients belonging to Group A (*n* = 20), monopolar cautery was used for cutting and coagulation and hemoclips or ligations to obstruct the blood vessels. In the patients of Group B (*n* = 20), an open surgery using UltraCision shears, 10 mm diameter were used in all steps of the dissection (Figs. 8.**1**, 8.**2**). Here, hemoclips were applied only in blood vessels >3 mm in diameter. All patients were treated preoperatively by TPN infusion for six days (40 calories per kg body weight per day) and anemia correction (epoetin A 10 000 IU/day plus iron intravenously 100 mg/day for five to seven days) when necessary. In cases of pyloric stenosis, a nasogastric tube was placed during the TPN infusion. Otherwise, the nasogastric tube was placed the day before surgery.

Total gastrectomy was performed in 16 patients of Group A (splenectomy in 14). Total gastrectomy was performed in 14 patients of Group B (splenectomy in 12), while subtotal gastrectomy was performed in four and six patients, respectively. The surgically related events are shown for the two groups of patients in Table 8.**1**. All the parameters of this table are significantly better in the UltraCision group (B) than in the monopolar cautery group (A).

In Fig. 8.**3** the daily amounts of the abdominal drainage during the first four postoperative days are shown. During these days, a statistically significantly higher fluid amount was drained in Group A than in Group B, every day. After the fifth day, the number of patients requiring drainage was too small for statistical analysis. The mean number of units of blood transfused (Fig. 8.**4**) and the number of patients with drainage in place, for each day, during the early postoperative period (Table 8.**1**), were higher in Group A than in Group B. The major postoperative complications were about the same in both groups, while none of the patients died during the first 30 postoperative days. These results suggest that the use of UltraCision shears in all steps of the extended lymphadenectomy is

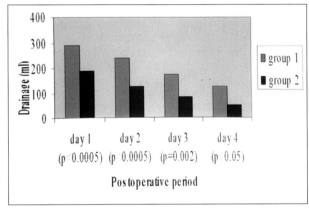

Fig. 8.**3**   Mean values of daily postoperative abdominal drainage (ml of fluid) during postoperative days one through four. A statistically significant higher amount of fluid was drained in Group A than in Group B.

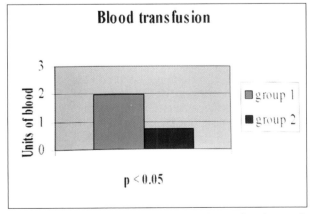

Fig. 8.**4**   Mean number of units of blood transfused in each group. The difference is statistically significant.

Table 8.1   Surgically related events in two groups of patients (mean ± SD)

Parameter	Group A	Group B	P Value
Operative time (min)	190 ± 18 (162–223)	184 ± 15 (154–205)	n.s.
Operative blood loss (ml)	580 ± 198 (250–980)	318 ± 163 (150–720)	<0.001*
Postoperative abdominal drainage (ml)	985 ± 602 (300–2 050)	460 ± 242 (230–1 080)	<0.002*
Postoperative day for drain removal	9.7 ± 2.9 (6–17)	5.6 ± 1.2 (4–8)	<0.001*
Number of units transferred	1.95 ± 1.7 (0–4)	0.7 ± 0.9 (0–2)	<0.01*
Number of patients transfused	11	7	>0.1**
Postoperative hospital stay (days)	12.5 ± 5.5 (12–20)	9.3 ± 4.3 (10–14)	<0.05*

* t test; ** χ^2 test

a safe method that reduces blood loss, postoperative lymphorrhea, blood transfusion, and length of stay.

Discussion

Surgical resection is the only curative treatment for gastric carcinoma presently available, while extended lymphadenectomy or D2 dissection can improve survival (3, 6, 8), especially in patients with stage II or IIIA disease (3, 6, 8, 12). The operation is based on knowledge of the regional lymphatic drainage of the stomach. In accordance with the basic tenets of oncological resection for epithelial cancers, surgical treatment requires wide excision of the primary gastric tumor and en bloc removal of the draining lymphatic network, including the regional lymph nodes and the intervening lymphatic vessels (13, 14).

D2 gastric resections are accompanied by higher morbidity and mortality rates than D1 resections (2, 3). Prospective trials indicate that the higher morbidity in the D2 dissection is not due to the extended lymphadenectomy, but instead largely to pancreatic resection and splenectomy (2, 3). The prolonged retention of intra-abdominal fluid or lymphorrhea probably originates from the cut end of the retroperitoneal lymphatic vessels (5). Meticulous ligation of lymphatic vessels may be essential when these nodes are removed (5), but this procedure is of longer duration. Electrosurgery is a faster procedure than meticulous ligation, but electrosurgery is not effective in lymphatic vessels since the vessel wall is usually not coapted (1).

According to our experience, the use of UltraCision shears in D2 gastric resection for stage II or IIIA gastric cancer led to a significant decrease of the blood loss and the drained fluid from the dissection areas compared with electrosurgery dissection. UltraCision led to the earlier postoperative drain removal, the lower blood transfusion, and the reduced postoperative hospital stay. In conclusion, the use of UltraCision shears in total or subtotal gastrectomy followed by extended lymphadenectomy or D2 dissection is a safe method that reduces the operative blood loss and the postoperative lymphorrhea, leading to decreased blood transfusion and hospital stay.

References

1. Amaral JF. Laparoscopic cholecystectomy in 200 consecutive patients using an ultrasonically activated scalpel. Surg Laparosc Endosc 1995; 5: 255–62.
2. Bonenkamp JJ, Songun I, Hermans J, et al. Randomised comparison of morbidity after D1 and D2 dissection for gastric cancer in 996 Dutch patients. Lancet 1995; 345: 745–48.
3. Cuschieri A, Fayers P, Fielding J, et al. Postoperative morbidity and mortality after D1 and D2 resections for gastric cancer: preliminary results of the MRC randomized controlled surgical trial. Lancet 1996; 347: 995–999.
4. Laycock WS, Trus TL, Hunter JG. New technology for the division of short gastric vessels during lasparoscopic Nissen fundoplication. Surg Endosc 1996; 10: 71–73.
5. Maeta M, Yamashiro H, Saito H, et al. A prospective pilot study of extended (D3) and superextended para-aortic lymphadenectomy (D4) in patients with T3 or T4 gastric cancer managed by total gastrectomy. Surgery 1999; 125: 325–31.
6. de Manzoni G, Verlato G, Guglielmi A, Laterza E, Genna M, Cordiano C. Prognostic significance of lymph node dissection in gastric cancer. Br J Surg 1996; 83: 1604–07.
7. Robertson CS, Chung SCS, Woods SDS, et al. A prospective randomized trial comparing R1 subtotal gastrectomy with R3 total gastrectomy for antral cancer. Ann Surg 1994; 220: 176–82.
8. Roder JD, Bonenkamp JJ, Craven J, et al. Lymphadenectomy for gastric cancer in clinical trials: Update. World J Surg 1995; 19: 546–53.
9. Rosin RD. Tumors of the stomach. In. Zinner MJ, Schwartz SI, Ellis H (eds), Maingot's Abdominal Operations. 10 th ed. Stamford, Conn., USA: Appleton & Lange; 1997. Vol. I: pp. 999–1028.
10. Siewert JR, Bottcher K, Roder JD, Busch R, Hermanek P, Meyer H and the German Gastric Cancer Study Group. Prognostic relevance of systematic lymph node dissection in gastric carcinoma. Br J Surg 1993; 80: 1015–18.
11. Siewert JR, Fink U, Sendler A et al. Gastric cancer. Curr Probl Surg 1997; 34: 835–42.
12. Siewert JR, Bottcher K, Stein HJ, Roder JD, and the German Gastric Carcinoma Study Group: Relevant prognostic factors in gastric cancer: Ten-year results of the German Gastric Cancer Study of gastric cancer. Ann Surg 1998; 228: 449–61.
13. Smith JW, Shiu MH, Kelsey L, Brennan MF. Morbidity of radical lymphadenectomy in the curative resection of gastric carcinoma. Arch Surg 1991; 126: 1469–73.
14. Sunderland D, McNeer G, Ortega L, Pearse L. The lymphatic spread. Cancer 1953; 6: 987–91.
15. Tsimoyiannis EC, Jabarin M, Glantzounis G, Lekkas ET, Siakas P, Stefanaki-Nikou S. Laparoscopic cholecystectomy using ultrasonically activated coagulating shears. Surg Laparosc Endosc 1998; 8: 421–24.
16. Tsimoyiannis EC, Jabarin M, Tsimoyiannis JC, Betzios J, Tsilikatis C, Glantzounis G. Ultrasonically activated shears in extended lymphadenectomy for gastric cancer. International Surgical Week, ISW99. Vienna, Austria, 1999: 46.

9 Laparoscopic Assisted Right Hemicolectomy for Crohn's Disease

A. D'Hoore

Over half the patients with Crohn's disease present with distal ileal involvement with or without extension into the adjacent colon. Recent progress in conservative treatment of active Crohn's disease relies on immunosuppressive drugs. Once the disease becomes symptomatic, it tends to progress and develop the well-recognized complications of obstruction, local sepsis, and fistulas. Within ten years of diagnosis, between 80 and 90% of the patients will face surgery (1).

Indication and Preoperative Management

Ileocaecal resection is indicated in complicated Crohn's disease for: obstructive disease; perforating disease (free perforation is rare); internal fistula formation; and failure of medical therapy.

Laparoscopic mobilization and resection may be difficult or impossible in patients with large, fixed masses; multiple complex fistulas with abscesses; or recurrent Crohn's disease (3). Clear contraindications represent emergency indications (e.g., toxic colitis, free perforation with peritonitis).

Timing of surgery can have a decisive effect on outcome: the nutritional status of the patient should be assessed and if necessary improved.

> Editor's tip: To avoid heavy septic complications, the time point of the operation should be determined after two to three months of unsuccessful intensive drug therapy in symptomatic patients. The chronic inflammation is the reason for the often substantial catabolic state. (9)

Anemia and dehydration must be corrected. If possible, immunosuppressive therapy should be tapered for as long as possible before surgery. Adequate perioperative steroids are to be administered.

All patients should undergo a preoperative colonoscopy to rule out active Crohn's colitis. Radiological small bowel examination will give some indication on the extent of the disease and/or the presence of internal fistulas. If necessary, abscesses should be drained percutaneously (guided by sonography or CT scan).

Preoperative bowel preparation must be adapted to the patient's condition (e.g., obstructive disease). We routinely use prophylactic parenteral antibiotics (cefazolin and metronidazole). Therapeutic antibiotics are advocated in patients with local septic disease.

Operation

The patient is installed in a supine position. Steep Trendelenburg and left-sided tilting are efficient in obtaining a good initial exposure. We only recommend a modified Lloyd-Davies position if an ileosigmoidal or ileovesical fistula are suspected.

The following instruments are routinely used:
- Two 10 mm ports (one blunt-tip trocar)
- One or two 5 mm ports
- 25° or 30° optics
- UltraCision 5 mm LCS shears
- Two 5 mm atraumatic grasping instruments
- One 5 mm endo-dissecting instrument

An "open" laparoscopy (Hasson technique), especially in the lean patient with a palpable mass, is performed to create the pneumoperitoneum and insert the optics. The peritoneal cavity is inspected and the feasibility for laparoscopic resection evaluated. Secondary ports are placed under direct visual control: a 10 mm port in the left iliac fossa, lateral from the inferior epigastric vessels; two 5 mm ports, in the right iliac fossa and the right subcostal position, respectively. The optic is now repositioned to the left lower port (Fig. 9.1). The surgeon and first assistant stand to the left of the patient. To lift the small bowel out of the pelvis, the operating table is placed in steep Trendelenburg. The extent of the disease is evaluated. With two atraumatic graspers, the small bowel is completely inspected to identify skip areas or unexpected internal fistulas.

> Editor's tip: Frequently, the presence of inflammatory or postoperative adhesions around the bowel and the thickened mesentery with a conglomerate of bowel loops make dissection very difficult. Therefore, the dissection has to begin with the healthy intestine and should go on to the critical part of the bowel.

The caecum and the mesenterium of the terminal ileum are elevated at the inferior borders. With the UltraCision 5 mm LCS (inserted through the right inferior port), the peritoneal reflection is incised obliquely above the right common iliac artery (Fig. 9.2). A broad retroperitoneal avascular dissection plane is created (Fig. 9.3). Using this maneuver, the gonadal vessels and ureter can be released from the dorsal aspect of the right colon. Some smaller vessels (especially present in inflammatory bowel disease) can easily be controlled without the use of clips. Dissection progresses up to the inferior border of the duodenum.

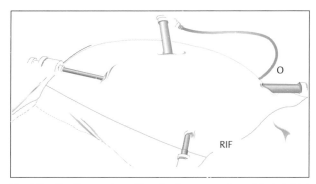
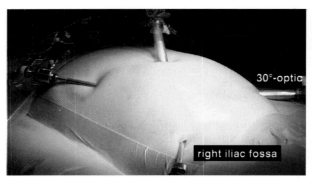

Fig. 9.**1**   Routine port position for laparoscopic assisted right hemicolectomy. *O* 30° optic, *RIF* right iliac fossa.

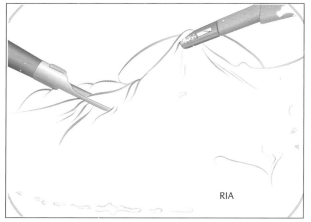
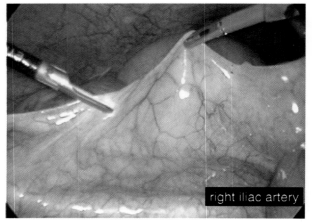

Fig. 9.**2**   Opening of the peritoneal reflection. *RIA* right iliac artery.

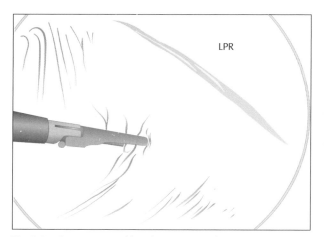
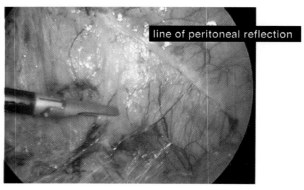

Fig. 9.**3**   Cavitation enables the creation of an avascular plane between the mesentery of the ascending colon and the retroperitoneum. *LPR* line of peritoneal reflection.

In a second step, the lateral attachments to Gerota's fascia are severed using the UltraCision instrument. The caecum and ascending colon are now retracted to the left and progressively the mesentery is further liberated from the upper border of the duodenum (Fig. 9.**4**).

This mobilization enables an en bloc exteriorization of the diseased ileocaecal segment. If there is extension to the caecum or ascending colon, the hepatic flexure has to be liberated as well. Therefore, the optic is re-introduced via the umbilical port. The operating table is further tilted to the left and in a slight Fowler position. Retraction of the hepatic flexure is done from the two

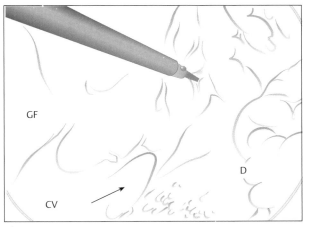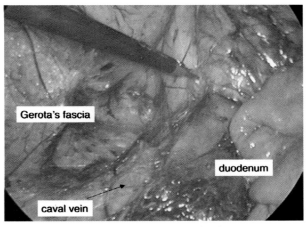

Fig. 9.**4** The mesentery is completely mobilized from the duodenum. *GF* Gerota's fascia, *CV* caval vein, *D* duodenum.

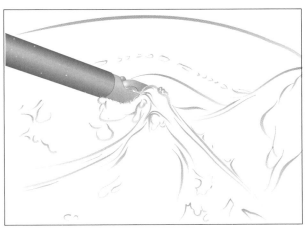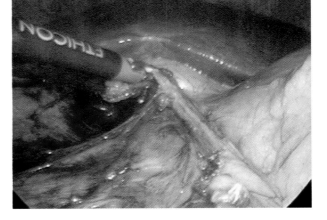

Fig. 9.**5** Transection of the hepatocolic ligament.

lower ports. The UltraCision LCS is now introduced through the right subcostal port to open the hepatocolic ligament (Fig. 9.**5**) and eventually open the omental bursa. To exteriorize the diseased ileocaecal segment, we extend the sub-umbilical incision and make a fascial incision through the midline (Figs. 9.**6a, b**; 9.**7**).

Editor's tip: To mobilize the right flexure, the preparation from the opened lesser sac is an alternative, easy step. The surface of the duodenum serves as a guide plane; trauma of the pancreas can be avoided with clear anatomical conditions.

A small wound-protector is inserted. Gradual traction should be applied so as not to tear the mesentery and to prevent mesenterial hematoma formation. Vascular control of the mesentery and transection of the small bowel and ascending colon are performed extracorporeally using standard techniques.

Editor's tip: A conservative attitude still persists regarding the question of the extent of resection. Resections have to be performed sparingly to protect as much of the bowel as possible. A histological infiltration of the resection margin is not important prognostically.

Progressive suture ligation of the inflammatory thickened mesentery is performed. We routinely make an oblique end-to-end manual anastomosis and close the mesenterial defect with single sutures (Fig. 9.**8**). Alternatively, a functional end-to-end anastomosis using stapling devices can be constructed.

The anastomosis is gently reduced and a suction drain can be placed in the right paracolic gutter through the right inferior port.

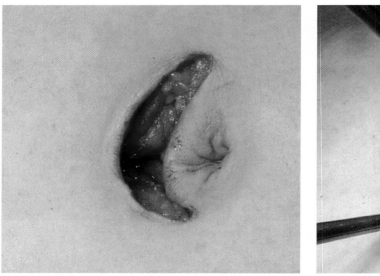
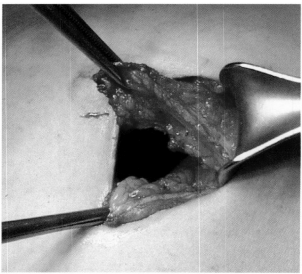

Fig. 9.**6 a, b**   Sub-umbilical incision and midline fascial opening to exteriorize the ileocaecal segment.

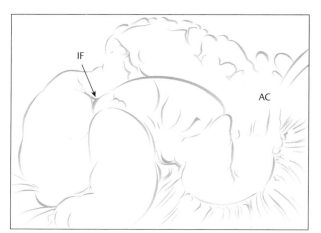
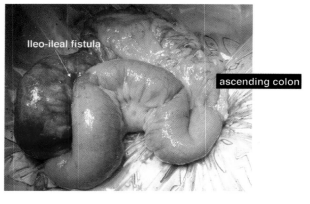

Fig. 9.**7**   The exteriorized ileocaecal segment. *IF* ileo-ileal fistula, *AC* ascending colon.

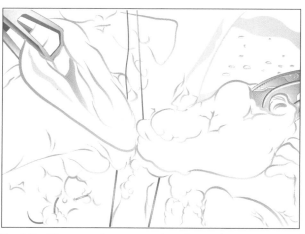
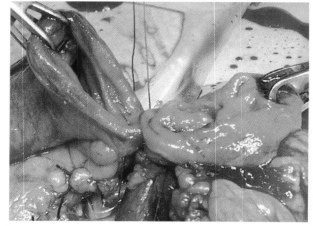

Fig. 9.**8**   After resection a manual, end-to-end anastomosis is fashioned.

Hints and Pitfalls

- Presence of skip-areas with occluding strictures: if there is a suspicion during laparoscopy, it is mandatory to unroll the complete small bowel through the sub-umbilical incision to have a tactile sensation of the bowel wall (mesenterial aspect). If present close to the diseased terminal segment, it is reasonable to include it in the resection; if more proximal, an additional stricturoplasty should be performed extracorporeally.
- To avoid fecal soiling during the laparoscopic mobilization, internal fistulas to the small bowel and ascending colon should be controlled after en bloc exteriorization.
- Deep pelvic fixation of an inflammatory mass is very difficult to mobilize in a controlled and safe way and is the main reason to abandon the laparoscopic approach.
- Be aware of an unexpected rectal fistula if a severe pelvic fixation is present.
- The presence of a ileosigmoidal or ileorectal fistula is not an absolute contraindication for laparoscopy. If no sigmoidal disease is present, the fistula can be controlled using an endostapler device performing a transverse wedge excision. If segmental colorectal disease is present, a combined segmental colectomy should be performed.
- A fistula to the bladder should be closed with sutures.

Personal Experience

All medical charts of patients who required primary surgery for ileocaecal Crohn's disease between 1996 and 1999 were analyzed (Table 9.1). In total, 69 patients out of 168 had a laparoscopic approach. Both groups are not matched, however, since more patients with obstructive disease (65 % of them) could benefit from a laparoscopic resection in comparison with patients with perforating disease (15 %).

In our series, 15 % of all patients had some additional surgery when ileocaecal resection was performed (Table 9.2).

Major complications included anastomotic leaks (2.8 %), with subsequent bleeding. In the open group, six patients (6 %) suffered from an important abdominal wall problem (Table 9.3).

Median postoperative hospital stay was seven days for the laparoscopic assisted group and nine days for the open resections.

Table 9.1 Indications for right hemicolectomy in Crohn's disease (1996–1999)

	Laparo-scopic	Open	Total
Therapy resistance	7	13	20
Obstructive	53	32	85
Perforating	4	28	32
Internal fistula	5	26	31
Total:	**69**	**99**	**168**

Table 9.2 Additional surgery

	Lap. assisted group	Open group
Stricturoplasty	3	2
Segmental enterectomy	1	1
Wedge resection recto-sigmoid	3	4
Sigmoid resection		4
Anterior resection		4
Abscess drainage		2
Cholecystectomy	1	

Table 9.3 Major morbidity after right hemicolectomy for Crohn's disease

	Laparo-scopic (n=69)	Open (n=99)	Total (n=168)
1. Septic complications Anastomotic leak	2 (=2.8 %)	4 (=4 %)	6 (=3.5 %)
– ileostomy	1	2	3
– re-suturing	1		1
– re-resection		1	1
– conservative treatment		1	1
Missed rectal fistula		1	1
Pelvic abscess	1	2	3
2. Bleeding	1 (hemo-perit.)	1 (trans-fusion)	2
3. Abdominal wall problems	0	6	6
Evisceration		1	
Eventration		1	
Important wound infection		4	

Discussion

Laparoscopic colorectal resections have some particularities that make them more complex than other laparoscopic procedures (e.g., laparoscopic cholecystectomy). The surgical field is multiquadrant; different larger vessels within a mesenterium must be secured; and, in most cases, an anastomosis has to be fashioned.

A laparoscopically assisted approach, as in ileocaecal resection for Crohn's disease, is a pragmatic approach to make the laparoscopic approach easy, reproducible, and feasible within an acceptable operating time limit. In this way, all laparoscopic difficulties with vascular control in an inflammatory thickened mesenterium are avoided. Different authors have published their initial experience with this approach (2, 3, 4, 5). The position of the angled optic and the installation of the patient allow an excellent visual control of the dissection field.

The introduction of the UltraCision LCS 5 mm instrument provided additional advantages: the depth of energy spread is more gradual and controllable than in HF electrosurgery (6), and the cavitation properties allow for a bloodless dissection between the retroperitoneum and mesentery. The minor lateral spread of energy and the design of the instrument having an inactive blade allow a safe dissection close to precious structures such as the ureter and duodenum (7). Especially in inflammatory bowel disease, the different adhesions with the retroperitoneum, Gerota's fascia, and the hepatocolic ligament are often substantially more vascular than in oncologic disease. The progressive coaptation and cutting effect obtained results with a perfect hemostasis and the omission of clips in the surgical field. In our series, intraoperative bleeding or problematic hemostasis was never a reason for conversion. The multiple properties of the instrument (grasping, dissecting, vascular sealing, and cutting) makes unnecessary the frequent changeover of different instruments. Moreover, the size (5 mm) of the instrument allows a more dynamic use from different ports.

Patients with obstructive Crohn's disease can now be offered a laparoscopically assisted approach resulting in a reduction of surgical trauma and stress response and, in most instances, a faster recovery of bowel function and shorter hospital stay (8). The impact on the immune system is not exactly known; nevertheless, this could influence early recurrence or flare-up of the disease. The cosmetic benefit, of far less importance in oncologic resections, has an impact on quality of life and self-perception in the young patient already stigmatized by the chronic disease.

 # References

1. Michelassi F, Balestrucci T, Chappell R, Block GE. Primary and recurrent Crohn's disease. Ann Surg 1991; 214: 230–40.
2. Hildebrandt U, Ecker KW, Feifel G. Minimal-invasive Chirurgie und Morbus Crohn. Chirurg 1998; 69: 915–21.
3. Bauer JJ, Harris MT, Grumbach NM, Gorfine SR. Laparoscopic assisted resection for Crohn's disease. Dis Colon Rectum 1995; 38: 712.
4. Ludwig KA, Milsom JW, Church JM, Fazio VW. Preliminary experience with laparoscopic intestinal surgery for Crohn's disease. Am J Surg 1996; 171: 52.
5. Reissman P, Salky BA, Edye M, Wexner SD. Laparoscopic surgery in Crohn's disease. Surg Endosc 1996; 10: 1201.
6. Amaral JF, Chrostek C. Depth of thermal injury: Ultrasonically activated scalpel vs. electrosurgery. Surg Endosc 1995; 9: 226.
7. Nduka CC, Super PA, Monson JRT, Darzi AW. Cause and prevention of electrosurgical injuries in laparoscopy. J Am Coll Surg 1994; 2: 161–70.
8. Chen HH, Wexner SD, Iroatulam AJN, et al. Laparoscopic colectomy compares favorably with colectomy by laparotomy for reduction in postoperative ileus. Dis Colon Rectum 2000; 43: 61–65.
9. Ecker KW, Hulten L, Operative Konzepte bei Morbus Crohn des terminalen Ileums und des Kolons. Zentralbl Chir 1998; 123: 331.
10. Zacherl J, Függer R, Imhof M, Bischof G, Jakesz R, Herbst F. Minimal invasive Chirurgie bei Morbus Crohn. Minimal Invasive Chirurgie 1998; 7: 42–44.

10 Open Colorectal Surgery

H. R. Nürnberger

According to the data of the German Cancer Register, colorectal cancer (7) is the second most frequent cancer cause of death for both sexes in Germany. The portion of the total cancer mortality amounts to about 12% for males and about 14% for females. The estimated numbers for the annual incidence of colon cancer are 14000 men and 19000 women; those for rectal cancer are 8800 men and 8700 women. That adds up to 50000 new cases per year in Germany.

Most colorectal carcinomas are sporadic, and the risk during one's life span to become afflicted amounts to 6%. Since about 70–80% of all patients with average risk will be diagnosed over the age of 50, precautionary and screening programs are recommended (7).

Accordingly, the surgical therapy for this major health problem must be standardized for quality assurance, and be performed following generally accepted guidelines for the improvement of the patient outcome (15, 22). The therapeutic objectives are to perform a wide anatomic resection with sufficient safety margins and with attendant mesentery, vascular, and lymphatic supply. In particular, rectal carcinoma should be operated by careful preparation and execution of the total mesorectal excision (TME). In this way, the rate of local recurrences can be reduced to 5–10% (1, 10, 11, 12, 17). These results place the question of the necessity for an adjuvant therapy in a new light (25). Furthermore, the danger of postoperative complications under multimodal adjuvant therapies must not be underestimated (4, 16, 20, 21).

Indication and Preoperative Management

After histological confirmation of the diagnosis of a colorectal carcinoma, radical anatomic resection of the tumor with the attendant lymphovascular pedicle is the only option for a possible curative treatment (15, 22). No evidence-based data exists, however, supporting the myths of colorectal surgery, such as: the no-touch isolation technique, tying the resection margins, early identification and high ligation of the blood vessels, flushing of the intestine with cytotoxic solutions (9, 14). All other additional procedures are indicated as (neo-) adjuvant modalities or for palliation.

The patient with a carcinoma often has weakness secondary to anemia from occult blood loss (ascending colon), vague lower abdominal pain or distention of the belly, and inability to evacuate due to obstruction of passage (left-sided colorectal carcinoma). Identification and localization of the primary tumor by endo-

scopic or radiological means must exclude the presence of other tumors or adenomas.

As part of the preoperative evaluation, all patients undergoing potentially curative colorectal resections are seen by a member of the stoma nursing team. Patients undergo presurgical marking of the abdominal wall for possible stoma sites along with an educational program about stoma care. The history and physical examination should assess anal sphincter function, because disturbances of continence may suggest that a sphincter-saving approach would not be appropriate.

Bowel preparation is performed using cathartics, osmotic agents, enemas, and (preferably) by peroral colonic lavage with an iso-osmotic solution when no high obstruction (ileus) is present. Recently, the dogma of mechanical bowel preparation has been challenged (2, 3, 23). Notwithstanding recent publications, however, it is still our practice to have our patients undergo a thorough mechanical preparation.

Adequate hydration and alimentation must be assured preoperatively during this preparation. In most cases, a central intravenous catheter should be placed in addition. Intravenous antibiotics are given just before the operation, and blood transfusions are avoided if possible.

Operation

Make a midline incision from below the xiphoid to the pubis and, after protection of the wound margins, insert the plastic ring-drape to protect the incision from contamination, and the retractor to exposure to the abdominal cavity. Explore the abdomen for hepatic, pelvic, peritoneal, and nodal metastases. The primary tumor should be inspected, though manipulation of it should be avoided at this stage. If one plans a left-sided or rectal resection, then exteriorize the small intestine and retract it to the patient's right.

Right and Left Hemicolectomy

Using the 10 mm UltraCision shears, make an incision in the peritoneum of the paracolic gutter and continue this dissection on the right side until the hepatic flexure is free of lateral attachments (blunt blade, level 5). It is important with the preparation using UltraCision to proceed in small steps in the loose tissue in order to avoid unnecessary bleeding.

Editor's tip: Avoid rough, blunt dissection around the gallbladder or the retroperitoneal duodenum, so as not to inadvertently lacerate it.

On the left side, incise the peritoneum between the descending colon and the white line of Toldt and continue the dissection until the splenic flexure is reached. The key to safely taking down the splenic flexure is sharp dissection under direct vision (blunt blade, level 3). Mobilization is approached alternatively from both the descending and transverse colon side. The peritoneal incision must be moved close to the colon. Then release the ligaments, which are one continuous membrane with multiple areas of attachment to the kidney, spleen, and pancreas, in repeated small steps from caudal-lateral without any tension. Divide the gastrocolic ligament and open the lesser sac with its attachments (blunt blade, level 5; larger vessels level 3). As these structures are fragile, gentle dissection is necessary. Finally, the transverse mesocolon is prepared up to the inferior border of the pancreas.

Editor's tip: Pay close attention to the tissue in the tip of the blade. Insure that everything is split and does not bleed. This includes the parenchyma of the pancreas.

Now mark the resection line in extension of the middle colic artery, which often divides very early. If the artery does divide, one can utilize the left lateral branch for the right hemicolectomy and the right lateral branch for the left hemicolectomy. Identify the renocolic ligament and, after dissection, gently sweep the fascia of Gerota from the posterior aspect of the mesocolon. Identify precisely the ureter in the retroperitoneum, without wide medial clearing. Typical peristalsis should occur when the ureter is compressed with sponges or forceps.

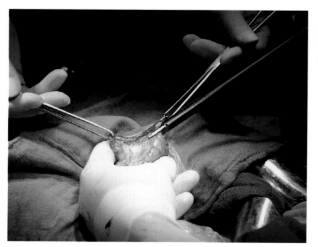

Fig. 10.**1**   Resection of the linear clip row at the colon with the UltraCision shears.

Finally, dissect on the right side the adhesions of peritoneum to the cecum and ileum so that the entire right colon is mobilized completely (blunt blade, level 5). Define the proximal resection line 5 to 10 cm in front of the ileocecal valve. On the left side, complete the dissection in the caudal direction, liberating the sigmoid colon from its lateral attachments down to the rectosigmoid region. After lifting up the colon and under direct vision (with transillumination), one can easily identify the central artery and vein (right vessels: colica dextra and ileocolica; left vessels: inferior mesenteric). Now divide and ligate them. Divide the mesenterium until the wall of the ileum and colon has been encountered (blunt blade, level 5; greater vessels at the arcades, level 3).

Editor's tip: Be sure to avoid unintentional injury to the intestine wall. Directly at the intestine wall, the tissue can be loaded with an Overhold clamp and then divided safely with UltraCision.

Resect the greater omentum lengthwise up to the marked resection line on each side and, after protection of the abdomen with large gauze pads, remove the whole specimen en bloc.

The resection of the transversum is a combination of both procedures with resection of the right and left flexure of the colon and complete resection of the greater omentum. A separate ligature of the branches of the colica media vessels and a lymphadenectomy at the inferior border of the pancreas and at the central root of the mesentery are then performed.

Before any anastomosis is begun, the blood supply should be carefully evaluated. Align both cut ends facing each other, so that their mesenteries are not twisted. Often the diameter of the ileum is narrower than that of colon. A slit of 1 or 2 cm is made on the antimensenteric border of the ileum to help equalize these two diameters.

Editor's tip: The opening of the intestine can also be performed without problems and with excellent hemostasis using UltraCision. To avoid the cavitation effect at the loose submucosa layer, the duration and the level of the power to the blade is decisive (Fig. 10.**1**).

The anastomosis is carried out with a 4–0 PDS seromuscular running suture, first at the posterior aspect of the anastomosis and then to the anterior border. The suture should always be done from the mesentery to the antimensentery side, so as to have a safe supply of the critical corner under good vision. After completion of the anastomosis, the mesenteric window is closed with a 3–0 Vicryl running suture. Take care to avoid occluding important vessels running in the mesentery in the course of the continuous suture.

Low Anterior Resection

In a modified lithotomy position, the first steps correspond to those of the left hemicolectomy. After mobilization of the descending colon and presentation of the left ureter, the peritoneum below and right-sided, the promontory of the sacrum is incised and prepared cranial to the left-sided central vessels (inferior mesenteric artery and vein). Make a lymphadenectomy around the artery without skeletonizing the aorta (Fig. 10.2) to protect the sympatic nerve bundles (blunt blade, level 3). Define the proximal line of resection and then divide the mesocolon sequentially and the vessels of the arcades until the wall of the colon has been reached (blunt blade, level 5; greater vessels at the arcades, level 3 and protection with a Overhold clamp) (Fig. 10.3). After dividing the sigmoid, the presacral shifting layer is prepared and then the total mesorectal excision is accomplished. With the lower sigmoid and rectum under steady upward retraction, it becomes evident that there is a dense band with only areolar tissue extending from the sacrum to the posterior mesorectum.

Any tendency on the part of the surgeon to insert a hand into this presacral space should be stoutly resisted. Through the cavitation effect of the UltraCision shears and by gently elevating the mesorectum, the proper presacral plane will be entered. The thin layer of fibroareolar tissue covering the sacrum, without presenting naked presacral veins or deep nerve bundles, is the correct plane of resection. Prepare in a forward direction dorsal and lateral on both sides. After completion of the preparation dorsolaterally, incise the peritoneum of the cul de sac ventrally, in order to stretch the rectum more effectively and to have greater mobility for the next step. Dissect at the rectum with the Dennoviller fascia as a guiding plane, preserving the vesicles and the prostate glands in men (blunt blade, level 3) (Fig. 10.4). Then divide the fascia of Waldeyer, which extends from the coccyx to the posterior rectal wall, to ensure that no coning of the mesorectum has occurred. Divide the vascular tissue around the rectum until the wall of the rectum is visible circumferentially (protection with an Overhold clamp) and divide the rectum after applying a clamp on the proximal rectum to avoid contamination (Fig. 10.5).

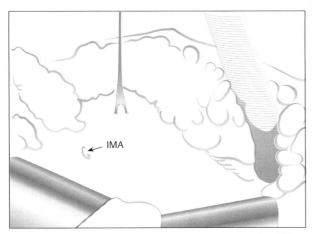
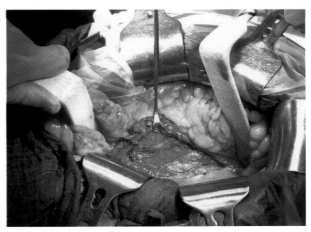

Fig. 10.**2** View of the prepared retroperitoneum and withdrawn inferior mesenteric artery (*IMA*).

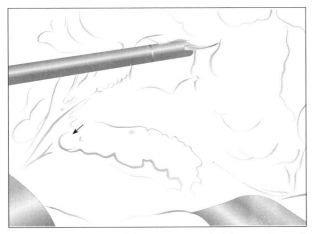
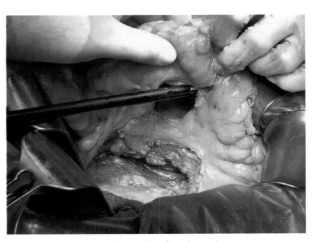

Fig. 10.**3** Preparation of the mesosigmoid with central vessel pedicle on to the proximal resection line (*arrow*).

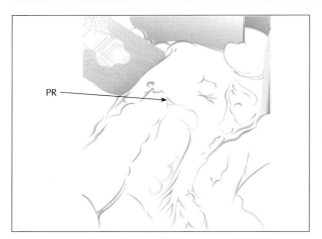
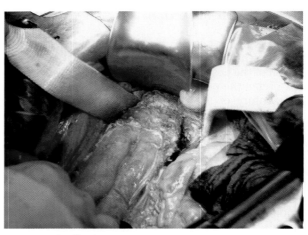

Fig. 10.**4** Ventral completion of the preparation of the rectum. *PR* peritoneal reflection.

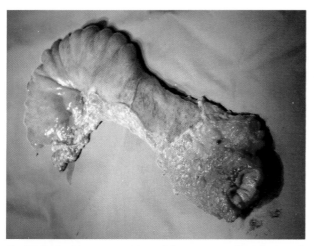

Fig. 10.**5** En bloc preparation of the rectum with intact peritoneal layer.

Suction and flushing the rectum frees it of any contents and with distilled water as a cytotoxic solution. The same procedure is undertaken at the colon, and after implantation of the anvil, the anastomosis can be accomplished without tension with the largest circular stapler. With complicated anastomosis a protecting ileostomy is established for six weeks.

Irrigate the abdominal cavity completely with Ringer's lactate, place an easy-flow drainage in the retroperitoneum or to the pelvis, and, after replacing the small bowel in a normal fashion to avoid any strangulation, close the wound in routine technique.

⚠ Hints and Pitfalls

- **Trauma of the ureter** Intraoperative injury of the ureter can occur, particularly when there are severe adhesions in that region from multiple previous operations, a malignancy, an inflammatory process, or previous radiation. Intraoperative injuries are uncommon during colorectal operations; however, most injuries result from gynecologic procedures and occur at the pelvic brim. Repair of ureteral injuries is a delicate matter that requires good judgment, experience, and skill. In general, injuries detected intraoperatively in a stable patient should be repaired immediately. When the patient is unstable or the detection is delayed for several days or weeks, the patient should undergo immediate proximal urinary diversion by placement of a percutaneous nephrostomy catheter followed by delayed repair. The principles of ureteral repair include debridement of viable tissues, tension-free anastomosis, and mucosa-to-mucosa reapproximation. Partial transection often can be managed by primary closure with interrupted 5–0 absorbable sutures (Vicryl). Complete transections and ischemic injuries can usually be repaired by resection of the injured segment followed by ureteroureterostomy. All repairs should be drained extraperitoneally and stented, such as with a double J stent for two weeks. To lower the pressure from the urinary system, it is effective to implant a transurethral bladder catheter (e.g., Foley catheter) immediately.
- **Injury to spleen** Operative injury to the spleen accounts for 20 to 40% of all splenectomies. Neither the incidence of this mishap nor its complications have lessened appreciably in recent decades. It has been shown that splenectomy is associated with a significant decrease in survival at five years in patients with Dukes' stage C colorectal cancer (6). The injury is invariably a small capsular lesion on the anterior or medial aspect of the lower pole of the spleen caused by tearing the normal splenic attachments, or it may be caused by traction on the greater omentum. For safe exploration of the left upper quadrant and mobilization of the splenic flexure, particularly in obese patients, it is important to have adequate exposure and the help of an

assistant. For this reason it is helpful to elevate the left costal margin additionally with a retractor. Most capsular tears can be managed by compressing the bleeding points using a temporary packing around the spleen with a hemostyptic fleece in place. Electrocautery is unsatisfactory for maintaining splenic parenchymal hemostasis. We have particularly good experience with the application of the argon beamer, since this non-contact technique makes good hemostasis possible. A splenectomy is undertaken only as a last resort. However, in an unstable situation one has to plan a splenectomy promptly so as not to lose too much time. The patient should be immunized with a currently available polyvalent pneumococcal vaccine as soon as possible after recovery from the operation and before discharge from the hospital (26).

- **Presacral hemorrhage** During mobilization of the rectum, presacral bleeding can occur if the presacral fascia is stripped and the presacral veins are torn. Although the bleeding is brisk, it can be controlled with packing. In some severe cases, the packing is placed for one or two days and removed, when conditions are favorable, with relaparotomy. For permanent arrest of hemorrhage, a thumbtack can be driven through the point of bleeding into the sacrum to achieve occlusion. This potentially fatal complication can be avoided by preserving the presacral fascia during mobilization of the rectum. Sharp dissection of the posterior mesorectum (e.g., by UltraCision) in the presacral areolar tissue plane is recommended rather than blunt dissection by hand.

- **Failure of anastomosis** An anastomotic leak usually becomes apparent after two to three days if technical errors are present, and later on (five to seven days) if blood circulation disturbances at the anastomosis arise postoperatively. Early dehiscence is usually serious since adhesions have not developed. Fecal spillage gives rise to generalized peritonitis. If a generalized peritonitis is obvious, along with other signs of sepsis, an urgent or emergency exploratory relaparotomy is indicated. Investigations to confirm the diagnosis are unnecessary and only delay treatment. The management should be directed at dismantling the anastomosis, with the proximal end brought out as a colostomy or ileostomy, and the distal end closed or brought out as a mucous fistula. Due to the existing peritonitis, programmed relaparotomies must be performed until the peritonitis is controlled. In most cases it is not appropriate to repair the anastomotic dehiscence or to reanastomose at this time. For late anastomotic leaks, pus or fecal material may be apparent if a drain is still in place. If the leak is not apparent but suspected, a gentle Gastrographin enema is the most accurate method of identifying the dehiscence. A CT scan cannot be used to determine the location of the leak, but the presence of accumulated fluid may suggest that a leak has occurred. In this situation, a diverting transverse colostomy or ileostomy and placement of a drain (e.g., CT guided) near the anastomoses in the detected fluid accumulation should be performed.

Personal Experience

We were very critical of UltraCision at first, but for the past few years we have worked almost exclusively with the UltraCision shears. We routinely use the long 10 mm shears (CS 10 mm) with "scissor handle" in the open procedure, because in this way we have the smallest conversions in the manual technique. In principle, we have worked satisfactorily with two different energy levels and different blade positions.

On the one hand, we use the conventional technique (blunt blade and level 3 or 5 depending on whether more coagulation or better cutting is demanded) and, on the other hand, the modification (sharp blade and only level 3). Both settings are similarly quick and lead to a bloodless preparation. A clear representation of the tissue planes is important, however. If necessary, in certain situations a preparation with shears or an Overhold has to be done first (e.g., near the wall of the intestine).

After going through the learning phase (about two weeks), we believe that preparation with UltraCision does not last longer than with the conventional technique. In contrast, one must compare the period of the tissue cutting with UltraCision and, on the other hand, the time for dividing and execution of ligatures on both sides in the conventional technique. We now are convinced that one can, particularly in adipose patients, prepare with the UltraCision even faster and with more security anatomically (18, 19). This is also shown during the release of the left flexure which, in most cases, is risky. Spleen cap lesions are to be avoided with careful gradual preparation, because after division of the ligaments, ligatures are no longer necessary. The lesion can often be provoked when imprudent knotting under tension is done.

As one particular point of risk, especially with adipose patients, the representation of the tail of the pancreas must be mentioned. At this location, one should divide the tissue in small steps only, so as not to risk a laceration of the parenchyma after a typical bleeding at the inferior border. The bleeding vessels must be ligated surely with a fine suture (4–0 or 5–0), in order to ensure clear anatomic conditions.

A characteristic advantage is the cavitation effect for preparation in the loose areolar tissue (e.g., with the rectum). The TME can be accomplished by the extension of the preparation in more distinct and anatomically exactly defined tissue layers without traumatic or thermal damage of the plexus of presacral nerve bundles (Fig. 10.**6**). Thus, the security for the patient in relation to postoperative functional disturbances of the sphincter apparatus (anal and bladder) can be increased and the postoperative quality of life improved.

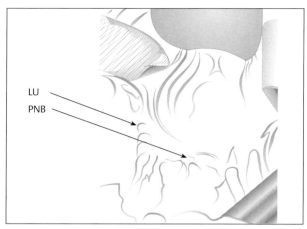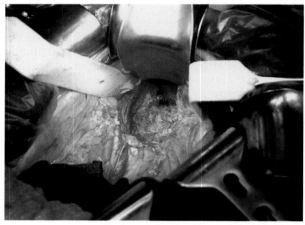

Fig. 10.**6**   View from cranial into the pelvis following a total mesorectal resection. *LU* left ureter, *PNB* presacral nerve bundles.

We always apply ligatures to the central vessels, although they can also be safely occluded the UltraCision alone. The large vessels have to be coagulated with the flat position of the blade in several locations along the length (1 cm) before final division without any tension (19).

 Discussion

The introduction of UltraCision to open colorectal surgery has led to the fact that, in most cases, one can prepare without any electric cauterization. The initial impression of the slow speed occurs in most cases at the beginning of an application. One has to wait for safe hemostasis before the tissue can be split completely. Early opening of the shears or tearing of the tissue leads to immediate bleeding, which is then managed in a usually complex manner. On the other hand, a careful blunt preparation in the tissue planes can be implemented very well when one uses the back of the active blade for this technique.

Because of the bloodless preparation we can achieve, particularly in rectal surgery, there has been a clear decrease in the number of transfused blood units. Though a current, ongoing clinical study has not yet been evaluated, this fact must be viewed as a particular advantage, especially for tumor-biological and immunological reasons, since in many studies it has been proven that the transfusion is related to a decreased prognosis (5, 8, 13).

The preparation of the splenic flexure with UltraCision is also substantially improved and leads only rarely to a spleen injury—which always represents an uncertain situation. In this way, the rate of accidental splenectomies can perhaps be reduced. From studies on TME it is well known that the rate of local recurrences is crucially related to the clean and complete preparation in the pelvis (10, 12). Especially in this region, the anatomically secure and clear preparation appears as a substantial requirement that is further improved by the cavitation effect of UltraCision.

Since lateral thermal damage is clearly less in comparison to the usual electrical surgery (24), one can assume that a substantially better preservation of the presacral plexus is reached, which would also lead in the late postoperative phase to fewer malfunctions. For this reason, thermal injuries of the ureter, which can only be identified by visual representation, are rather improbable in the close dissecting preparation in the retroperitoneum. To avoid such a serious complication, an exact preparation in the correct anatomic layers is particularly important.

If the initial high costs of the shears are set against the expenditure for blood products and saved thread material, then the costs probably balance. A primary, unexpected side effect is a substantially lower occurrence of problems in the operation theater. The surgeon armed with UltraCision can also use the same instrument for the management of a bleeding vessel. This leads to the fact that (with the exception of a few situations) special threads or different thread sizes are no longer required. The OR personnel have more time, can better follow the course of the operation, need have fewer instruments and suture material on the scrub nurse's table, and can concentrate on maintenance and cleaning of the UltraCision device.

In conclusion, we are sure the UltraCision is an innovative advance in surgical technology.

References

1. Aitken RJ. Mesorectal excision for rectal cancer. Br J Surg 1996; 83: 214–6.
2. Brownson P, Jenkins SA, Nott D, Ellenbogen S. Mechanical bowel preparation before colorectal surgery: Results of a prospective randomized trial. Br J Surg 1992; 79: 461–462.
3. Burke P, Mealy K, Gillen P, Joyce W, Traynor O, Hyland J. Requirement for bowl preparation in colorectal surgery. Br J Surg 1994; 81: 907–910.

4. Camma C, Giunta M, Fiorica F, Pagliaro L, Craxi A, Cottone M. Radiotherapy for resectable rectal cancer: A meta-analysis. JAMA 2000; 284: 1008–15.

5. Chiarugi M, Buccianti P, Disarli M, Galatioto C, Cavina E. Effect of blood transfusions on disease-free interval after rectal cancer surgery. Hepatogastroenterology 2000; 47: 1002–05.

6. Davis EJ, Ilstrup DM, Pemberton JH. Influence of splenectomy on survival rate of patients with colorectal cancer. Am J Surg 1988; 155: 173–79.

7. Deutsche Arbeitsgemeinschaft Bevölkerungsbezogener Krebsregister. In: Ed, Krebs in Deutschland: Häufigkeiten und Trends, Braun-Druck, Riegelsberg, Saarbrücken, 1997.

8. Edna TH, Bjerkeset T. Perioperative blood transfusions reduce long-term survival following surgery for colorectal cancer. Dis Colon Rectum 1998; 41: 451–59.

9. Gastinger I, Marusch F. Evidence-based surgery in colon carcinoma. Zentralbl Chir 2001; 126: 283–88.

10. Hall NR, Finan PJ, Al-Jaberi T, Tsang CS, Brown SR, Dixon MF, Quirke P. Circumferential margin involvement after mesorectal excision of rectal cancer with curative intent. Dis Colon Rectum 1998; 41: 979–83.

11. Heald RJ, Husband EM, Ryall RDH. The mesorectum in rectal cancer surgery: the clue to pelvic recurrence? Br J Surg 1982; 82: 1297–99.

12. Heald RJ, Moran BJ, Ryall RD, Sexton R, MacFarlane JK. Rectal cancer: the Basingstoke experience of total mesorectal excision, 1978–1997. Arch Surg 1998; 133: 894–99.

13. Heiss MM, Mempel W, Delanoff C, Mempel M, Jauch KW, Schildberg FW. Clinical effects of blood transfusion-associated immune modulation on outcome of tumor surgery. Infusionsther Transfusionsmed 1993; 20 (Suppl 2): 25–29.

14. Köhler L, Eypasch E, Paul A, Troidl H. Myths in management of colorectal malignancy. Br J Surg 1997; 84: 248–51.

15. Kolonkarzinom. Interdisziplinäre Leitlinie der Deutschen Krebsgesellschaft und ihrer Arbeitsgemeinschaften, der Deutschen Gesellschaft für Chirurgie und der Deutschen Gesellschaft für Verdauungs- und Stoffwechselkrankheiten. Kurzgefasste Interdisziplinäre Leitlinien 2000, B5, pp. 124 ff.

16. Lehnert T, Herfarth C. Multimodale Therapie des Rectumcarcinoms. Chirurg 1998; 69: 384–92.

17. MacFarlane JK, Ryall RDH, Heald RJ. Mesorectal excision for rectal cancer. Lancet 1993; 341: 457–60.

18. Maruta F, Sugiyama A, Matsushita K et al. Use of the harmonic scalpel in open abdominoperineal surgery for rectal carcinoma. Dis Colon Rectum 1999; 42: 540–42.

19. Msika S, Deroide G, Kianmanesh R, Iannelli A, Hay JM, Fingerhut A, Flamant Y. Harmonic scalpel in laparoscopic colorectal surgery. Dis Colon Rectum 2001; 44: 432–36.

20. Nelson H, Sargent DJ. Refinement multimodal therapy for rectal cancer. N Engl J Med 2001; 345: 690–92.

21. Ooi BS, Tjandra JJ, Green MD. Morbidities of adjuvant chemotherapy and radiotherapy for resectable rectal cancer: an overview. Dis Colon Rectum 1999; 42: 403–18.

22. Rectumkarzinom. Interdisziplinäre Leitlinie der Deutschen Krebsgesellschaft und ihrer Arbeitsgemeinschaften, der Deutschen Gesellschaft für Chirurgie und der Deutschen Gesellschaft für Verdauungs- und Stoffwechselkrankheiten. Kurzgefasste Interdisziplinäre Leitlinien 2000, B6, pp. 139 ff.

23. Santos JCM, Batista J, Sirimarco MT, Guimaraes AS, Levy CE. Prospective randomized trial of mechanical bowel preparation in patients undergoing elective colorectal surgery. Br J Surg 1994; 81: 1673–6.

24. Feil W, Lippert H, Lozaćh P, Palazzini G. editors. UltraCision: das harmonische Skalpell in: Atlas chirurgischer Klammernahttechniken. Heidelberg: Verlag Johann Ambrosius Barth; 2000.

25. Willett CG, Badizadegan K, Ancukiewicz M, Shellito PC. Prognostic factors in stage T3N0 rectal cancer. Do all patients require postoperative irradiation and chemotherapy? Dis Colon Rectum 1999 42: 167–73.

26. Working party of the British Committee for Standards in Hematology, Clinical Hematology Task Force. 1996 Guidelines for the prevention and treatment of infection in patients with an absent or dysfunctional spleen. Br Med J 1996; 312: 430–33.

11 Laparoscopic Treatment of Left Colon Diverticulitis

F. Psalmon

Laparoscopic colon resection is an elegant but difficult surgical procedure with many technical demands. One's experience in the field of laparoscopic surgery must be quite advanced to perform it in its entirety and safely.

Before the development of laparoscopic surgery and even up to the present time, the indication for colon resection for diverticulitis has often been delayed, except in cases of emergency, not only because of the operative risk but also because of the heavy consequences and damage to the abdominal wall due to heavily septic surgery with many chances of parietal abscesses, evisceration, postoperative hernias, and poor cosmetic results. All of these consequences seemed to be out of proportion for a benign disease, even if its evolution could lead to dramatic complications.

With increasing surgeons' experience, laparoscopic surgery achieves results equal to those of conventional surgery in terms of security with the well-known advantages such as postoperative comfort, short hospital stay, limited parietal damages, and some other positive results.

> Editor's tip: Proponents believe that these considerations are sufficient reasons to support adoption of the new technology. However, attempts to quantify these parameters have not been unequivocal and clear-cut indications for such an approach are far from accepted.

Laparoscopic surgery in the curative treatment of the colorectal carcinoma cannot be judged conclusively. These patients should be evaluated in controlled studies, and in the future we should be able to find a generally accepted consensus when the long-term results of the current studies of this technique are presented.

For the treatment of benign illnesses, laparoscopic technology has now been introduced in numerous centers and most of the operations are performed for the treatment of the diverticulitis.

It was sometimes difficult to perform an open left colectomy in patients coming to surgery after a long-term evolution and with a history of many acute attacks: we all know that long-term evolution (if not complicated by peritonitis requiring emergency treatment) causes huge local inflammatory adhesions to the surrounding peritoneum, abdominal wall and many other organs such as bladder, small intestine, left fallopian tube, ovaries, etc.

Therefore, in such conditions, laparoscopic left colon resection may be a true surgical challenge. The situation is now changing for three main reasons:

Table 11.1 Proposal of a new grading system

Grade 1
Inflammation limited to the colon or the mesocolon; few adhesions around; possibility of small abscesses enclosed in diverticles or mesocolon.

Grade 2
Pseudo-tumoral lesions of the sigmoid colon with huge inflammation and dense adhesions to the iliac and posterior abdominal wall.

Grade 3
Old chronic lesions with known or unknown fistula or dense adhesions to the surrounding organs such as ileum, bladder, Fallopian tubes, etc.

1. The proven good results of laparoscopic colectomy. These results lead to an earlier indication for surgery than previously, thus facilitating the laparoscopic treatment.
2. The use of the UltraCision shears whose inherent advantages lead to much more comfort and facility for the surgeon and much less operative risk for patients because of the total lack of electrical damage.
3. The reliable ability for dissection and hemostasis—especially in inflammatory tissues.

So many possibilities of local lesions may be encountered that it is not easy classify them. Nevertheless, we suggest a classification based on strictly technical and surgical points of view (Table 11.1).

Preoperative findings of examinations such as colon opacification with colloids and CT scan rarely lead to a complete anatomic diagnosis; nevertheless, CT scans are useful for the diagnosis of pericolic or pelvic abscesses and assessment of treatment by percutaneous drainage prior to surgery.

Most of the time (with the exception of the Grade 1 situation), however, the true lesions and potential surgical difficulties are, in fact, discovered at the time of operation.

In any case, we know now that the objectives of surgery should be:

- To resect the pathologic part of the colon and the rectosigmoidal junction. More recently, the length of bowel resection and necessity to preserve the arterial and nervous supply of the remaining rectal stump have been subject of much discussion.

> Editor's tip: The crucial step in decompressing the colon is the resection of the rectosigmoidal high pressure zone.

- To resect where required (in the case of close adhesion or fistula) the organ concerned: bladder, small intestine, left internal genital organs in women, etc.
- To create an anastomosis between the descending colon and the rectal stump with or without protection colostomy.

> Editor's tip: Whenever possible, the creation of a diverting colostomy should be avoided in the elective situation.

Indication and Preoperative Management

From a strictly technical surgical point of view the best indication is chronic diverticulitis with previous recurrent attacks *before* the time of severe complications. Preparation, depending on one's experience, has to provide at the time of operation with an empty and flat colon; otherwise, exposition might be extremely difficult, possibly leading to an impossible or dangerous laparoscopic treatment.

In emergency situations, indications for laparoscopic treatment, are actually unclear and will therefore not be discussed. Of course, if colon resection is to be considered, even in emergency conditions, the following technical description is of interest, with or without anastomosis (Hartmann procedure).

Operation

The patient is placed exactly as for a colon cancer resection, in a double team position, the so-called "French position."

The operating table must be shaped with the possibility to put the patient in heavy Trendelenburg and right rotation position.

The surgeon and the first assistant holding the camera stand on the right side of the patient, the second assistant takes a position between the patient's legs.

Usually four ports are necessary:
- One 10 mm port, 2 cm on the right side and above the umbilicus (camera)
- One 10–12 mm port in the inferior right quadrant (LCS 10 or 5 mm shears, staplers)
- Two 5 mm ports: one in the right upper quadrant (grasping instrument), one on the midline just above the pubic arch (probe)
- An additional 5 mm port may be placed, if necessary, for left angle taking down, at the left side of the left rectus muscle at the site of the forthcoming mini-laparotomy for specimen extraction and anvil placement

Naturally, the definitive placement of each port is decided after creation of the pneumoperitoneum and close examination of the abdominal cavity according to intra-abdominal geography and patient morphology.

The following choice of instruments is recommended:
- UltraCision 5 mm or 10 mm shears (We usually take the 5 mm LCS shears which allows positioning in different ports.)
- Two 5 mm atraumatic grasping instruments
- One 5 mm probe with possible angulation of the extremity
- Suction-irrigation device

> Editor's tip: The use of larger grasping instruments (Babcock clamps) with atraumatic jaws is safer and prevents damage to the colonic wall during retraction.

Strategy

From a surgical tactical point of view, two kinds of resection are to be considered:

- Large "cancer-like resection" with early ligation of the IMA and IMV. At the start, mobilize the left Toldt fascia above the inflammatory lesions and then the upper rectal stump. To find the safe path between the three major anatomic structures we absolutely have to preserve the left ureter, left iliac vessels, and hypogastric nerves.
- Limited sigmoid resection with preservation of the inferior mesenteric artery, leading to a trans-mesocolic dissection and hemostasis, often including the necessity to work through inflammatory tissues.

Large Resection

Dissection starts on the aorta with ultrasonic treatment of the inferior mesenteric artery (IMA): here the use of LCS shears is a true help, periarterial tissues often being inflammatory and containing lymph nodes. They provide a clean, non-bleeding dissection with an excellent lymphostasis.

Even if hemostasis of the inferior mesenteric artery is perfect, we think that it is necessary to put a safety clip on the aortic side, especially at start of one's experience and certainly in large and very inflammatory inferior mesenteric pedicles.

Dissection continues upward to the inferior mesenteric vein (IMV) which is not immediately transected, its back side being the best key point to open the plane of the left fascia of Toldt. In this place, there is no inflammation and it is easy to open the fascia, leaving posteriorly the hypogastric nerves, the spermatic or lombo-ovarian veins and, of course the left ureter which, at this place, is deeply situated between the left side of the aorta and the inferior pole of the left kidney.

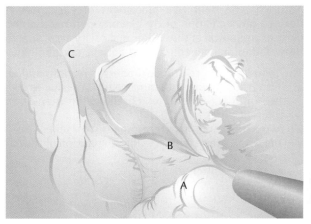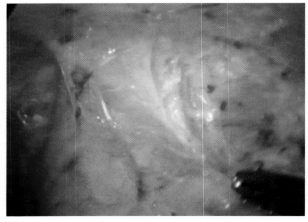

Fig. 11.**1** Parietal adhesions. *A* colon, *B* vas deferens, *C* adhesions.

Working this way, these elements are seen "along the way" and not *truly* dissected; dissection is not necessary.

The opening of the Toldt's fascia is conducted, as far as possible, laterally and in the direction of the left angle, while realizing for the first time the taking down of the left angle.

At this stage of the dissection, the LCS shears are being used like a dissecting clamp, allowing simultaneous hemostasis of the very small vessels and thus keeping a very clear and clean operating field. The activated back side of the shears may be used as a cutting blade, providing a quick, dry, and effective opening of the planes of dissection.

The next step is the opening of the right flap of the mesosigmoid down to the upper part of the rectal stump at the site of the future rectal section, always using the LCS shears. The rectal stump is easily separated from the sacral plane.

> Editor's tip: If the diverticulitis involvement is located in the middle or upper part of the sigmoid, the reverse procedure, starting distally at the rectosigmoid junction could be of advantage. The strategy is to start the preparation of the mesocolon in non-infiltrated tissue and then to proceed to the risky, involved part of the sigmoid.

This being done, we are ready to dissect the sometimes inflammatory mesosigmoid root from iliac vessels and left ureter.

It may be difficult at this time not to lose the good plane of dissection; the use of the LCS shears is now dramatically advantageous, combining perfect hemostasis and the cavitation effect. It enables a much easier and safer progression through sometimes dense and inflammatory tissues, helping, thanks to a clear and clean vision of the dissection field, to remain in the correct path. The cavitation effect that gently blows the planes of dissection provides a great security at this sometimes dangerous step of the dissection by allowing a perfect identification of anatomic structures.

Once separated from the noble posterior anatomic structures, the colon has to be divided from the lateral abdominal wall, which is much less dangerous even if dense and inflammatory adhesions make the planes of dissection unclear. Here again the LCS shears are very efficient (Fig. 11.**1**).

After complete mobilization of the colon, the mesorectum is divided with the LCS shears without any need for clips or stapler. Then, the upper rectum is transected just under the rectosigmoidal junction using an EZ 45 mm or EZ 35 mm endoscopic stapler.

Control of the rectal closure is routinely made by air injection into the remaining rectum.

The specimen is then pulled out through a short, left lateral laparotomy (5 cm ± 1 cm) protected by a circled plastic wound protector in order to minimize further parietal septic complication.

> Editor's tip: It is better to enlarge the wound than to tear the specimen and contaminate the abdominal cavity.

Once the pathologic colon is resected, the anvil of a CDH stapler is inserted and ensured in the proximal colon which is then reinserted in the abdominal cavity. The short laparotomy is closed in two layers of PDS 2/0.

Returning to laparoscopy, we check if the remaining colon goes down gently—without any tension—to the anastomotic site; if not, it is necessary to take down the left colon angle.

> Editor's tip: The proximal colon segment is also reviewed to ensure that the mesentery is well aligned.

This is performed by dividing the great omentum from the left part of the transverse colon and transecting the root of the left transverse mesocolon from the inferior board of the pancreatic tail, always working with the LCS shears.

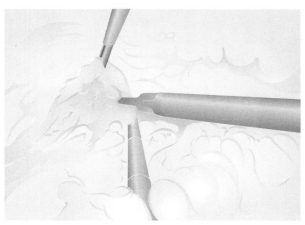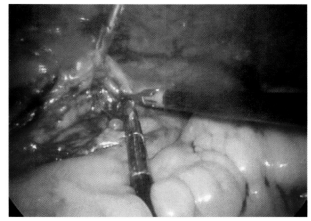

Fig. 11.**2**   Inferior mesenteric artery dissection: exposing step by step the sigmoid arteries.

Especially in obese patients, separation of the greater omentum from the colon might be tedious with a lot of different situations in terms of adhesions between the omentum, the left transverse colon, the left angle, the lower pole of the spleen and the descending colon.

We find that it is always easy to work with the LCS shears along the colonic wall, obtaining a perfect hemostasis without any danger to the colon wall.

The colo-rectal anastomosis is then performed with the CDH stapler applied transanally. The anastomosis is controlled by air injection.

> Editor's tip: If the stapler resists removal, the distal side of the anastomosis may be gently held with a Babcock.

The closure of the right-sided retroperitoneum by a running Lahotni suture of the mesentery is recommended.

A suction drainage is inserted through the sub-pubic 5 mm port and placed in the pelvis before exsufflation and closure of the 10 mm ports holes. In military parlance, we can say that we used an "encircling" strategy which is safe and easy in our experience.

Limited Resection

Some will prefer a limited resection with conservation of the inferior mesenteric vessels and less possible damage to hypogastric nerves: this leads to a trans-mesocoloic dissection by creating a window through the mesosigmoid in order to find the Toldt fascia. One then identifies the left ureter and transects above and below the mesosigmoid using the LCS shears.

This is an elegant technique when lesions are of short length and limited to the colon wall and without consequent inflammation of the mesocolon (Grade 1): if not, finding the Toldt fascia and identification of the left ureter might be hazardous, even unsafe.

Furthermore, in severe inflammatory conditions, limited resection might lead to an insufficient colon resection with the risk of performing the anastomosis on a non-perfect colon wall, thus increasing the chances of postoperative leakage.

Another way to preserve the inferior mesenteric artery and hypogastric nerves is to start the dissection by discovering the inferior mesenteric vein. Then the left Toldt fascia is opened downwards, which leads to the back side of the mesenteric inferior artery which is to be followed in its course. This allows a progressive dissection of the sigmoidian arteries which are, one by one, transected using the UltraCision shears with no need for clips or ties (Fig. 11.**2**).

The inferior mesenteric artery is most of the time rather easily followed in Grade 1 situations. Dissection is continued on to the upper part of the rectal stump which is, at the same time, prepared for transection. In this kind of dissection, fat, veins, and hypogastric nervous branches following arteries are easily identified and transected: recognition of these elements is certainly facilitated by the cavitation effect.

The use of 5 mm curved UltraCision shears is at this time very efficient but it is necessary to preset the variable power at level 1 or 2 to obtain a definite hemostasis before resection.

Difficult Conditions

The most difficult conditions are mainly Grade 3 situations. The success of laparoscopic treatment depends at the start on the possibilities for exposure: if exposure is too difficult to obtain, to be secure, or if the space for work is highly insufficient, it might be safer to go back to open surgery where, it should be noted, the laparotomic UltraCison scalpel is also a true help for the surgeon.

Colo-bladder fistula UltraCision helps the dissection by providing a good hemostasis, especially in the bladder wall which is afterwards sutured endoscopically.

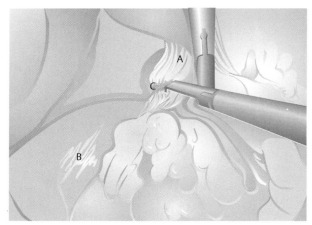
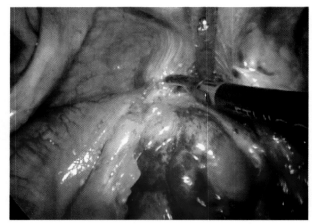

Fig. 11.**3**   Colo-vaginal fistula. *A* vaginal wall, *B* colon, *C* colo-vaginal fistula.

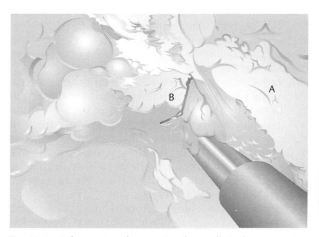
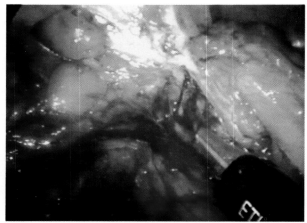

Fig. 11.**4**   Colo-ovarian abscess. *A* colon wall, *B* abscess cavity.

We have found that bladder wall damage was less important in laparoscopy than in conventional dissection. Dissection with UltraCision appears to be more precise, working nicely in the dense tissues surrounding the fistulic zone. In our experience, we never had to resect the bladder wall. Closure of the fistula, which is usually small, with one or two stitches and bladder drainage for a few days have been sufficient to obtain a good healing without urinary complications.

Editor's tip: In order to achieve a complete decompression of the bladder, a transurethral catheter is preferred.

Colo-vaginal fistula Communication between the lumen of the colon and vagina is most of the time easy to dissect. The vagina does not need to be sutured (Fig. 11.**3**).

Adhesions to left genital organs If not easily cleavable, incident annexectomy might be a good choice. This procedure can be carried out entirely with the UltraCision scalpel for section of the Fallopian tube, treatment of uterine ligaments, and hemostasis and transection of lumbo-ovarian veins (Fig. 11.**4** and Fig. 11.**5**).

Colo-enteric fistula Difficulties of presentation make these fistulas difficult to treat laparoscopically but, if one decides to do so, the small bowel resection, which is often necessary, is facilitated by using the UltraCision shears for section and hemostasis of the mesentery. The small bowel is then transected with staplers at each side of the fistula. The small bowel anastomosis is performed endoscopically or through the laparotomy created to take out the colon specimen. Here again, the use of UltraCision facilitates and shortens the procedure.

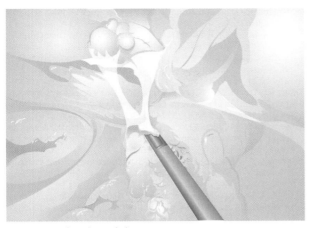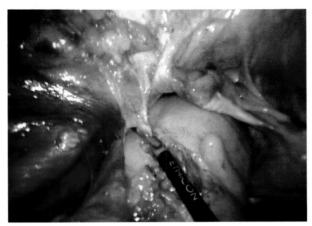

Fig. 11.**5**   Colo-adnexial dissection.

Hint and Pitfalls

If correctly manipulated, UltraCision shears are perfectly secure, especially in inflammatory conditions. The key point is to achieve a perfect balance between the tension and pressure delivered on the tissues within the jaws of the shears and to read and interpret properly the image of tissue changes so as to get the best control possible by letting the ultrasonic effect take its course.

With 5 mm curved scissors, section might be rather quick; therefore, it is recommended to set the lower power in the generator at level 1 or 2 at most.

In our experience small bleedings are always the consequence of a too quick manipulation with too much tension on the tissues.

It is often interesting, in these inflammatory tissues, to work with the back side of the activated blade manipulated as a blunt dissector: in this way blunt dissection is safe and dry.

Personal Experience

Since starting work with the UltraCision devices, we can report on 52 cases of left colon laparoscopic resections for diverticulitis using the 10 mm LCS shears at start and the 5 mm LCS shears for the 20 last patients.

In this time, 72 patients were proposed for surgery; 8 of them were not considered, at the start, as being suitable for a laparoscopic procedure.

The 64 remaining patients were explored laparoscopically and 12 of them quickly converted to conventional surgery for technical reasons such as insufficient space to work, unclear vision or accompanying difficulties leading to an extended time of surgery, which would probably have been questionable depending on the patient's status.

Of the 52 patients totally operated laparoscopically, 25 were Grade 1, 18 were Grade 2 and nine were Grade 3.

Among the latter nine patients, four required a left annexectomy, two had a bladder fistula dissected and closed laparoscopically, one had a fistula between a diverticle and a vaginal scar from a previous hysterectomy, one had a fistula with the seminal vesicle and the last one had a fistula between the small bowel and the left colon dissected laparoscopically, the small bowel being resected and anastomosed through the mini-laparotomy used for the specimen extraction.

The mean operating time was 180 minutes (150–310 minutes).

All patients were operated solely with the UltraCision for dissection and hemostasis, no clip was used except on the aortic side of the IMA.

Only two patients required the use of stapling devices on the inferior mesenteric artery because of an enlarged pedicle surrounded by heavy inflammatory tissues.

In all cases, the inferior mesenteric vein was transected using the LCS shears with no additional clip.

None of the 52 patients required intra- or postoperative transfusion; blood loss was estimated in all cases to be less than 100 ml.

The mean volume of irrigation was 300 ml: irrigation has been essentially used to check the rectal stump closure and the anastomosis.

We had no intraoperative complications with the surrounding organs.

Discussion

The use of ultrasonic instruments and particularly of UltraCision devices brings comfort and safety. It allows a significant reduction of operating time, 30 % in our experience, by using a single instrument for dissection and hemostasis. By the way, it also diminishes costs of stapler use.

In difficult situations, even if the working space is tight, the lack of electrical and thermal danger to surrounding structures allows a more confident work. This certainly increases the possibilities for laparoscopic treatment of sigmoid diverticulitis even in severe local conditions.

Suggested Reading

Bernhart W. [Sigmoido-uterine fistula, an uncommon complication in sigmoid diverticulitis]. Zentralbl Gynakol 1967 Apr 8; 89(14): 499–502 (German).

Bertero D, Buzio M, Albertino B, Giaccone M, Ricci E, Gagna G. [A case of ureteral stenosis and ureterorectal fistula secondary to sigmoid diverticulitis]. Minerva Chir 1992 Oct 15; 47(19): 1567–9 (review Italian).

Berthou JC, Charbonneau P. Elective laparoscopic management of sigmoid diverticulitis. Results in a series of 110 patients. Surg Endosc 1999 May; 13(5): 457–60.

Berthou JC, Charbonneau P. [Results of laparoscopic treatment of diverticular sigmoiditis. Apropos of 85 cases]. Chirurgie 1997; 122(7): 424–9 (French).

Bruce CJ, Coller JA, Murray JJ, Schoetz DJ Jr, Roberts PL, Rusin LC. Laparoscopic resection for diverticular disease. Dis Colon Rectum 1996 Oct; 39(10 Suppl): 1–6.

Chen HH, Wexner SD, Weiss EG, et al. Laparoscopic colectomy for benign colorectal disease is associated with a significant reduction in disability a compared with laparotomy. Surg Endosc 1998 Dec; 12(12): 1397–400.

Heili MJ, Flowers SA, Fowler DL. Laparoscopic-assisted colectomy: a comparison of dissection techniques. JSLS 1999 Jan–Mar; 3(1): 27–31.

Junghans T, Bohm B, Schwenk W, Grundel K, Muller JM. [Progress in laparoscopic sigmoid resection in elective surgical therapy of sigmoid diverticulitis]. Langenbecks Arch Chir 1997; 382(5): 266–70 (German).

Kockerling F, Schneider C, Reymond MA, et al. Laparoscopic resection of sigmoid diverticulitis. Results of a multicenter study. Laparoscopic Colorectal Surgery Study group. Surg Endosc 1999 Jun; 13(6): 567–71.

Kohler L, Rixen D, Troidl H. Laparoscopic colorectal resection for diverticulitis. Int J Colorectal Dis 1998; 13(1): 43–7.

Lacy AM, Garcia-Valdecasas JC, Delgado S, et al. Postoperative complications of laparoscopic-assisted colectomy. Surg Endosc 1997 Feb; 11(2): 119–22.

Leung KL, Yiu RY, Lai PB, Lee JF, Thung KH, Lau WY. Laparoscopic-assisted resection of colorectal carcinoma: five-year audit. Dis Colon Rectum 1999 Mar; 42(3): 327–32; discussion 332–3.

Libermann MA, Phillips EH, Carroll BJ, Fallas M, Rosenthal R. Laparoscopic colectomy vs. traditional colectomy for diverticulitis. Outcome and costs. Surg Endosc 1996 Jan; 10(1): 15–8.

Reissman P, Agachan F, Wexner SD. Outcome of laparoscopic colorectal surgery in older patients. Am Surg 1996 Dec; 62(12): 1060–3.

Schiedeck TH, Schwandner O, Bruch HP. [Laparoscopic sigmoid resection in diverticulitis]. Chirurg 1998 Aug; 69(8): 846–53 (German).

Schlachta CM, Mamazza J, Poulin EC. Laparoscopic sigmoid resection for acute and chronic diverticulitis. An outcomes comparison with laparoscopic resection for nondiverticular disease. Surg Endosc 1999 Jul; 13(7): 649–53.

Sher ME, Agachan F, Bortul M, Nogueras JJ, Weiss EG, Wexner SD. Laparoscopic surgery for diverticulitis. Surg Endosc 1997 Mar; 11(3): 264–7.

Siriser F. Laparoscopic-assisted colectomy for divderticular sigmoiditis. A single-surgeon prospective study of 65 patients. Surg Endosc 1999 Aug 13(8): 811–3.

Smadja C, Sbai Idrissi M, Tahrat M, et al. Elective laparoscopic sigmoid colectomy for diverticulitis. Results of a prospective study. Surg Endosc. 1999 Jul; 13(7): 645–8.

Stevenson AR, Stitz RW, Lumley JW, Fielding GA. Laparoscopically assisted anterior resection for diverticular disease: follow-up of 100 consecutive patients. Ann Surg. 1998 Mar; 227(3): 335–42.

Tancer ML, Veridiano NP. Genital fistulas caused by diverticular disease of the sigmoid colon. Am J Obstet Gynecol. 1996 May; 174(5): 1547–50.

Troiani F, Attardo S, Del Papa M, Paolucci G, Mobili M, Braccioni U. [Complications of colonic diverticular disease: a rare case of sigmoid-vaginal fistula]. G Chir 1993 Jul; 14(6): 305–8. Italian.

12 Laparoscopic Colorectal Surgery for Cancer

H. R. Nürnberger

Laparoscopic surgery should be recognized as a technique-based concept and not as a new therapy in itself. Instead, laparoscopic surgery involves minimal access, the technical support to accomplish the same result, and hopefully leads to a decreased morbidity for the patient. The indications for surgical interventions are the same, but the technique for entry differs. Nevertheless, the final product should be the same whether performed as an open surgery or laparoscopically (15). Colorectal procedures require advanced laparoscopic skills. This is related to the need to work in multiple quadrants of the abdomen, division of major blood vessels in the mesentery, extraction of a bulky specimen, and anastomotic restoration of bowel continuity. Many surgeons perform a laparoscopic-assisted procedure with laparoscopic mobilization of the specimen, division of blood vessels and bowel intracorporeally, before extraction of the specimen. Others exteriorize the mobilized bowel and perform the resection and the anastomosis extracorporeally (most right-sided resections).

Indication and Preoperative Management

The reputed advantages of laparoscopic operations have been widely discussed, but clear-cut indications for such an approach are far from accepted. Some protagonists forge ahead, whereas some conservative surgeons only grudgingly concede its existence. In general, the laparoscopic technique is accepted in the context of a curative approach only with T1–T2 (T3) tumors. Wall-exceeding T4 tumors cannot be managed under curative objectives laparoscopically. Peritoneal dissemination of malignant cells must be considered to have an eventual fatal outcome.

The preoperative diagnostic measurements are not different to the open procedure. However, a safe evaluation of the intestine wall infiltration should be performed (colon: CT, rectum: CT and/or endosonography). Similarly, a possibly necessary stoma creation should be discussed with the patient and be prepared (see Chapter 9).

The patient should be informed that intraoperative circumstances may mandate conversion of the technique to an open procedure. In particular, no increase of risk due to the laparoscopic technology may be accepted. From the outset, concern about patient security rather than about conversion is advised. Patient selection is critical for obtaining good results. Short, obese patients make laparoscopic surgery difficult, while tall, slender patients are ideal candidates. Frail, elderly patients with extensive comorbidity, who would benefit most, often suffer from the pulmonary and hemodynamic sequelae of the pneumoperitoneum.

Operation

The description of the operation technique will consider first the left-sided operations. The right hemicolectomy is described in detail by D'Hoore in chapter 9. Characteristics of tumor surgery are emphasized.

The patient is placed in a modified lithotomy position and must be secured to the table to prevent sliding under extreme tilting. The operating surgeon stands on the right side.

The following instruments are routinely used:
- The assistant robot (Aesop) for optic guidance (if available)
- An angled 25°/30° laparoscope
- 4 × 1 0–11 mm trocars
- 2 × blunt Babcock clamps
- 10 mm UltraCision Shear (LCS)
- Ring drape protection
- 1 × endo-dissecting instrument

General operative guidelines (1):
- Determine ideal patient positioning,
- Determine ideal port placement,
- Cleanse scope frequently,
- Keep instruments in view at all times,
- Withdraw instruments/scope with loss of pneumoperitoneum,
- Convert to open procedure when safe dissection is impossible (45 minute rule).

The pneumoperitoneum is achieved for safety with the open technique. It is performed through an incision immediately above the umbilicus and the dense fascia is grasped with a Kocher clamp and pulled cephaled. After opening the abdominal cavity, the first trocar is placed under direct vision. For colorectal surgery, usually four additional ports are needed: two for the surgeon's instruments, two for the assistant's instruments. Port placement must be planned so that the ports are directed at the pathology in a semicircle. The strategic placement permits their incorporation into a later incision for specimen retrieval or stoma creation, if needed. Now the patient is placed in a steep, head-down position and the table is rotated to the right, causing the small bowel to fall away from the left lower quadrant. Incise the peritoneum medial and right-

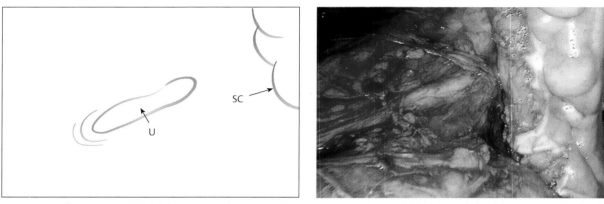

Fig. 12.**1**   Wide exposure of the left ureter in the prepared retroperitoneum (view from the medial side). *SC* sigmoid colon (retracted), *U* ureter.

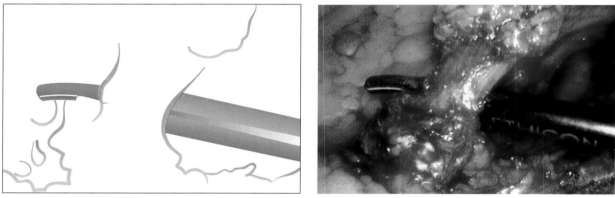

Fig. 12.**2**   Central preparation of the inferior mesenteric artery before ligation.

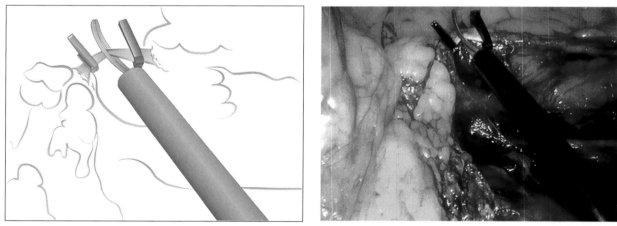

Fig. 12.**3**   Exposure of the inferior mesenetric vein in the mesentery and high withdrawal by clips.

sided below the promontorium. Proceed to identify the presacral shifting layer (a dense band with only areolar tissue extending from the sacrum to the posterior mesorectum) and separate the left ureter (Fig. 12.**1**) in the retroperitoneum from the specimen clearly (blunt blade, level 3). Prepare the mesentery cranial to expose the vessels centrally (Figs. 12.**2**, 12.**3**); then the inferior mesenteric artery (IMA) is divided with a vascular stapler. We clip the prepared vein proximal and distal.

Some times in obese patients, the inferior mesenteric vein is unrecognized transsected with the UltraCision without any complication. The sigmoid is retracted medially, exposing the left lateral attachments of the descending colon. Usually the UltraCision shears (blunt blade, level 5) are used to incise the white line of Toldt and to mobilize the colon from the loose areolar retroperitoneal tissue.

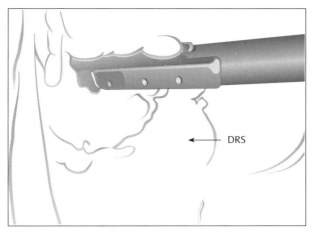 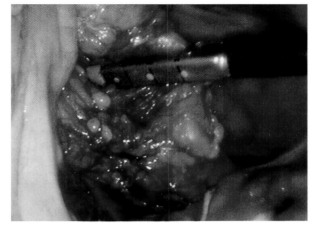

Fig. 12.**4**   Cleavage of the rectum with the linear cutter after preparation of the mesorectum. *DRS* distal rectal stump

> Editor's tip: The mesentery should rarely be grasped to retract or manipulate the bowel, because it may result in bleeding that is difficult to control.

Right hemicolectomy is performed mostly as a laparoscopically assisted procedure. In contrast to the operation with inflammatory bowel disease, (Chapter 9), the mandatory safety margins must be followed with tumor operations and the central lymphadenectomy has to be performed without any changes. After release of the ascending colon, the trocar canal in the right upper quadrant is extended and the widely mobilized bowel can be easily luxated in front of the abdominal wall. In an extracorporeal manner, mark the lines of resection at the intestine and incise the parietal peritoneum with the UltraCision down to the central vessels at the root of the mesentery (ileocolic, right colic, right-sided branches of the middle colic artery and vein). Under transillumination, the vessels are prepared and managed with suture ligation. Remove the en bloc preparation with the central lymph nodes and perform an end-to-end ileotransversostomy in the usual technique using a seromuscular 4–0 PDS running suture (see Chapter 9).

If an anterior resection or left hemicolectomy is necessary, the splenic flexure has to be mobilized. The team must change position, and the monitors must be realigned. The operating surgeon usually stands between the patient's legs and uses the left sided ports for his instruments. The assistant moves to the right upper quadrant to grasp the bowel. The table is shifted to a head-up position to cause the small bowel to slide down and to the right. Careful traction on the splenic flexure exposes the attachments. A layer after layer preparation (blunt blade, level 3) is necessary just like in the open technique to avoid laceration of the spleen and pancreas. Dissection close to the transverse colon along the omentum and opening the lesser sac is relatively bloodless.

Dissection into the pelvis is performed under direct vision (blunt blade, level 5). The rectum is pulled anterior to enter the presacral dissection plane over the sacral prominence.

> Editor's tip: Transanal placement of a blunt instrument (e.g., EEA sizer) can provide additional retraction to the rectum and distal sigmoid colon.
> Using the magnification of the laparoscopic optic together with the small size of the equipment, an amazingly good overview can be obtained of the preparation field.

The subsequent preparation is the same as in the conventional technique. When the two sides of transection are decided upon, the rectum mesenteric fat is dissected off in preparation for an anastomosis.

In comparison to the open procedure, the anastomosis is performed in the double-stapling technique. The rectum can be transected with a linear stapler (Fig. 12.**4**) (often two magazines are necessary) and, after decompression of the pneumoperitoneum, the planned short incision in the left lower quadrant for specimen removal is made.

> Editor's tip: Before firing the stapler, the surgeon should confirm its proper positioning. Both sides and the tip of the stapler should be clearly visualized.

The plastic ring drape is inserted and the mobilized colon drawn out of the wound. Then the proximal transection line is determined, the mesenterium prepared, and a standard end-to-end stapler anvil is inserted. To ensure a sufficient length and to perform a tension-free anastomosis, the proximal colon must be long enough to reach over the symphysis. The proximal colon is replaced back into the abdominal cavity and the fascia sutured. After the pneumoperitoneum has been reestablished a lavage of the operation area and the pelvis should be accomplished, in order to avoid an unintentional contamination.

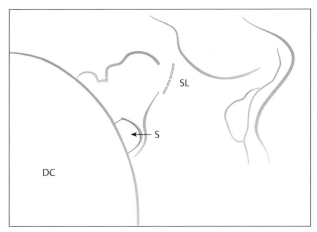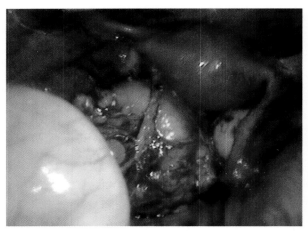

Fig. 12.**5**   Anastomosis (double stapling) after deep anterior resection of the rectum for reestablishment of continuity. *DC* descending colon, *SL* stapling line, *S* spike.

Editor's tip: Even with the fascia securely closed, there still is escape of gas. To avoid subcutaneous emphysema, the skin should be left open until the termination of the pneumoperitoneum.

Inspect the peritoneal cavity for correct orientation of the mesentery and if adequate hemostasis is present.

The stapler is introduced via the anus and the stapler trocar opened to penetrate the linear staple line ventrally. The anvil and stapler are connected, the stapler closed and fired and, after withdrawal, the rings of excisional tissue are inspected for completeness (Fig. 12.**5**). The anastomosis can be tested by introducing air under pressure and bubbles in the rinsing liquid in the pelvis will be seen if there is a leakage. Another very helpful tool is to inspect the anastomosis with a rectoscope to control the anastomotic ring and, if needed, one can make an additional stitch to approximate the resection lines surely. After complete irrigation of the operative field with Ringer's solution, place an easy-flow drain down to the pelvis and close the retroperitoneum medially with a running suture.

If a diversionostomy is necessary, in most cases a loop ileostomy is the simplest method. The mobile segment of the distal ileum is drawn up to determine whether the loop will reach though the abdominal wall. The pneumoperitoneum is released and the bowel is pulled through the wound. The bowel may be fixed to the fascia with interrupted sutures and the prominent asymmetric ileostomy is created as for a loop ileostomy in the conventional fashion. The last step of the procedure is again the control of the correct placement of the ileum with the camera observing from the abdominal side.

⚠ Hints and Pitfalls

Apart from the well-known complications from the open technique, some special problems of the laparoscopic technique have to be mentioned.

- **Access** A significant proportion of complications of laparoscopic surgery occur during creation of the pneumoperitoneum (e.g., vascular, intestinal lesions). For this reason, today the open, safe technique is generally recommended. Also, broad adhesions can be quickly recognized and predict the indication to conversion (5).

- **Instrumentation** The choice of bowel graspers is especially important. The need for effective traction to mobilize and dissect the colon must be balanced with the tendency for these instruments to cause serosal or full-thickness bowel tears. Inadvertent torsion or excessive compression may result in an intramural hematoma, leading to ischemia and necrosis with resultant perforation at the site, or an injury at the initial operation that remains unrecognized. For this reason, atraumatic laparoscopic clamps are preferred (e.g., Babcock clamps).

- **Hemorrhage** Vascular injuries to the abdominal wall are a relatively infrequent occurrence, although its true incidence is probably underreported (0.05–2.5%, (3)). The source of bleeding is usually the inferior epigastric artery or one of its branches. The surgeon should attempt to identify these vessels using the transillumination of the laparoscope from inside out before inserting the accessory ports. The trocar incision site should be located lateral to the rectus muscle. At the end of the operation, the removal of the trocars should be done under direct vision in order to be able to recognize bleedings from the trocar canal.

Personal Experience

Before availability of UltraCision, laparoscopic resections of the colon were a complex and technical demanding procedure. The introduction of UltraCision in the laparoscopic surgery is a new advance in quality. Without any electrical cauterization, dissection and tissue division are easily performed and the hemostasis is very effective.

In particular, the preparation of the mesorectum in the loose areolar presacral layer can be performed very surely and rapidly. However, we still continue to suture the central vessels with the vascular stapler.

In a comparison of costs, one must consider that otherwise additional (and expensive) multifire clip appliers are needed, in order to achieve a safe hemostasis in the mesocolon. With the use of the UltraCision it is not necessary to change the instrument frequently during the same operation.

In some studies, repeated instrument changes were a substantial factor for the emergence of trocar site metastases. By the way one can prepare for the operation without undue stress.

Discussion

In Germany at present 15 % of all surgical units operate 1–2 % of all colorectal carcinomas laparoscopically. Right-sided hemicolectomy (20%), resection of the sigma (30%) and low anterior resection (45%) are accomplished predominantly (9, 17). The mortality rates range between 0–2.1 % and thus do not differ significantly in comparison to those for open resection. The morbidity rate for the laparoscopic technique ranges between 7–31 % and for the conventional operation between 15–31 %, whereby only few examiners can indicate a significantly lower morbidity rate (11). The insufficiency rates of the anastomosis as the most important complication do not differ significantly (laparoscopic. 0–6%, open 10%).

For all procedures, the sometimes rather steep learning curve must be passed before the benefits can be achieved. The learning curve appears to require more than 50 cases for the laparoscopically skilled surgeon to become proficient. Technological innovations allow surgeons to resect colorectal malignancies, but the propriety of performing such an operation has strongly been questioned. At present it is recognized that the extent of the lymphadenectomy is comparable to that with the conventional procedure. In the same way, the safety of wide resection and free distal resection margins correspond between the two methods (2, 6, 7, 16).

Concerns arose regarding the extent of lymph node dissection and reports of implantation of malignant cells at trocar sites, incision sites, and drain sites. The number of lymph nodes retrieved in a resected specimen has been equated with the adequacy of resection.

Furthermore, it is unclear whether the difference in lymph node count is clinically significant because the number of lymph nodes harvested has not been shown to affect survival. The number of nodes found in surgical specimens varies substantially (4). A number of studies have reported that lymphovascular clearance in laparoscopic-assisted colectomy is similar to that of an open operation (8).

Knowledge of port site metastases is the first step in prevention, and the most effective precaution is simply to avoid any injury to the tumor. Recent updates of excellent centers indicate a port site recurrence rate of about 1 % (6, 11, 12). These data are nearly identical to the incidence of recurrences of the laparotomy wound (14). In spite of many studies, so far no generally recognized causal explanation for the trocar site recurrences is available (18).

In a non-randomized prospective study (13) the UltraCision shears were found to be technically easy and fast to use and the results of coagulation and division were reliable. No postoperative bleeding was observed although the central artery and vein were coagulated with the flat position of the blade along the length (1 cm) before final division without tension. UltraCision has been shown to shorten operative time in this series and to eliminate the need for other instruments. The technically easy management and safe procedure may shorten the learning curve.

References

1. Bailey WB. General Considerations. In: Bailey RW, Flowers JL. editors. Complications of laparoscopic surgery. St. Louis: Quality Medical Publishing; 1995. p. 19.
2. Bokey EL, Moore JWF, Keating JP, Zelas P, Chapuis PH, Newland RC. Laparoscopic resection of the colon and rectum for cancer. Br J Surg 1997; 84: 822–25.
3. Boswell WC Odom JW, Rudolph R, Boyd CR. A method for controlling bleeding from abdominal wall puncture site after laparoscopic surgery. Surg Laparosc Endosc 1992; 6: 169–76.
4. Canessa CE, Badia F, Fierro S, Fiol V, Hayek G. Anatomic study of the lymph nodes of the mesorectum. Dis Colon Rectum 2001; 44: 1333–6.
5. Chandler JG, Corson SL, Way LW. Three spectra of laparoscopic entry access injuries. J Am Coll Surg 2001; 192: 478–90.
6. Fleshman JW, Nelson H , Peters WR, Kim HC et al. Clinical outcomes of surgical therapy (COST) study group: Early results of laparoscopic surgery for colorectal cancer: retrospective analysis of 372 patients treated by clinical outcomes of surgical therapy (COST) study group. Dis Colon Rectum 1996; 39: 53–8.
7. Franklin ME Jr, Rosenthal D, Abrego-Medina D, Dorman JP, Glass JL, Norem R, Diaz A. A prospective comparison of open vs. laparoscopic colon surgery for carcinoma: five year results. Dis Colon Rectum 1996; 39 (Suppl): 35–46.
8. Hartley JE, Mehigan BJ, Qureshi AE, Duthie GS, Lee PW, Monson JR. Total mesorectal excision: assessment of the laparoscopic approach. Dis Colon Rectum 2001; 44: 315–21.
9. Herold A, Shekarriz H, Casper L, Schiedeck T. Current status of laparoscopic colorectal surgery national census. Langenbecks Arch Chir (Suppl/Kongressband) 1997; 114: 1185–7.
10. Lacy AM, Garcia-Valdecasas JC, Castells A, Pique JM, Delgado S, Campo E, Bordas JM, Taura P, Grande L, Fuster J, Pacheco JL, Visa J. Short outcome analysis of randomized stud comparing

laparoscopic vs. open colectomy for cancer. Surg Endosc 1995; 9: 1101–5.

11. Lacy AM, Delgado S, Garcia-Valdecasas JC, Castells A, Pique JM, Grande L, Fuster J, Targaroma EM, Pera M, Visa J. 1998 Port site metastasis and recurrence after laparoscopic surgery. A randomized trial. Surg Endosc 1998; 12: 1039–42.

12. Milsom JW, Böhm B, Hammerhofer KA, Fazio V, Steiger E, Elson P. A prospective, randomized trial comparing laparoscopic versus conventional techniques in colorectal cancer surgery: a preliminary report. J Am Coll Surg 1998; 187: 46–54.

13. Msika S, Deroide G, Kianmanesh R, Iannelli A, Hay JM, Fingerhut A, Flamant Y. Harmonic scalpel in laparoscopic colorectal surgery. Dis Colon Rectum 2001; 44: 432–36.

14. Reilly WT, Nelson H, Schroeder G, Wieand HS, Bolton J, O'Connell MJ. Wound recurrence following conventional treatment of colorectal cancer. A rare but perhaps underestimated problem. Dis Colon Rectum 1996; 39: 200–07.

15. Schiedeck TH, Schwandner O, Baca I, Baehrlehner E, Konradt J, Kockerling F, Kuthe A, Buerk C, Herold A, Bruch HP. Laparoscopic surgery for the cure of colorectal cancer: results of a German five-center study. Dis Colon Rectum 2000; 43: 1–8.

16. Stage JG, Schulze S Moller P, Overgaard H, Andersen M, Rebsdorf-Pedersen VB, Nielsen HJ. Prospective randomized study of laparoscopic versus open colonic resection for adenocarcinoma Br J Surg 1997; 84: 391–96.

17. Tittel A, Schumpelick V. Laparoscopic surgery: expectation and reality. Chirurg 2001; 72: 227–35.

18. Zmora O, Weiss EG. 2001 Trocar site recurrence in laparoscopic surgery for colorectal cancer. Myth or real concern? Surg Oncol Clin N Am 2001; 10: 625–638.

13 Laparoscopic Cholecystectomy using the 10 mm UltraCision Blade (DH 010)

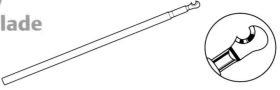

R. Perunović

Laparoscopic cholecystectomy has a unique place in surgery and even medicine at the current time. Not only the fact that merely a few years after its introduction it now represents the "gold standard" for the treatment of gallstone disease, but it has also become a paradigm of the era of minimally invasive approaches, opening the door wide for a whole range of different procedures in every field of operative medicine. In the history of medicine there is no other example of a procedure for which, only a few years after its establishment, the scientific literature offers papers on its history.

 ## Indication and Preoperative Management

The indications for laparoscopic cholecystectomy are identical to those for open cholecystectomy—symptomatic gallbladder calculosis being by far the most frequent. Contraindications present at the beginning of the laparoscopic era (acute cholecystitis, gallbladder empyema, liver cirrhosis, morbid obesity, previous abdominal operations, etc.) have diminished in importance or even vanished with the improvement of operative techniques for laparoscopic cholecystectomy, increasing surgical experience, and global technological advances.

Preoperative management consists of standard laboratory tests, hepatogram (serum bilirubin, alkaline phosphatases, SGOT, SGPT), and abdominal ultrasound (US), all being mandatory. A useful tool for the preoperative visualization of the intra- and extrahepatic biliary tree in the first years was intravenous cholangiocholecystography (IVCC), but this is now being occasionally replaced by magnetic resonance cholangiography (MRC), a more specific and sensitive method. However, availability and price are still limiting factors for the routine use of the latter technique.

In patients with suspected stones in the common bile duct (CBD), (history, laboratory parameters, US), preoperative endoscopic retrograde cholangiopancreatography (ERCP) is performed. ERCP can also be used as a therapeutic tool when needed.

Editor's tip: Using various combinations of clinical history (jaundice, dark urine, cholangitis or pancreatitis), liver function tests, and common bile duct size, one is still unable to get a positive predictive value for the presence of stones in the CBD high enough to justify preoperative CBD imaging with ERCP. The cost of ERCP to the patient (morbidity 5–8% and mortality 0.5%) and to the health system is too great when the PPV is at best around 60–70% with most systems. Accepted indications for preoperative ERCP are jaundice, cholangitis and severe gallstone pancreatitis.

 ## Operation

After orotracheal intubation, a nasogastric tube is placed and patient is positioned in anti-Trendelenburg position (20–30°) combined with left decubitus (10–20°).

The following choice of instruments is recommended:
- 2 × 10 mm ports (camera, UltraCision, Maryland preparation forceps, Ligaclip, scissors, suction/irrigation tube, grasping forceps claw type)
- 2 × 5 mm ports (grasping forceps, scissors, suction/irrigation tube)
- reduction 10/5 mm
- UltraCision 10 mm blade spatula (sharp, blunt)
- 1 × 1 mm Maryland preparation forceps
- 1 × 5 mm scissors
- 2 × 5 mm grasping forceps
- 1 × 10 mm grasping forceps claw type
- 1 × Ligaclip (ER 320 or ER 420)

Editor's Tip: Routine laparoscopic cholecystectomy can be easily accomplished with three 5 mm ports and one 10 mm port for the camera. The development of 5 mm clip appliers, both disposable and reusable has allowed the epigastric port to be down sized to 5 mm.

Establishment of the pneumoperitoneum for laparoscopic procedures may be followed by potentially fatal complications. In order to stratify the risk factors the patients can be divided in 3 categories:

- Group I: Patients with no history of previous intra-abdominal operations.
- Group II: Patients having previous intra-abdominal operations in the lower abdomen.
- Group III: Patients having previous intra-abdominal operations in the upper abdomen and/or major incisions.

For Groups I and II the patient is positioned in an anti-Trendelenburg position combined with left decubitus, the pneumoperitoneum is created in a closed manner.

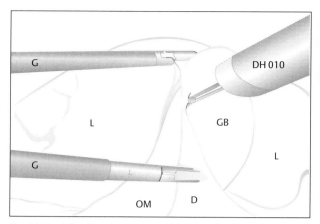 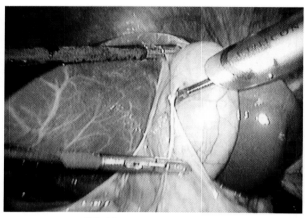

Fig. 13.**1**   Adhesions between gallbladder, duodenum and greater omentum. *GB* gallbladder, *D* duodenum, *OM* greater omentum major, *L* liver, *G* grasper, *DH 010* laparoscopic dissecting hook 10 mm.

For Group I an umbilical incision to the fascia is made and the Veress needle is directed upright towards the right medioclavicular line and the right costal margin crossing. Once adequate intra-abdominal pressure has been achieved, the primary trocar is directed towards the gallbladder, using the same directional landmarks.

For Group II the Veress needle is introduced on the right rectal abdominal muscle at the lateral margin and then directed upright. Once adequate intra-abdominal pressure has been achieved, the primary trocar is introduced in the midline, approximately 2 cm subxiphoidally towards the gallbladder.

For Group III, the standard open technique—Hasson procedure—is used.

> Editor's tip: The open technique of establishing a pneumoperitoneum (Hasson) has been shown to be faster than the blind Veress technique. Most surgeons use the open approach for previously operated and other difficult abdomens, which demonstrates the technique's greater standardization and safety.

In order to maintain stable cardiocirculatory parameters the pneumoperitoneum is initially created with low-level flow of 1 l/min until an intraperitoneal pressure of 12–14 mmHg is achieved.

The primary port is used for introducing the optics (30°) in order to explore the abdominal cavity prior to introduction of secondary ports under direct vision.

Two 10 mm ports are introduced, one through umbilicus and another in the mid-abdominal line, approximately 2 cm subxiphoidally, directed downwards to the right, the tip entering the intra-abdominal cavity laterally just right from the falciform ligament.

Two 5 mm trocars are introduced as lateral as possible at the level of the umbilicus, near to the right anterior axillary line and with a distance of approximately 2 cm between one another.

A modified double two-hand technique is used, the surgeon and assistant being positioned to the patient's left. Using the grasping forceps introduced through the most lateral 5 mm port, the gallbladder fundus is grasped by the assistant. Secured at the junction point of the gallbladder fundus and the liver, the gallbladder is directed to the anterior abdominal wall and cephalad to the right hemidiaphragm, for obtaining optimal visualization and exposure of the porta hepatis and Calot's triangle.

Adhesions to the omentum, duodenum, and transverse colon may need to be freed by use of an UltraCision blade spatula introduced through the subxiphoid port (level 3 or 5). The assistant grasps the gallbladder and directs it to the anterior abdominal wall and cephalad. Adhesions to the omentum and duodenum are to be freed by use of the UltraCision blade spatula (level 3 or 5). (Fig. 13.**1**).

Once the gallbladder is freed from adhesions, the surgeon grasps the infundibulum with a grasper thus enabling an adequate approach to dissection of the elements of Calot's triangle.

Dissection starts with the stripping of serosa from the lateral aspect of Calot's triangle. Dissection is directed downwards, starting from the gallbladder wall and may be done bluntly using a dissector or started by serosal incision using the UltraCision (level 3 or 5) (Fig. 13.**2**).

The same principle is used for freeing elements from the surrounding fibroareolar tissue, cautiously avoiding injury to the posterior cystic branch, occasionally positioned in this region. Successfully completed dissection allows clear vision of the gallbladder infundibulum-cystic duct junction. Further serosal dissection is applied along the medial aspect of Calot's triangle in the same manner, by retracting the grasped infundibulum anterolaterally. This dissection may be complicated by enlarged cystic lymph nodes.

Once the peritoneal coverage is dissected off the cystic triangle, the cystic duct and cystic artery are iden-

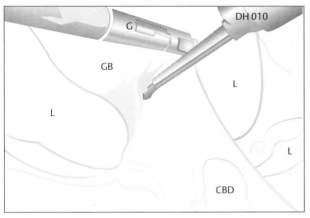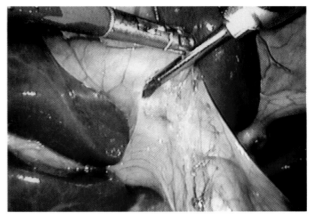

Fig. 13.**2** Serosal incision of Calot's triangle, lateral aspect. *GB* gallbladder, *L* liver, *CBD* common bile duct, *G* grasper, *DH 010* laparoscopic dissecting hook 10 mm.

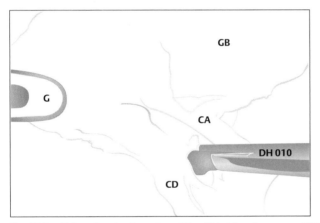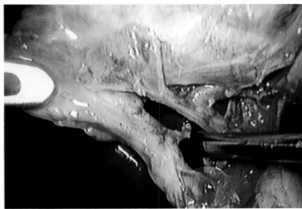

Fig. 13.**3** Calot triangle dissection. *GB* gallbladder, *G* grasper, *DH 010* laparoscopic dissecting hook 10 mm, *CA* cystic artery, *CD* cystic duct.

tified utilizing blunt dissection within the cystic triangle.

> Editor's tip: To reemphasise the author's comments regarding dissection, a safe cholecystectomy requires careful dissection and subsequent skeletonization of structures in the hepatocholecystic triangle. The dissection always starts on the gallbladder and moves down. Thereby, the surgeon is always "above" any biliary anatomical variations. The demonstration of one biliary structure entering the neck of the GB and a free GB edge to liver-bed ensures safety. Identification of T-junctions is potentially misleading.

The principal aim of the dissection of Calot's triangle is to open two "windows", one between the cystic duct and the cystic artery and another between the cystic artery and the gallbladder bed. Use of the UltraCision for freeing the gallbladder out of the distal part of its bed is essential for creating a sufficient and secure

"window" between the cystic artery and the gallbladder bed (level 3).

In order to free the whole circumference of the cystic duct, branches of the cystic artery (Calot's arteries) have to be cut, whenever encountered. The UltraCision blade spatula can be successfully used for completing this procedure (level 3) (Fig. 13.**3**).

After completed dissection and prior to any clipping, a clear identification of the cystic duct and the cystic artery or its branches is mandatory. The cystic duct is not routinely dissected to its junction at the common bile duct.

Once the cystic duct and cystic artery are identified and dissected, intraoperative cholangiography may be performed—but not as a routine procedure. If an operative cholangiogram is obtained through the cystic duct, a single clip is used to occlude the neck of the gallbladder and scissors are used to open the cystic duct on its anteromedial surface. The cystic duct is then "milked" back, away from the junction with the common hepatic duct. Various percutaneously inserted cholangiogram catheters can be used.

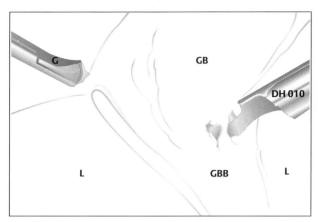

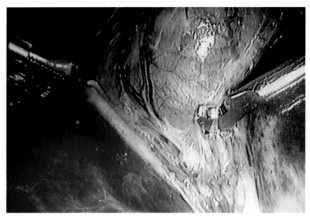

Fig. 13.**4**   Gallbladder dissection from gallbladder bed. *GB* gallbladder, *GBB* gallbladder bed, *G* grasper, *DH 010* laparoscopic dissecting blade 10 mm, *L* liver.

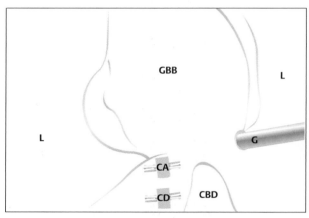

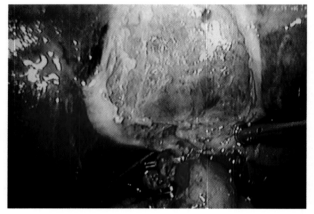

Fig. 13.**5**   Operative field inspection. *GB* gallbladder, *GBB* gallbladder bed, *G* grasper, *L* liver, *CBD* common bile duct, *CA* cystic artery, *CD* cystic duct.

> Editor's tip: The controversy of routine versus selective cholangiography will never be resolved. What is known is that a selective policy can be done with acceptable results. However, even if a selective approach is adopted, the surgeon will still be required to perform cholangiograms when indicated by clinical history, LFTs and CBD size and also when there is unclear anatomy. It would, therefore, seem logical (at least in the training phase) to practice routine intraoperative cholangiography so that when an X-ray is needed it can be done with reproducible quality and interpretation.

Clipping of the cystic artery and cystic duct should be done if the cholangiogram reveals no evidence of injury or choledocholithiasis. Three clips are applied on the cystic artery, two proximally and one distally, while further three clips are applied to the cystic duct, one on the gallbladder side and two in the direction of the common bile duct. Both structures are divided using scissors or the UltraCision (level 5). The cystic artery is always cut first.

The gallbladder is then dissected from its bed using the UltraCision blade spatula (level 3 or 5), first dividing serosa 1–1.5 cm from the liver margin, both medially and laterally, followed by dissection of the gallbladder. This process is facilitated by the vibrating tip of the UltraCision blade, splitting tissue layers within the gallbladder bed (Fig. 13.**4**).

The UltraCision can also be used to control low to moderate venous bleeding from the gallbladder bed, by applying the blunt outer radius of the blade spatula.

Before the fundus of the gallbladder is detached from the liver bed, the operative field should be inspected for hemostasis and secure closure of the cystic duct and cystic artery. Prior to final extraction of the trocars, the operative field is inspected (Fig. 13.**5**).

For removal of the gallbladder through the umbilicus, the surgeon and the camera operator must reverse their positions. For gallbladder removal, the neck is grasped with a crocodile grasper and pulled into the trocar. The trocar and gallbladder are then pulled out together through the umbilical incision. Once the neck of the gallbladder has been withdrawn, the gallbladder can be incised, bile can be aspirated, and stones can be extracted or crushed.

> Editor's tip: With three 5 mm ports, the GB is removed as follows. The most lateral 5 mm port grasps the neck of the GB. This port then intubates the Hasson cannula under vision. The neck of the GB then enters the Hasson cannula as the camera is simultaneously withdrawn a short distance. The 5 mm port and attached GB neck then follows the Hasson cannula out of the umbilicus as the Hasson cannula is withdrawn.

Prior to final extraction of the trocars, the operative field is irrigated with saline solution and inspected. No drain is placed within the abdominal cavity. Fascial stitches are applied only on the umbilical port while the other ports are approximated or closed only with skin stitches.

Summary of the laparoscopic cholecystectomy:
- Gallbladder adhesions are bluntly removed.
- Serosa is stripped in the lateral aspect of Calot's triangle.
- Serosa is stripped in the medial aspect of Calot's triangle.
- Dissection of Calot's triangle and creation of two "windows", one between the cystic duct and the cystic artery and another between the cystic artery and the gallbladder bed.
- Clipping and cutting of the cystic artery and cystic duct after clear identification.
- The cystic artery is cut first.
- Dissection of the gallbladder from the liver bed in the proper plane.
- Extraction of the gallbladder through the umbilical incision.

⚠ Hints and Pitfalls

- The lateral ports should be introduced after the umbilical port. The gallbladder is grasped and retracted to the anterior abdominal wall and cephalad in order to choose the optimal position for insertion of the subxiphoid port, in accordance with the individual anatomic conditions of the patient, thus facilitating operative manipulations.
- The standard use of 30° optics is recommended in order to achieve better visualization of the operative field, especially in dissecting the lateral aspect of Calot's triangle and the gallbladder.
- Cutting of the cystic artery and the cystic duct between clips should be done using scissors or the UltraCision and never with electrocautery which bears the risk of postoperative necrosis of the structures due to the energy dissipation.
- A 30° optic, suction/irrigation "roller" pump, and UltraCision are essential in the management of complicated inflammatory cases for better visualization, more frequent and efficient irrigation and suction, easier and more accurate dissection, diminished injury risk, and shortening of the operative time.
- In cases of gallbladder distention (hydrops, empyema) which reduces its mobility and makes element dissection difficult or impossible, gallbladder punction should be done percutaneously and the content removed.
- In cases of gallstones spillage from the gallbladder into the abdominal cavity, in most cases they can be identified and removed laparoscopically, presenting no reason for immediate conversion.
- In cases of excessive inflammatory changes of the gallbladder wall and/or perforation, use of an endobag is recommended in order to facilitate extraction and avoid contamination of the umbilical incision.
- The standard place for gallbladder extraction is umbilicus since the abdominal wall is thinner there than in other positions, thus being easiest for eventual widening of the incision.
- Meticulous dissection and clear visualization of the elements of Calot's triangle (cystic artery and cystic duct) are of utmost importance for a safe procedure.

🦉 Personal Experience

Starting from January 1993, in an 8-year period, 3854 consecutive patients underwent laparoscopic cholecystectomy in our institution. Preoperative US was routinely used in all patients as well as laboratory analyses including hepatogram (serum bilirubin, alkaline phosphatases, SGOT, SGPT). The vast majority of the patients (98.3%) underwent preoperative intravenous cholangiocholecystography. Asymptomatic, "silent", common bile duct stones were detected in 1.93% of the patients undergoing i.v. cholangiocholecystography. Those patients were referred to various types of interventional endoscopic procedures for CBD clearance preoperatively.

UltraCision was introduced in February 1997, and has been routinely used since then. It has now been employed in round 1528 laparoscopic cholecystectomies—the number is increasing constantly. It was used in 72% of total number of operations in 1997, 84% in 1998, 92% in 1999, and 100% in 2000.

From February to October 1997, a prospective study was carried out on two groups of 100 patients each, with gallbladder disease, homogeneous by sex, age, and degree of gallbladder inflammation.

In one group electrocautery was used for dissection while in the other group we employed UltraCision. The duration of operative procedure, coagulative ability, influence on visualization, and incidence of gallbladder wall lesions were followed and compared.

The average duration of the procedure was 54 and 57 minutes, respectively; no significant difference was observed. Coagulative ability was equal, visibility in four patients (4%) treated with electrocautery was reduced to the extent of needing repeated gas insufflation and desufflation with no statistical significance. The sole statistically significant difference was observed in the frequency of gallbladder wall perforation, being more frequent in the electrocautery group (11 vs. 7, $p < 0.05$). The conclusion of the study was that UltraCision represents a significant technological advance allowing easier, more efficient, and safer techniques.

Based on our experience with over 1500 patients we can conclude that the UltraCision blade spatula offers following advantages:

- Easier and safer dissection in Calot's triangle because of the avoidance of energy dissipation, thus sparing fine biliary and vascular structures from injuries.
- Better visualization since no smoke and char are produced enabling easier, safer, and faster dissection.
- Easier dissection based on vaporized fluid at low temperatures, separating tissue planes, being essential in excessive inflammation thus minimizing the risk of gallbladder wall perforation and injury to superficial vascular and biliary structures of the liver bed.

Discussion

The use of monopolar radio frequency electrical energy in surgery has a history of more than half a century.

Laparoscopic cholecystectomy introduced the era of minimally invasive surgery as a field where both electrocautery and laser found a renewed and indispensable position. Offering no essential efficiency and safety advantages, but being more expensive and less available, the use of the laser has declined substantially in comparison to electrocautery in recent years (16, 20).

The broadening operative spectrum of videoendoscopic surgery has, in general, shown certain limitations of electrocautery. These include an increasing number and type of electric injuries, accounting for a significant number of procedural complications varying in extent from minor to life-threatening (23). In practice, three mechanisms can be observed: insulation failure in the active electrode, direct coupling, and capacitive coupling (9, 10, 13, 16, 18, 21, 22, 23, 24). Smoke and char production were related to certain problems already existing in open surgery, ranging from reduced visibility to systemic effects, are even more exaggerated in minimally invasive surgery (12, 14, 19, 25).

The introduction of UltraCision represents a major advance through being close to the ideal form of energy for use in laparoscopic surgery. The numerous advantages can be divided into at least three categories:

- Mere technical improvements facilitating operative work like absence of smoke, cutting like a knife, coagulating like monopolar electrosurgery, absence of charring, absence of sticking to tissue, facility of self-cleaning, usable as a dissector
- Advantages regarding patient safety such as minimal tissue injury, the patient being out of the circuit
- Advantages regarding surgeon and industry such as minimum training needed for competent use, safety for the surgeon, inexpensive method, minimal setup needed, etc. (1, 2, 3, 7, 11, 15)

The mentioned advantages have been proven in laparoscopic cholecystectomy, in accordance with the frequency and importance of the procedure (4, 5, 6, 8, 17). Two essential improvements resulted from the routine use of UltraCision in a number of studies in recent years. Firstly, precise dissection in the immediate vicinity of vascular and biliary structures is possible to a greater extent than ever before using any previously known form of energy. Secondly, in cases with excessive inflammatory changes, use of the UltraCision enables easier, faster, and safer dissection.

References

1. Amaral JF. Ultrasonic dissection. End Surg 1993; 2: 181–5.
2. Amaral JF. Laparoscopic application of an ultrasonically activated scalpel. Gastrointest Endosc Clin North Am 1993; 3: 381–92.
3. Amaral JF. Ultrasonic energy in laparoscopy surgery. Book extract: Surgical Technology International III, 155–61.
4. Amaral JF. The experimental development of an ultrasonically activated scalpel for laparoscopic use. Surgical Laparoscopy & Endoscopy 1994; 4: 92–9.
5. Amaral JF. Laparoscopic cholecystectomy in 200 consecutive patients using an ultrasonically activated scalpel. Surgical Laparoscopy & Endoscopy 1995; 5: 255–62.
6. Amaral JF. Prospective randomized trial of electrosurgery vs. ultrasonically activated scalpel for laparoscopic cholecystectomy. Paris: World Hepatobiliary Society, 1993.
7. Amaral JF, Chrostek C. Depth of thermal injury: Ultrasonically activated scalpel vs. electrosurgery. Surg Endosc 1995; 9: 226.
8. Amaral JF, Chrostek CA. Experimental comparison of the ultrasonically-activated scalpel to electrosurgery and laser surgery for laparoscopic use. Min Invas Ther & Allied Technol 1997; 6: 324–31.
9. Ata AH, Bellemore TJ, Meisel JA, Arambulo SM. Distal thermal injury from monopolar electrosurgery. Surg Laparosc Endosc 1993; 3: 323–7.
10. Berry SM, Ose KJ, Bell RH, Fink AS. Thermal injury of the posterior duodenum during laparoscopic cholecystectomy. Surg Endosc 1994; 8: 197–200.
11. Fowler DL. Use of the ultrasonically activated scalpel and shears in endoscopic surgery. Third International Congress on New Technology and Advanced Techniques in Surgery, Luxemburg, 1995.
12. Giordano BP. Don't be a victim of surgical smoke. AORN J 1996; 63: 520–2.
13. Grosskinsky CM, Ryder RM, Pendergrass HM, Hulka JF. Laparoscopic capacitance: A mystery measured experiments in pigs with confirmation in the engineering laboratory. Am J Obstet Gynecol 1993; 169: 1632–5.
14. Lanfranchi JA. Smoke plume evacuation in the OR. AORN J 1997; 65: 627–33.

15. Markovicz S, Chrostek C, Amaral JF. Surgical laparoscopic energy and lateral thermal damage. Society for Minimally Invasive Therapy, SMIT, Berlin, 1994.
16. McAnena OJ, Wilson PD. Diathermy in laparoscopic surgery. Br J Surg 1993; 80: 1094–5.
17. Moreno F, Fernandez-Cebrian V, Capela J, Fernandez I, Perez de Oteyza J, Martinez Molina E, et al. Laparoscopic cholecystectomy: Initial experience and results in 400 patients. Minimally Invasive Surgery and New Technology. St. Louis: Quality Medical Publishing, Inc.; 1994. p. 123–30.
18. Nduka CC, Super PA, Monson JRT, Darzi AW. Cause and prevention of electrosurgical injuries in laparoscopy. J Am Coll Surg 1994; 179: 161–70.
19. Ott D. Smoke production and smoke reduction in endoscopic surgery: Preliminary report. End Surg 1993; 1: 230–2.
20. Schurr MO, Wehrmann M, Kunert W, Melzer A, Lirici MM, Buess G. Histologic effects of different technologies for dissection in endoscopic surgery: Nd:YAG laser, high frequency and water-jet. End Surg 1994; 2: 195–201.
21. Tucker RD, Voyles CR, Silvis SE. Capacitive coupled stray currents during laparoscopic and endoscopic electrosurgical procedures. Biomed Instrum Technol 1993; 26: 303–11.
22. Tucker RD, Voyles CR. Laparoscopic electrosurgical complications and their prevention. AORN J 1995; 62: 51–71.
23. Tucker RD, Laparoscopic electrosurgical injuries: Survey results and their implications. Surg Laparosc Endosc 1995; 5: 311–7.
24. Willson PD, Walt van der JD, Moxon D, Rogers J. Port site electrosurgical (diathermy) burns during surgical laparoscopy. Surg Endosc 1997; 11: 653–4.
25. Wu JS, Luttmann DR, Meininger TA, Soper NJ. Production and systemic absorption of toxic byproducts of tissue combustion during laparoscopic surgery. Surg Endosc 1997; 11: 1075–9.

14 Laparoscopic Cholecystectomy using the 5 mm UltraCision Curved Shears (LCSC 5)

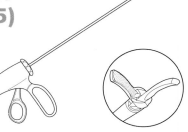

E. C. Tsimoyiannis

Laparoscopic cholecystectomy (LC) has rapidly become the operation of choice for symptomatic cholelithiasis because no disadvantages, other than the learning curve for this procedure, have been consistently reported in the literature. To achieve adequate hemostasis during LC, electrosurgical units as well as lasers are usually used. But these devices generate considerable smoke during their use, making them less than optimal (5). The ideal energy form for LC should be characterized by minimal tissue injury, little or no smoke to obscure the visual field, cutting ability equal to or superior to that of a conventional scalpel, coagulating ability equal to or greater than that of monopolar electrosurgery, lack of danger to the patient such as from stray energy, no need for special preparation of the patient (grounding pad) or surgeon (glasses), and no need for special training (2).

UltraCision shears or scalpels have been used in experimental porcine cholecystectomy (3), in human LC (2, 15), in laparoscopic Nissen procedures (14), in laparoscopic splenectomy (13), as well as in several open surgery procedures (16).

Indications and Preoperative Management

The indication for LC includes, nowadays, every patient with acute or chronic cholecystitis with or without choledocholithiasis. Contraindications are severe cardiac and lung problems, cancer of the biliary tract, and inability to recognize the anatomy of the extrahepatic biliary tree. The use of UltraCision is indicated in every LC.

The general preoperative assessment and complete anesthesiological evaluation are not different from that done for patients who have to face a surgical procedure under general anesthesia. In studies aiming to reveal a concomitant biliary pathology, ultrasonography of the intrahepatic and extrahepatic biliary tract and liver function tests are included for all patients. Elevated liver function tests and an increased diameter of the common bile duct are indications for preoperative ERCP and possibly for endoscopic sphincterotomy. When ERCP is not available or contraindicated, MRCP is an excellent alternative or intraoperative cholangiography must be scheduled in these cases.

Operation

The patient under general anesthesia can be positioned supine with his legs spread or straight. We usually prefer a modified 4-trocar technique (two 10 mm and two 5 mm ports) as described by Reddick and Olsen (12). In young women and children without severe cholecystitis, we prefer a 10 mm (for camera), a 5 mm (working), while the other two are 2 mm ports.

In all cases we use:
- 2 × 5 mm or 2 mm grasping instruments
- UltraCision shears 5 mm
- 1 × endoscopic hemoclips instrument 10 mm or 5 mm
- 10 mm telescope of 0° or 30°

Having prepared and draped the abdomen, the pneumoperitoneum is instituted. For the closed technique, the Veress needle is inserted at 90° to the abdominal wall and is held upright by the surgeon and assistant. Usually this will be at the lower border of the umbilicus through a small incision, but previous surgery may dictate another insertion point. A 10 ml syringe filled with saline is attached to the needle, followed by aspiration, to determine whether proper entry has been achieved into the abdominal cavity. Tubing from the CO_2 insufflator is attached, and insufflation commences, initially at no more than 1.5 l/min. This ensures that if, for example, the needle is in a vessel, the anesthesiologist will have the opportunity to detect a problem before fatal air embolus occurs. If a good flow rate is maintained, we try to achieve an intra-abdominal pressure of 12–13 mmHg. Then the needle is removed, the incision is enlarged and a 10 mm port is introduced. Some surgeons routinely prefer the open Hasson trocar technique, especially if the patient has an umbilical hernia that will require repair, a previous abdominal operation, or in cases where Veress needle insertion has failed. In our department we prefer the Hasson trocar technique in all cases, believing that this technique is safer than the Veress technique for the avoidance intra-abdominal visceral injury.

The pre-warmed laparoscope 0° or 30° is introduced, the patient is placed in the reverse Trendelenburg position with the right side tilted up. A vertical incision is made in the midline below the xiphisternum, and a

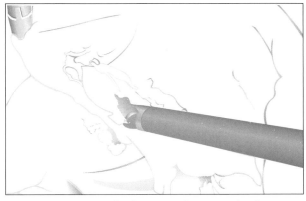

Fig. 14.**1** Dissection of Calot's triangle using only UltraCision.

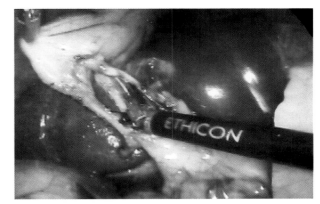

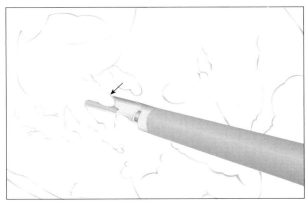

Fig. 14.**2** The cutting of the cystic artery using UltraCision without clips. The *arrow* shows the arterial stump.

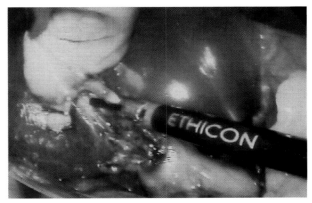

10 mm or 5 mm trocar is introduced under direct vision through the midline but just to the right of the falciform fat. The third trocar, a 5 mm or 2 mm instrument, is introduced under direct vision, generally, in the midclavicular line below the right costal margin, and it is this that will provide medial and lateral retraction of Hartmann's pouch. The fourth trocar, a 5 mm or 2 mm instrument, is introduced in the anterior axillary line above the anterior superior iliac spine. Through this trocar, a grasping forceps is used to hold the fundus of the gallbladder up and over the liver. Immediately before the performance of the incisions of all trocars, 15 ml of a bupivacaine solution are infiltrated in the trocar wound areas. There may be adhesions to the gallbladder, which should be teased down toward (never up away from) the common bile duct to avoid avulsing the cystic duct from the common bile duct. Attention should be turned to the area of Hartmann's pouch and Calot's triangle. Careful maneuvers, with limited or no electrosurgery, should free up the attachments, lateral and medial to the gallbladder.

To avoid injuries, smoke, and to have better hemostasis, it is preferable that all steps of the dissection and shearing be performed with the UltraCision shears (Fig. 14.**1**). The cystic artery is divided without clips (Fig. 14.**2**), while the cystic duct is divided between clips (Fig. 14.**3**). The dissection of the bed of the gallbladder is completely performed with the UltraCision shears.

Editor's Tip: Arcing injuries due to insulation failure of a diathermy hook as well as capacitive and direct coupling injuries are specific to monopolar diathermy and therefore an inherent risk of the instrument. The safest approach is to avoid all energy sources when dissecting in the hepatocholecystic triangle. If coagulation energy is needed, then ultrasonic technology may represent a more controllable risk than diathermy with well-defined limited collateral injury and no chance of arcing injuries.

After removal of the gallbladder through the umbilical incision, the umbilical trocar is reinserted, a final review of the trocar insertion sites and cholecystectomized area is performed. Then, with the patient in a 30° Trendelenburg position, normal saline at 37 °C is infused under the right hemidiaphragm until the liver is covered. The suction instrument is placed above the liver, and the fluid is suctioned after the pneumoperitoneum has been deflated (17). A solution of bupivacaine (1.5 mg/kg B.W.) is infused under the right

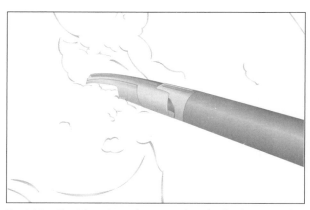
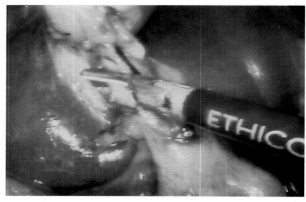

Fig. 14.**3**   The UltraCision shears used to divide the cystic duct between clips. No scissors are needed.

hemidiaphragm through the suction instrument, after the end of the fluid suction (18). In cases where oozing or leakage of bile is likely, a subhepatic closed drainage is left for 24 hours. In these patients after post-deflation fluid suction, no subdiaphragmatic bupivacaine infusion is required (18). The subdiaphragmatic infusion of normal saline and bupivacaine significantly reduces the postoperative abdominal and shoulder pain after LC (17, 18).

⚠ Hints and Pitfalls

- LC is the treatment of choice for emergency or elective symptomatic cholelithiasis, with reduced contraindications in increased experience.
- A great deal of attention has been paid to the different techniques of removing the gallbladder from the liver bed. It is likely that the skill of the surgeon and familiarity with the chosen method is more important than the inherent characteristics of any of the modalities.
- Monopolar electrosurgery, bipolar electrosurgery, free beam laser, contact laser, hydrodissection, CUSA, and harmonic scalpel are the energy sources used in LC. Each has its advantages and disadvantages.
  UltraCision has the ability to dissect without smoke and blood, less tissue injury, less bile leakage. The use of only one instrument in all steps of the procedure leads to a shorter operative time, while the complete replacement of scissors and dissectors, decreases the cost. We believe that UltraCision is the ideal energy form for LC.
- The use of the 5 mm UltraCision shears is more ergonomic than the 10 mm. The UltraCision shears are preferable to the UltraCision blade, because they achieve easier dissection, better hemostasis, and safer coaptation and sealing of the accessory bile ducts, preventing postoperative bile leaks.

 ## Personal Experience

During the last three years we have used UltraCision in more than 1000 LCs. During the initial phase we used the 10 mm UltraCision shears and the 5 mm UltraCision blade. During the last two years we have come to prefer the 5 mm shears, because they are more ergonomic, while dissection and shearing abilities are about same as those of the 10 mm shears. We believe that the UltraCision shears are better than the blade in dissection, hemostasis, and sealing of the assessor bile ducts.

In a prospective randomized study performed in our department (15) comparing UltraCision with monopolar electrosurgery, we have found that:

1. UltraCision is able to complete all steps of every LC, emergency or elective.
2. The median operating time is shorter in UltraCision than in monopolar cautery group (Table 14.**1**).
3. The mean postoperative hospital stay and the mean blood loss are significantly lower in the UltraCision group (Table 14.**1**).
4. In the monopolar cautery group, the bile leakage from the bed of the gallbladder is 3%, while in the UltraCision group it is 0%.
5. The histological findings of the cystic artery and the narrow cystic ducts divided by UltraCision are shown in Figs. 14.**4** and 14.**5** and illustrate the superiority of UltraCision versus monopolar electrocautery.
6. In patients bearing a pacemaker, there was no dysfunction from the use of UltraCision.

Our three-year experience shows that UltraCision can safely and completely replace monopolar or bipolar electrosurgery in all laparoscopic cholecystectomies.

Discussion

Previous studies on LC in animals (3) and in humans (2) have demonstrated no differences in operative time, postoperative hematological values, or hospital stay between the use of electrosurgery, laser surgery, or the ultrasonically activated scalpel. In our department (15), we found shorter operative times and hospital stay and less blood loss in patients operated on by UltraCision than in those operated on by electrosurgery. We believe that this difference from the previous studies is due to the use, in our study, of shears and not a scalpel as was previously used (2, 3). Before beginning the present study, we observed in our operating theater, during the learning period of UltraCision and the ultrasonically activated scalpel, a superiority of the shears versus scalpel in coagulation and operative time. This superiority is due to the clamping of the coagulated and cut tissue (2) and to the use of shears for all steps of the procedure so that no conventional dissectors or scissors are needed, whereby the cystic artery can be divided without clips. The results of our (15) and previous (14) studies demonstrate the safety of small vessel division using UltraCision, without clips.

Bile leakage, defined as a clinically significant biliary fistula, fluid collection, or peritonitis, is one of the complications that may follow LC. Most attention to bile leakage after LC has focused on injury to the bile ducts, but bile leakage without bile duct injury was found in 1% to 3% of the cases (1, 4, 7, 8, 11, 15). It has been suggested that the use of electrosurgery to mobilize the gallbladder out of its bed causes necrosis of ducts lying just deep to the gallbladder (1). Thus, when injury to a major bile duct is excluded and the cystic duct stump is well closed, a leak from the accessory hepatic duct of Luschka or from the gallbladder bed constitutes the next step of bile leak investigation (1, 10).

In our study (15) the absence of bile leak in the UltraCision group, as well as the histological findings of the small diameter cystic ducts cut by UltraCision (Figs. 14.4, 14.5), suggest that the UltraCision shears could safely obstruct the narrow accessory ducts. It is well known that coagulation with UltraCision relies on coaptation of the bleeding site. Pressure and coaptation of the vessel walls seals them together during activation (2). This coaptation was observed in the studied bile ducts (Fig. 14.5). By contrast, the vessels are usually not coapted significantly with electrosurgery because of the concomitant reduction in current density as the surface area of contact increases and because of the need for establishing arcs for fulguration (9).

Table 14.**1** Demographic data and operative variables (Mean ± SD)

	Group A	Group B
Age (y)	55±6	52±9
Weight (kg)	61±5	62±6
Height (cm)	163±8	162±6
Mean operative time (min)	45±7	37±9*
Mean postoperative hospital stay (days)	1.9±0.8	1.6±0.7*
Bile spill (no. of patients)	15	9
Mean blood loss (ml)	14±9	2±1.8*

* Statistically significant difference vs. Group A (t-test)

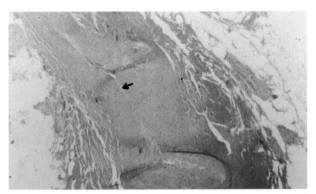

Fig. 14.**4** Histological section of a cystic artery. The lumen of the artery is closed (*arrow*) because the coapted vessel walls were well sealed during activation of UltraCision (hematoxylin and eosin stain, ×200).

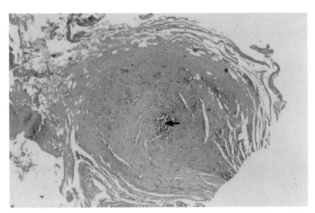

Fig. 14.**5** Histological section of a narrow cystic duct. The lumen of the cystic duct is closed (*arrow*) because the coapted walls of the duct were well sealed during activation of UltraCision (hematoxylin and eosin stain, ×100).

Editor's tip: While described as a minor bile leak, these injuries can lead to complicated and prolonged hospitalization and therefore are not minor in a clinical context. It has been suggested that some of these leaks are due to diathermy heat injury resulting in biliary peritonitis on day 3–5 after surgery when the burn eschar sloughs off. This suggestion fits in with the clinical time course for these patients. The UltraCision shears and scalpel may minimize this complication due to a more limited collateral thermal injury. A randomized prospective trial to test such a hypothesis on a clinical problem

> with a 1–2% incidence will need to be very large to be authoritative. If a properly sized trial demonstrated a clear benefit of the UltraCision shears, it may justify the added expense of using these on-off instruments routinely.

Less tissue injury when using UltraCision in comparison with electrosurgery or laser surgery is well documented in skin incisions (6) and in procedures involving the liver and stomach (2). Its ability to dissect with better visualization (no smoke, no blood) and less tissue injury minimizes the necrosis of ducts lying just deep to the gallbladder (1). This fact, combined with the safe obstruction of the small accessory bile ducts (15), could reduce bile leakage in the broad application of this technique to LC. The complete coaptation of the narrow cystic ducts cut by UltraCision (15) did not lead us to divide cystic ducts without clips. We believe that putting clips in the cystic duct stump is an easy and safe way to prevent bile leaks.

The elimination of electrosurgery from LC not only obviates the need for grounding and the risks of injury from grounding pad failures but also greatly reduces the risk of inadvertent injury to the common bile duct and the adjacent organs during the procedure (2). In addition, in replacing electrosurgery, UltraCision could also replace scissors and dissectors and thus act as a strong blunt dissector, reducing both cost and operative time.

We can conclude that UltraCision is a safe and effective energy form for cutting and coagulating. Its advantages include no smoke, a clear visual field, no need for grounding, lower blood loss, lower incidence of bile leakage, shorter operative time, shorter hospital stay, and complete replacement of scissors and dissectors, thus decreasing the costs.

References

1. Albasini JLA, Aledo VS, Dexter SPL, Morton J, Martin IG, McMahon MJ. Bile leakage following laparoscopic cholecystectomy. Surg Endosc 1995; 9: 127–48. Corbitt J. Laparoscopic cholecystectomy: Laser versus electrosurgery. Surg Laparosc Endosc 1991; 1: 85–8.
2. Amaral JF. Laparoscopic cholecystectomy in 200 consecutive patients using an ultrasonically activated scalpel. Surg Laprosc Endosc 1995; 5: 255–62.
3. Amaral JF. The experimental development of an ultrasonically activated scalpel for laparoscopic use. Surg Laparosc Endosc 1994; 4: 92–9.
4. Brooks DC, Becker JM, Connors PI, Carr-loke DL: Management of bile leaks following laparoscopic cholecystectomy. Surg Endosc 1993; 7: 292–5.
5. Corbitt J. Laparoscopic cholecystectomy: Laser versus electrosurgery. Surg Laparosc Endosc 1991; 1: 85.
6. Hambley R, Hebda PA, Abell E, Cohen B, Jegasothy BV. Wound healing of skin incisions produced by ultrasonically vibrating knife, scalpel, electrosurgery, and carbon dioxide laser. J Dermatol Surg Oncol 1988; 14: 121–37.
7. Hawasli A. To drain or not to drain in laparoscopic cholecystectomy: Rationale and technique. Surg Laparosc Endosc 1992; 2: 128–30.
8. Moosa AR, Easter DW, Van Sonnenberg E, Casola G, D'Agostino H. Laparoscopic injuries to the bile duct. Ann Surg 1992; 215: 203–8.
9. Pearce JA. Cutting and coagulating processes. In: Pearce JA. editor. Electrosurgery. New York: Wiley; 1981. pp. 621–28.
10. Peters JH, Olliva D, Nichols KE et al. Diagnosis and management of bile leaks following laparoscopic cholecystectomy. Surg Laparosc Endosc 1994; 4: 163–70.
11. Quinn SF, Sangster W, Standdage B, Schuman E, Gross G. Biliary complications related to laparoscopic cholecystectomies. Radiologic diagnosis and management. Surg Laparosc Endosc 1992; 2: 279–86.
12. Reddick EJ, Olsen DO. Laparoscopic laser cholecystectomy. Surg Endosc 1989; 3: 131–4.
13. Rothenberg SS. Laparoscopic splenectomy using the harmonic scalpel. J Laparoendosc Surg 1996; 6(suppl. 1): 61–3.
14. Swanstrom LL, Pennings JL. Laparoscopic control of short gastric vessels. J Am Coll Surg 1995; 181: 347–51.
15. Tsimoyiannis EC, Jabarin M, Glantzounis G. Lekkas ET, Siakas P, Stefanaki-Nikou S. Laparoscopic cholecystectomy using ultrasonically activated coagulating shears. Surg Laparosc Endosc 1998; 8: 421–4.
16. Tsimoyiannis EC, Jabarin M, Tsimoyiannis JC, Betzios J, Tsilikatis C, Glantzounis G: Ultrasonically activated shears in extended lymphadenectomy for gastric cancer. International Surgical Week, ISW99, Vienna, Austria, 1999.
17. Tsimoyiannis EC, Siakas P, Tassis A, Lekkas ET, Tzourou H, Kambili M. Intraperitoneal normal saline infusion for postoperative pain after laparoscopic cholecystectomy. World J Surg 1998; 22: 824–8.
18. Tsimoyiannis EC, Glantzounis G, Lekkas ET, Siakas P, Jabarin M, Tzourou H. Intraperitoneal normal saline and bupivacaine infusion for reduction of postoperative pain after laparoscopic cholecystectomy. Surg Laparosc Endosc 1998; 8: 416–20.

15 Hepatic Resection with the UltraCision 10 mm Shears with Rotating Blade for Open Surgery (CS 150 Pistol Grip or CS 6S Needle-Holder Grip) and the UltraCision Blade (DH 010)

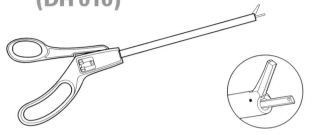 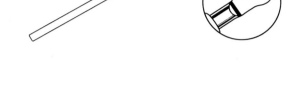

D. C. Broering, E.-G. Achilles, X. Rogiers

In the last 20 years, hepatic resections have advanced from a high-risk to a well-defined procedure with a calculable mortality. Modern, state-of-the-art liver surgery requires a profound knowledge of the anatomy of the liver. Here, an optimal exposure, control of the vascular inflow and outflow, as well as a safe parenchymal dissection technique are crucial.

Indication and Preoperative Management

Indications for anatomical or non-anatomical liver resections are benign or malignant primary or secondary liver tumors. Occasionally, living-related donors or liver cadaveric donors are enrolled in our transplantation program for procurement of the left lateral graft. The extent of preoperative evaluation is dependent on the indication for resection.

Operation

Procurement of the left lateral liver segment for living-related liver transplantation and in situ split technique

This operation is essentially a liver resection without any kind of vascular exclusion. Therefore, it illustrates the qualities of a typical resection technique.

The abdomen is opened through a transverse, upper abdominal incision with median extension to the xyphoid process. After opening, a thorough exploration of the abdominal cavity and the vascular anatomy of the liver are performed. An abdominal pad is placed behind the segments II and III. Now the left triangular ligament can be transected. The left hepatic lobe is lifted with a retractor and the lesser omentum is dissected using the UltraCision shears.

> Editor's tip: To avoid injuries to the caudate lobe when the lesser omentum is dissected, the inactive blade is turned towards the caudate lobe.

The anterior peritoneal sheath of the hepatoduodenal ligament is opened. The level of dissection is defined by the lower margin of segment IV and the left hepatic artery. The left hepatic artery is prepared until its course to the left liver can safely be identified and is marked with a vessel loop. In the following step, the parenchymal bridge between segments IV and III is dissected with the UltraCision shears. Occasionally, additional sutures may be necessary. Thereafter, the ligamentum teres hepatis is separated from peritoneal adhesions towards the quadrate lobe. The peritoneal sheath is opened on the right side of the umbilical recess. The delicate portal branches towards segment IV are prepared and suture-ligated with 50 sutures.

> Editor's tip: The vascular dissection in the hepatoduodenal ligament is facilitated with the new 5 mm curved shears turning the flat inactive blade towards the vessels.

The main branch of the left portal vein as well as the recess of Rex and the portal branches towards segment IV are exposed using UltraCision or an Overholt clamp. The middle hepatic artery should be spared if possible. Additional dissection of portal branches supplying segment IV is in the technique described earlier. A tape is slung around the left portal vein. After additional preparation, exposition of the main branch of the left portal vein is fulfilled.

The next vessel to be isolated is the left hepatic vein. After marking the liver capsule along the sulcus arantii the vein is prepared cautiously ventrocranially and dorsocaudally using an Overholt clamp. After control of the left hepatic vein is accomplished, dissection of the liver parenchyma can be started. The liver capsule is marked with electrocautery or ultrasound dissector.

Editor's tip: The sharp side of the UltraCision shears is excellent for scoring in all form of tissues.

The plane of transection is defined by the falciform ligament. Since there are only few vessels in this layer between segments II and IV, bleeding is limited.

Editor's tip: A large tributary of the left hepatic vein sometimes runs across the falciform ligament and can, when unrecognised, cause severe bleeding.

The dissection of the liver parenchyma is performed in small steps using the UltraCision shears. With this technique vessels are easily identified and can safely be occluded. Suture-ligation is necessary if the diameter exceeds 2 mm. The parenchyma is dissected down to the hilar plate. The hilar plate, containing the left main bile duct, is controlled with a right-angled clamp. Transection of the hilar plate is performed with a scalpel or vascular scissors. Any kind of electrocautery in this region has to be avoided. On the right side, suture-ligation of the stump of the left bile duct is performed using absorbable suture material.

Now the left end of the vessel loop, slung around the left hepatic vein, is passed below the left lateral lobe and anterior to the left portal vein and hepatic artery. After this maneuver, this vessel loop serves as a guide to maintain the right direction for transection of the liver between the left and middle hepatic veins (2). At this point a safe dissection of the remaining parenchyma is performed with the UltraCision shears. Again, small vein branches are isolated and clipped. Once the last part of the parenchyma is cut, the vessel loop comes free and division of the liver is accomplished. Throughout the entire preparation, the right part of the hepatoduodenal ligament has remained untouched.

Now the donor has two livers whose perfusion can be appreciated before harvesting. The left hepatic artery is clamped and cut. The left portal vein is cut immediately at the portal vein bifurcation. Once the left hepatic vein is clamped and transected, the left lateral graft is transferred to the back-table and flushed with preservation solution. The vascular stumps of the right liver are sutured. For safety reasons the venous stump is sutured twice. Arteries are suture-ligated. Complete biliostasis and hemostasis is crucial. Using the technique described above there is no need for compressing mattress sutures.

Immediately after explantation, perfusion of the graft with preservation solution via the artery, the portal vein, and the bile duct is started. The graft is weighed and stored on ice until implantation.

The described procurement technique has been proven in our department to be safe, reproducible, and easy to learn. In case of a cadaveric donor, the right liver is procured using the standard technique.

The living liver donor should stay on the ICU for 24 hours postoperatively. On average discharge from the hospital is possible after five days.

 ## Hints and Pitfalls

- To achieve complete hemostasis during parenchymal dissection, the control of the inflow vessels can be performed as a nonselective vascular exclusion such as the Pringle maneuver or extra- or intrahepatic selective preparation and clamping of the left or right pedicle (selective Pringle).
- The outflow is controlled by preparation of the hepatocaval ligament and selective clamping of the right, middle, or left hepatic vein.
- Depending on the extent of hepatic resection and expected blood loss as well as the quality of the parenchyma (normal versus cirrhotic liver), a temporary total vascular isolation (clamping of the infrahepatic and suprahepatic vena cava and the hepatoduodenal ligament) may be necessary.
- Usually a total clamping of the hepatoduodenal ligament (Pringle) or selective clamping of the pedicle (selective Pringle) in combination with a selective clamping of the outflow can be performed in non-cirrhotic livers as intermittent occlusions for 15 to 20 minutes followed by 5 to 10 minutes of perfusion.
- Extreme care must be taken in cirrhotic or fatty livers where vascular exclusion techniques may enhance the risk of postoperative liver failure.
- In addition an optimized central venous pressure (between 0–4 cm H_2O) reduces blood loss during dissection.

 ## Personal Experience

Since we began using the UltraCision instrument in 1997 in our living-related liver transplantation program, there were no cases of bile fistula, bleeding, or any other major complication in the 26 patients treated (unpublished results). Trupka et al. reported a series of 15 patients with successful liver resections through an open (13 patients) or laparoscopic (two patients) approach with UltraCision (20).

Most of the following authors have published data in the past two decades that recently developed methods for parenchymal dissection render in common a significant reduction in blood loss. However, differences exist mainly in terms of the resection time.

The first results of 33 liver resections performed with the CUSA published in 1984 (7) showed complications in only 18% of cases. Others reported in series of 34 patients and 70 patients, respectively, the advantage of a reduced intraoperative blood loss in comparison to the classic finger fracture technique (3, 5). This advantage and others (lower postoperative blood loss, reduced postoperative length of stay) were also reported by Hanna et al. (6) and Rees et al. (19).

Comparing the average blood loss and the time of operation in a series of patients undergoing hepatic resections, Izumi et al. (8) could not find a difference between the water-jet dissector and the CUSA. Others (17, 18) reported in two prospective studies on 116 and 60 patients, respectively, undergoing liver resection a significantly faster resection time concomitant with a lower blood loss using the water-jet dissector in comparison to the CUSA and the blunt dissection technique. Baer et al. (1) demonstrated a significant reduction of blood loss comparing the water-jet dissector and the finger fracture technique.

In a series (three-year period) of 232 patients undergoing liver resections for benign and malignant tumors in non-cirrhotic livers, we found a mortality rate of 0% (perioperative mortality until hospital discharge). In 83 patients with cirrhotic livers undergoing resections of malignant tumors we found a mortality rate of 2.4%. Other authors published similar data: in 1974 Lin (12) 3.8%, finger fracture technique, 104 patients; in 1996 Rees et al. (19) 0.7%, CUSA, 150 patients; and in 1998 Elias et al. (4) 2%, 147 patients.

Up to now the definite place for minimal invasive surgery on the liver, especially with the use of the UltraCision shears, remains to be further investigated. Besides this, there are first reports on series of laparoscopic partial hepatectomies using the UltraCision shears alone (20) or in conjunction with other instruments (10). Others (9, 13) reported the successful treatment of solid liver tumors or parasitic and dysontogenetic cysts using electrosurgical instruments or an ultrasonic surgical system from Olympus, respectively. All in all, there is still a need for larger prospective studies to document the place in liver surgery of UltraCision shears with its ability to safely occlude small vessels and bile ducts in conjunction with the diminished trauma through a laparoscopic approach.

According to our experience the UltraCision shears provide a reliable and safe transection instrument in liver surgery especially for parenchymal dissection. For this reason we use the UltraCision shears in our living-related liver transplantation program. Although further randomized studies are necessary, we noticed a reduced blood loss in liver resections for benign and malignant tumors as compared to classic techniques using clamps or finger fracture. The definitive place in comparison to the CUSA and other recently developed instruments remains to be demonstrated.

Discussion

The major complications of liver surgery are hemorrhage and the development of biliary fistula as well as pleural effusion, wound infections, and fatal liver insufficiency.

In 1896 Kousnetzoff and Pensky (11) described a coagulation of the resection margin with hot iron, elastic tourniquet, and suturing using blunt needles. Pringle described his occlusion of the hepatoduodenal ligament in 1908 (16). Later Ogilvie published blunt dissection using a finger fracture technique (14). Lin et

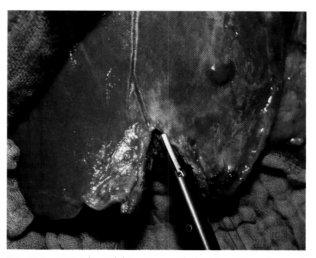

Fig. 15.**1**   Parenchymal dissection with the UltraCision shears of the left lateral lobe (segments II and III) in a patient with liver metastases of a colorectal carcinoma.

al. (12) introduced the resection clamp method in 1974 rendering the advantage of shorter resection times in combination with a lower blood loss as compared to the classic finger fracture technique. In the following three decades several transection techniques were established, to a certain extent, on the basis of totally different physical principles.

Hodgson and DelGuercio (7) published a series of hepatic resections using an ultrasonic dissection technique (CUSA, Valley Lab). A longitudinal oscillating titanium tip separates the parenchyma by imploding and fragmenting the hepatocytes on contact while, due to their high collagen content, sparing bile ducts and blood vessels. These structures could thereafter be selectively ligated and separated. This technique could reduce the usual blood loss from about 3000 ml to about 1000 ml and provided a lower risk of accidental damage to surrounding main structures due to a limited bleeding of the cut surface.

Papachristou and Barters (15) developed the water-jet dissector that is closely related to the CUSA in its functional result although operating according to a totally different physical principle. After creating a corridor through removal of hepatocytes without major blood loss, the skeletonized blood vessels and bile ducts can be selectively ligated or clipped.

Besides methods to achieve hemostasis during parenchymal dissection such as compressing mattress sutures ("U-sutures"), selective ligation, clipping, electrocoagulation, argon coagulation, infra-red coagulation, fibrin tissue glue, a further dissection technique (UltraCision) has been recently presented.

The UltraCision device, initially developed for laparoscopic surgery, occludes vascular structures by protein defragmentation induced via a longitudinally oscillating titanium blade or scissors that break up intracellular hydrogen bonds. Tissue dissection is performed through cellular wall destruction by rapid

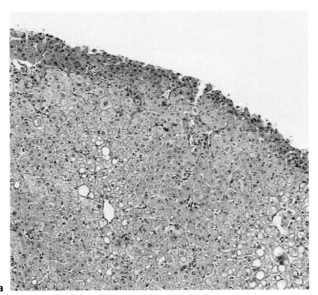
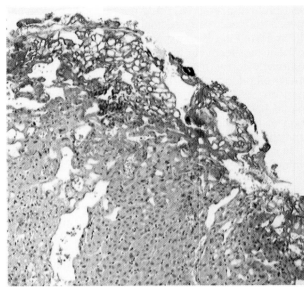

Fig. 15.**2 a** Histological section (hematoxylin and eosin staining, 100 fold magnification) of hepatic parenchyma dissected with the UltraCision shears. The tissue denaturation is limited to superficial regions of 50 to 100 μm thickness. **b** In comparison, the denaturation with electrocoagulation (hematoxylin and eosin staining, same magnification) is more severe at up to 200 μm depth, and there is confluent tissue necrosis.

changes of the intracellular volume. There is hardly any damage to deeper adjacent structures in the parenchyma since the defragmentation is mainly limited to the tissue between the blades of the scissors (Fig. 15.**2 a, b**).

The major advantages of UltraCision in liver surgery are a possible permanent occlusion of blood vessels and bile ducts up to a diameter of 12 mm, while larger vascular structures can safely be isolated. Therefore, the overall blood loss—although this remains to be demonstrated in controlled studies—seems to be reduced, especially in extended liver resections. In addition, the resection is facilitated through an optimal visibility of the cutting surface—as illustrated in Figure 15.**1**—as compared to the possible risk of accidental clamping of major structures during bleeding phases in classic parenchyma dissection techniques.

We conclude that ultrasonically activated instruments to dissect liver parenchyma are very helpful with regard to a reduced blood loss and that UltraCision is an alternative to the more expensive CUSA. According to our experience we can recommend the UltraCision shears in parenchymal dissection of the liver. However, in the regions of large vessels and bile ducts we prefer the UltraCision blade, as this device reduces the risk of accidental damage to these structures.

> Editor's tip: The blade is well designed also for the abdominal incision using the sharp edge for cutting and the flat side for hemostasis.

The additional use of the UltraCision blade tip does not seem to have any additional advantage in comparison to the shears or the blade. Moreover, most parts of the device can be reused. Further prospective studies are necessary to prove the value of the UltraCision shears in open and laparoscopic hepatic surgery.

References

1. Baer HU, Stain SC, Guastella T, Maddern GJ, Blumgart LH. Hepatic resection using a water-jet-dissector. HPB Surgery 1993; 6: 189–98.
2. Broering DC, Rogiers X, Malago M, Bassas A, Broelsch CE. Vessel loop-guided technique for parenchymal transection in living donor or in situ split-liver procurement. Liver Transpl Surg 1998; 4: 241.
3. Chou FF, Chen CL, Sheen-Chen SM, Chen YS, Chen MC. Ultrasonic dissection in resection of hepatocellular carcinoma. Int Surg 1995; 80: 105–7.
4. Elias D, Cavalcanti de Albuquerque A, Eggenspieler P, Plaud B, Ducreux M, Spielmann M, et al. Resection of liver metastases from a noncolorectal primary: indications and results based on 147 monocentric patients. J Am Coll Surg 1998; 187: 487–93.
5. Fasulo F, Giori A, Fissi S, Bozzetti F, Doci R, Gennnari L. Cavitron Ultrasonic Surgical Aspirator (CUSA) in liver resection. Int Surg 1992; 77: 64–6.
6. Hanna SS, Nam R, Leonhardt C. Liver resection by ultrasonic dissection and intraoperative sonography. HPB Surg 1996; 9: 121–8.
7. Hodgson WL, DelGuercio LR. Preliminary experience in liver surgery using the ultrasonic scalpel. Surgery 1984; 95: 230–4.
8. Izumi R, Yabushita K, Shimizu K, Yagi M, Yamaguchi A, Konishi K, et al. Hepatic resection using a water-jet dissector. Surg Today 1993; 23: 31–5.
9. Kaneko H, Takago S, Shiba T. Laparoscopic partial hepatectomy and left lateral segmentectomy: technique and results of a clinical series. Surgery 1996; 120: 468–75.
10. Katkhouda N, Hurwitz M, Gugenheim J, Mavor E, Mason RJ, Waldrep DJ, et al. Laparoscopic management of benign solid and cystic lesions of the liver. Ann Surg 1999; 229: 460–6.

11. Kousnetzoff M, Pensky J. Sur la résection partiélle du foie. Rev de Chir 1896; XVI: 501–21.

12. Lin TL. A simplified technique for hepatic resection. Ann Surg 1974; 180: 285–90.

13. Morino M, De Giuli M, Festa V, Garrone C. Laparoscopic management of symptomatic nonparasitic cysts of the liver. Ann Surg 1994; 219: 157–64.

14. Ogilvie H. Partial hepatectomy. Br Med J 1953; 2: 1136–8.

15. Papachristou DN, Barters R. Resection of the liver with a water jet. Br J Surg 1982; 69: 93–4.

16. Pringle JH. Notes on the arrest of hepatic hemorrhage due to trauma. Ann Surg 1908; 48: 541–9.

17. Rau HG, Schardey HM, Buttler E, Reuter C, Cohnert TU, Schildberg FW. A comparison of different techniques for liver resection: blunt dissection, ultrasonic aspirator and jet cutter. Eur J Surg Oncol 1995; 21: 183–7.

18. Rau HG, Meyer G, Jauch KW, Cohnert TU, Buttler E, Schildberg FW. Leberresektion mit dem Wasser-Jet: konventionell und laparoskopisch. Chirurg 1996; 67: 546–51.

19. Rees M, Plant G, Wells J, Bygrave S. One hundred and fifty hepatic resections: evolution of technique towards bloodless surgery. Br J Surg 1996; 83: 1526–9.

20. Trupka A, Hallfeldt K, Kalteis T, Schmidbauer S, Schweiberer L. Open and laparoscopic liver resection with a new ultrasound scalpel. Chirurg 1998; 69: 1352–6.

16 Hepatic Surgery with the UltraCision Blade for Open Surgery (DH 105)

P. Gertsch

Indications for hepatectomies have expanded to increasingly complex cases while at the same time mortality and morbidity have progressively decreased. Hepatectomies for centrally located tumors and for tumors in close contact with major intrahepatic vessels are not unusual. Liver resections limited to one or two segments are performed for patients with compromised liver function. These developments require precise and atraumatic separation of vascular and biliary structures from the surrounding liver parenchyma. Parenchyma transection has been performed using different techniques. Fracture using a clamp has largely replaced finger fracture and is adequate for most hepatectomies. However, since the resection plane frequently comes in close contact with large intrahepatic vessels, there is an increasing interest for using devices such as simple, strong aspiration of the liver parenchyma, ultrasonic aspirators, or water-jet cutters that allow precise and bloodless isolation of such structures (2, 3, 5).

Recently, an ultrasonically activated scalpel (UltraCision) has been developed and used in various procedures, mostly performed laparoscopically (1, 14, 17). This instrument has been used in open and laparoscopic liver resections whereby, in the latter, the UltraCision shears were used in a similar way as a crushing clamp (20). We use the UltraCision ultrasonically activated blade for dissection of intrahepatic structures and section of liver parenchyma in open liver surgery (4).

Indication and Preoperative Management

Patients with primary tumors localized in the liver are considered for surgery whenever malignancy is proven or cannot be ruled out. Benign tumors, with the exception of liver adenoma, are not operated on unless they clearly cause symptoms. Secondary tumors are resected whenever a curative resection seems possible.

Apart from an evaluation of the patient's general condition and operability, assessment of liver function according to Child-Pugh's criteria is carried out for patients with cirrhosis (15); only patients in the categories A and B are considered for surgery. Specialists in radiology, nuclear medicine, and gastrointestinal endoscopy may be involved to rule out extrahepatic dissemination or local tumor recurrence.

The localization and extent of disease in the liver and the characteristics of the main intrahepatic structures are studied in detail with radiological imaging. This, together with the estimated liver function, helps us to plan the margins for liver resection. Measurement of the volume of the assumed remaining liver after resection is obtained by computed tomography and three-dimensional reconstruction (7). Embolization of the portal branch of the pathological side of the liver is performed for inducing atrophy and contralateral hypertrophy whenever the volume of the remaining liver after resection might seem insufficient (6).

Operation

All patients are operated on under controlled hypovolemia and low central venous pressure to decrease back-bleeding from the hepatic veins and reduce blood loss during parenchyma transection (11). The operations are generally performed through a right subcostal incision extended to the left with upward midline extension when necessary. As an exception, when the tumor is localized high under the diaphragm, a thoraco-phreno-laparotomy may give better access for efficient working with the hand piece of the UltraCision blade. Intraoperative ultrasound is performed to rule out any disease undetected by preoperative imaging, to define the limits of the lesion to be removed, and to identify important intrahepatic anatomic landmarks.

Anatomic hepatectomies After hilar dissection, control of the ipsilateral branch of the portal vein and hepatic artery is obtained in patients submitted to hemihepatectomies while the extrafascial approach is used to isolate the portal triads of the segments to be resected in the other cases (8). The line of parenchymal transection is determined by the limit of ischemia on the surface of the liver when clearly visible after selective clamping, or according to the anatomic landmarks. Section of liver parenchyma is performed under intermittent vascular inflow occlusion. We use the UltraCision blade to cut the liver parenchyma and to dissect hilar or intrahepatic structures. The instrument is set on the highest level (level 5) of the scale with the possibility of choosing a lower power level with a pedal switch.

Editor's tip: The UltraCision blade is also appropriate for the abdominal incision, using the sharp edge for cutting and the flat side for hemostasis.

The section of the liver parenchyma is performed using either the sharp edge of the vibrating blade for cutting Glisson's capsule or small intrahepatic vessels, or its blunt edge or flat side to progress into the section of liver parenchyma or to coagulate vessels before section (Fig. 16.**1**).

> Editor's tip: The coagulating effect on vascular and biliary structures of less than 3 mm is excellent when the flat side of the blade is used together with level 2 on the generator and no tension on the tissues.

The hand piece is moved, producing small, slow lateral displacements of 1 cm in amplitude of the UltraCision blade with simultaneous, unhurried, forward progression until an intrahepatic structure or a bleeding point is encountered. Bleeding is controlled by application of the lateral side of the vibrating blade on the bleeding parenchyma for a few seconds. Vessels not exceeding 2 mm in diameter are coagulated with the blunt edge of the blade and subsequently cut with its sharp side. Larger intrahepatic structures are isolated by similar dissection and ligated or controlled with clips and cut with scissors (Fig. 16.**2**).

> Editor's tip: The ends of the sutures are easily cut with the sharp curvature of the blade. This is convenient and avoids the need for frequent instrumental changes.

Non-anatomic hepatectomies, tumorectomies

Bloodless and complete excision is obtained using the UltraCision blade as previously described. Planes of dissection are defined by intraoperative ultrasonography and by palpation.

 Hints and Pitfalls

- The technique of controlled hypovolemia and low central venous pressure, together with partial or total interruption of hepatic inflow, is an important complement to the use of the harmonic scalpel. Prevention of bleeding from the cut surface of the liver is essential for efficient working with the UltraCision blade: the presence of blood tends to obscure vision by an effect of spray confined to its tip.
- When planning the operation, care must be taken to figure out the plane of section within the liver. As the hand piece of the UltraCision blade measures 15 cm in length, sufficient space between the liver surface and the diaphragm is necessary to use it. Standard subcostal incision is adequate for major hepatectomies and for segmentectomies and bisegmentectomies; for segment VIII resection or for local excisions of tumors high under the diaphragm, thoracophreno-laparotomy may give better access (19).

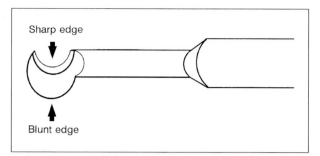

Fig. 16.**1** The 5 mm hook of the UltraCision scalpel with its sharp and blunt edge and flat lateral side.

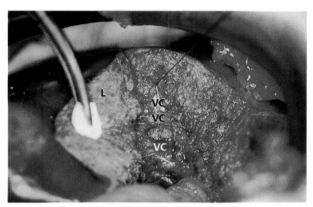

Fig. 16.**2** Cut surface of the liver showing intrahepatic tubular structures isolated with the UltraCision scalpel. *L* cut surface of the liver, *VC* intrahepatic vascular channels to be tied.

- Cirrhotic changes may, in some cases, reduce the efficacy of the UltraCision blade. Lowering the power of the instrument and slowing progression of the vibrating blade into the liver can improve the situation. If not, parenchyma fracture with a clamp might be preferable as bleeding from the cut surface prevents efficient use of the UltraCision blade.
- The UltraCision hand piece tends to transmit generated heat after continuous use exceeding 5 minutes; this may on occasion require wrapping the instrument's handle with a wet gauze to protect the surgeon's hand.

 Personal Experience

Forty-three hepatectomies were performed in 42 patients (27 male and 15 female) aged between 31 and 79 years (median age 65 years). Indications for hepatectomies are given in Table 16.**1**. Embolization of a portal branch was performed four weeks before surgery in three patients. Nine patients underwent a right and one a left hepatectomy; two patients underwent left hepatectomies extended to segment V and VIII (left trisegmentectomies) and two had right hepatectomies extended to segment IV and I (right triseg-

Table 16.**1**   Indications for hepatectomies

Pathologic diagnosis	Number of cases
Hepatocellular carcinoma	17
Primary biliary malignancy	3
Metastatic colorectal carcinoma	11
Other metastatic malignancies	6
Benign	5
Other	1

Table 16.**2**   Types of hepatectomies

Operations	Segments	Number
Right hepatectomy	V, VI, VII, VIII	9
Left hepatectomy	II, III, IV	1
Extended right hepatectomy	IV, V, VI, VII, VIII, & I	2
Extended left hepatectomy	II, III, IV, V, VIII	2
Left lobectomy	II, III	9
Right posterior sectorectomy	VI, VII	5
Resection of one segment	IV/V/VI/VII	6
Resection of two segments	V & VI/IVa & V/IVb & VIII	6
Resection of three segments	IV, V, VIII	1
Tumorectomy		2

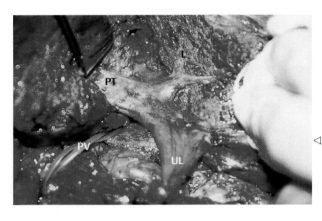

◁ Fig. 16.**3**   Resection of segments II and III. Dissection of the intrahepatic branches of the left portal vein with UltraCision. The branch to the segments II and III will be ligated while that to segment IV will carefully be spared. *PT* portal triad to segment IV, *PV* vessel loop around left portal vein, *L* cut surface of the liver (seg. II & III), *UL* umbilical ligament.

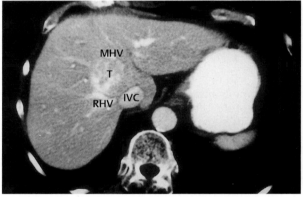

a

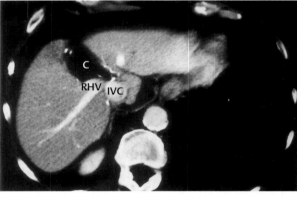

b

Fig. 16.**4**   **a** Hepatocellular carcinoma in segments VIII and IVb in close contact with the right hepatic vein and inferior vena cava, infiltrating the middle hepatic vein. The liver is cirrhotic with compromised function. *T* tumor, *MHV* middle hepatic vein, *RHV* right hepatic vein, *IVC* inferior vena cava. **b** Computed tomography 36 h after bisegmentectomy VIII and IVb. The upper parts of the right hepatic vein and inferior vena cava are opacified and free at the bottom of the cavity resulting from the bisegmentectomy. The volume of the cavity is reduced as segments II and VII collapse against each other. *C* collapsed cavity resulting from resection, *RHV* right hepatic vein, *IVC* inferior vena cava.

mentectomy). Three, two, and one segments were resected respectively in one, and 20, and six patients (Table 16.**2**). A metastatic tumor nodule was resected in segment I and an atypical resection for focal nodular hyperplasia in segment VII and VIII was performed through a thoraco-phreno-laparotomy.

The dissection and cutting effects of the UltraCision scalpel were satisfactory in most patients submitted to hepatectomies (4). Segments of the portal elements could be isolated for clamping and subsequent section in the patients undergoing segmentectomies (Fig. 16.**3**). When hepatectomy involved segment VI and VII, the right hepatic vein was preserved and its wall partially exposed on the surface of the resection plane. Similarly, dissection of tumors in close contact with hepatic veins or the inferior vena cava proved to be safe (Fig. 16.**4a, b**). The hemostatic effect was excellent in most patients, and the cut surface was bloodless at the end of the resection in all cases. The cutting and coagulating effect was less satisfactory in three out of 14 patients with cirrhosis. Median blood loss was 350 ml (range 03–400 ml) and 12 patients received a median number of 2 packed red cells (72% of patients operated without blood transfusions). Median operative time was 300 minutes (range 80–720 minutes).

There was one hospital death due to portal vein thrombosis and postoperative liver failure after left trisegmentectomy. One patient underwent resection of segment VII for ischemic necrosis 36 hours after segmentectomy VI for HCC, and another patient presented a biliary fistula that healed spontaneously within 12 days after percutaneous drainage. One patient submitted to bile duct exploration for concomitant stones presented a bile duct stenosis after removal of the T-drain. This stenosis was treated by balloon dilatation No single case of bleeding was observed in the postoperative period.

> Editor's tip: The reliability of the hemostatic function of the UltraCision scalpel is also the editor's experience—with no reoperations because of bleeding.

Patients were discharged within seven to 24 days (median hospital stay 14 days).

 ## Discussion

In spite of recent progress, hepatectomy remains an operation with important risks. Section of liver parenchyma or lesion of major vascular structures, particularly the hepatic veins and the inferior vena cava may cause significant blood loss. Inflow occlusion and section of parenchyma in anatomical intersegmental planes have contributed in reducing hemorrhage during parenchyma transection (9). Lowering central venous pressure further contributes to control bleeding in reducing back flow from the hepatic veins (11). With these techniques, blood loss is not influenced by the time required for parenchyma transection; finger fracture has largely been replaced by the more precise but slower technique of fracture with a forceps. Crushing the liver parenchyma results in selective destruction of hepatocytes and sparing of more resistant structures such as blood vessels and bile ducts that are subsequently either coagulated, or tied and cut. A similar effect is obtained in a less traumatic way with ultrasonic aspirators: the hepatocytes are destroyed, leaving intact all other structures for coagulation or tying before section. Ultrasonic aspirators may have contributed in reducing blood loss during hepatectomies in some centers (3). We use the UltraCision scalpel in a similar way as ultrasonic aspirators, for selective destruction of hepatocytes by the high-frequency vibrating blade that leaves intact vessels and bile ducts. In our experience, this destruction of hepatocytes is extremely selective, leaving unaltered thin-walled structures such as the hepatic veins. As with other ultrasonic dissectors, tissue disintegration is obtained essentially by cavitation and interfascial friction

resulting in destruction of the cell membranes and matrix (12). This cellular destruction has been demonstrated to be complete in an experimental model involving tumor dissection (13). On occasions, the performance of the UltraCision scalpel was less satisfactory in patients with cirrhosis (4). The high content of collagen in the liver may have prevented preferential destruction of cells and sparing of blood vessels. Tuning the instrument to a lower energy level and slowing the progression into the liver parenchyma improves the situation in such cases. Operative time may be prolonged by dissection with the UltraCision blade as previously observed with ultrasonic aspirators (3).

Coaptive coagulation is specific to the harmonic scalpel with sealing of vessels by a sticky coagulum resulting from denatured tissue proteins. Thermal injury is limited and the effect is obtained without smoke (1, 10). The surgeon holds, therefore, a very versatile instrument in his hand. Besides the destruction of hepatocytes, hemostasis of actively bleeding parenchyma is possible by gentle pressure of the lateral side of the vibrating blade. The instrument does not stick to tissues after coagulation, and hemostasis is achieved once the instrument is removed.

> Editor's tip: The UltraCision scalpel never sticks to the tissues if it is activated during withdrawal. This is one of the most appreciated characteristics of ultrasonically activated instruments and illustrates a sharp contrast to diathermy.

Vessels with a diameter of 1 to 2 mm may be sealed in a similar way and subsequently cut with the sharp edge of the blade.

Blood transfusions, given to only 26% of our patients, and median blood loss of 350 ml, compare favorably with data from centers of expertise (3, 11, 16, 18). We attribute this mainly to the technique of controlled hypovolemia and low central venous pressure, to the use of intermittent inflow occlusion during parenchyma transection, and to the precise and atraumatic dissection obtained with the UltraCision scalpel near large intrahepatic vascular channels. The hemostatic effect of the vibrating blade may also, to a lesser extent, have contributed to this.

In our experience, the UltraCision scalpel contributes to the safety of hepatectomies by allowing bloodless and precise dissection of intrahepatic structures. It represents more than an alternative to classically used ultrasonic aspirators, and has the advantage that transection of the liver parenchyma together with coagulation and section of small vessels can be done using a single instrument. Finally, the harmonic scalpel has a lower cost than an ultrasonic aspirator and can be used in a wider range of operations.

Acknowledgements

The following authors have contributed to this work: P. Gertsch, A. Pelloni, A. Guerra, A. Krpo.

References

1. Amaral JF. The experimental development of an ultrasonically activated scalpel for laparoscopic use. Surg Laparosc & Endosc 1994; 2: 92–9.
2. Baer HU, Stain SC, Guastella T, Maddern GJ, Blumgart LH. Hepatic resection using a water-jet dissector. HPB Surg 1993; 6: 189–96.
3. Fan ST, Lai ECS, Lo CM, Chu KM, Liu CL, Wong J. Hepatectomy with an ultrasonic dissector for hepatocellular carcinoma. Br J Surg 1996; 83: 117–20.
4. Gertsch P, Pelloni A, Guerra A, Krpo A. Initial experience with the harmonic scalpel in liver surgery. Hepatogastroenterology 2000; 47: 763–6.
5. Hodgson WJB, Morgan J, Byrne D, DelGuercio LRM. Hepatic resection for primary and metastatic tumors using the ultrasonic surgical dissector. Am J Surg 1996; 163: 246–50.
6. Kawasaki S, Makuuchi M, Miyagawa S, Kakazu T. Radical operation after portal embolization for tumor of hilar bile duct. J Am Coll Surg 1994; 178: 480–6.
7. Kubota K, Makuuchi M, Kusaka K, Kobayashi T, Miki K, Hasegawa K, Harihara Y, Takayama T. Measurement of liver volume and hepatic functional reserve as a guide to decision-making in resectional surgery for hepatic tumors. Hepatology 1997; 26: 1176–81.
8. Launois B, Jamieson GG. The importance of Glisson's capsule and its sheaths in the intrahepatic approach to resection of the liver. Surgery Gynecol and Obst 1992; 174: 7–10.
9. Man K, Fan ST, Ng IOL, Lo CM, Liu CL, Wong J. Prospective evaluation of Pringle maneuver in hepatectomy for liver tumors by a randomized study. Ann Surg 1997; 226: 704–13.
10. McCarus SD. Physiologic mechanism of the ultrasonically activated scalpel. J Am Assoc Gynecol Laparosc 1996; 3: 601–8.
11. Melendez JA, Arsalan VA, Fischer ME, Wuest D, Jarnagin WR, Fong Y, Blumgart LH. Perioperative outcomes of major hepatic resections under low central venous pressure anesthesia: Blood loss, transfusion, and the risk of postoperative renal dysfunction. J Am Coll Surg 1998; 187: 620–5.
12. Mueller W, Fritzsch G. Medicotechnical basics of surgery using invasive ultrasonic energy. End Surg 1994; 2: 205–10.
13. Nduka CC, Dye JF, Mansfield AO, Darzi A. Viability of airborne cancer cells released by ultrasonic cavitation and electrosurgery. Br J Surg 1997; 84: 720.
14. Ohtsuka T, Wolf RK, Hiratzka LF, Wurnig P, Flege JB. Thoracoscopic internal mammary artery harvest for MICABG using the harmonic scalpel. Ann Thorac Surg 1997; 63: S107–9.
15. Pugh RNH, Murray-Lyon IM, Dawson JL, Pietroni MC, Williams R. Transsection of the oesophagus for bleeding oesophageal varices. Br J Surg 1973; 60: 646–9.
16. Rees M, Plant G, Wells J, Bygrave S. One hundred and fifty hepatic resections: evolution of technique towards bloodless surgery. Br J Surg 1996; 83: 1526–9.
17. Rothenberg SS, Chang JH. Laparoscopic pull-through procedures using the harmonic scalpel in infants and children with Hirschprung's disease. J Pediatr Surg 1997; 32: 894–6.
18. Takano S, Oishi H, Kono S, Kawakami S, Nakamura M, Kubota N, Iwai S. Retrospective analysis of type of hepatic resection for hepatocellular carcinoma. Br J Surg 2000; 87: 65–70.
19. Takenaka K, Fujiwara Y, Gion T, Maeda T, Shirabe K, Shimada M, Yanaga K, Sugimachi K. A thoracoabdominal hepatectomy and a transdiaphragmatic hepatectomy for patients with cirrhosis and hepatocellular carcinoma. Arch Surg 1998; 133: 80–3.
20. Trupka A, Hallfeldt K, Kalteis T, Schmidbauer S, Schweiberer L. Offene und laparoskopische Leberresektion mit einem neuen Ultraschallskalpell. Chirurg 1998; 69: 1352–6.

17 Laparoscopic Splenectomy with the 5 or 10 mm UltraCision Shears (LCSC 5 or LCS 15)

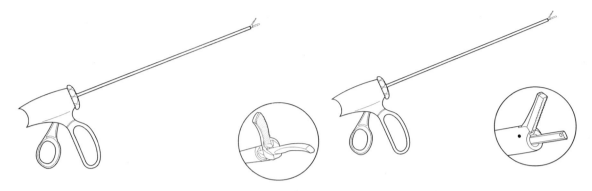

T. Reck

Laparoscopic splenectomy remains a technically demanding procedure. This is due mainly to the complexity of the vascular supply of the organ, and the associated danger of causing a life-threatening hemorrhage. Thus, numerous authors report a relatively high intra-operative blood loss (3, 5) and the operating time—at least in the learning phase—is considerably longer than in open surgery (7). According to the literature, the conversion rate approaches 20% (5), the reasons for conversion often being the complication of bleeding. This situation led to such developments as the so-called hand-assisted laparoscopic technique (1) or the attempt to achieve preoperative embolization of the splenic artery (9). In the last report, however, it has now been shown that the use of a lateral approach and the UltraCision scalpel facilitates dissection, shortens operating time, and reduces blood losses.

Indication and Preoperative Management

The indications for the laparoscopic technique are, in particular, benign hematological disorders with hypersplenism and mild-to-moderate splenomegaly, that is, a spleen weighing up to 500 g (normal dimensions: 12×8×4 cm, 120–200 g). Of clinical significance, therefore, are idiopathic thrombocytopenic purpura (ITP, Werlhof's disease) (62%), hereditary spherocytosis (9%), and autoimmune hemolytic anemias (5%) (4, 10).

Preoperative computed tomography serves both to assess the dimensions of the spleen and also the search for accessory spleens—prevalence roughly 15% (4). Antipneumococcal vaccination should be carried out at the latest two weeks prior to surgery. The prior medical treatment (cortisone, immunoglobulins) is continued until immediately before the operation, with the aim of maintaining a high number of platelets. Preoperatively the patients are given a single shot of antibiotics.

Operation

The patient is placed in a right lateral decubitus position and supported in such a way that rotation of the operating table about the longitudinal axis through approximately 30° to the left is possible (placement of the optic trocar, conversion). The surgeon and camera assistant stand to the right of the operating table and both look across the operating area to view the monitor placed above and to the left of the patient.

The following choice of instruments is recommended:
- 4 × 12 mm ports (camera, UltraCision, swab, linear stapler)
- Ultracision 5 mm or 10 mm LCS shears
- Two swabs and a curved grasping forceps
- Endoscopic vascular stapling device

The following devices may be needed either additionally or alternatively:
- Vessel clips (titanium)
- 5 mm grasping instrument

The optic trocar is inserted left-lateral to the umbilicus using the open technique (Hasson trocar), and three further working trocars are placed under direct visual control as far apart as possible, roughly along a line running oblique to the costal arch in the left upper abdomen. The larger the spleen to be removed, the further caudally and to the right this line is placed. This pattern of placement of the trocars and the use of two 12 mm trocars ensures maximum flexibility for the subsequent use of the linear stapler. Because of the right lateral position of the patient, the spleen is exposed "spontaneously" and traction applied thereby to the ligamentous attachments. In a first step, the splenocolic and splenorenal ligaments are divided using the UltraCision scalpel exclusively (Fig. 17.1). In contrast to electrocoagulation, the latter permits dissection close to the wall of the colon with a relatively small risk of injury.

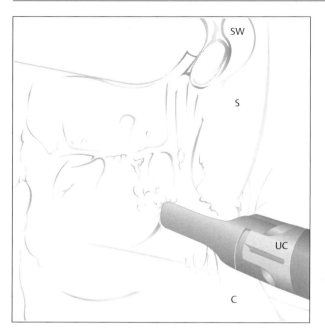

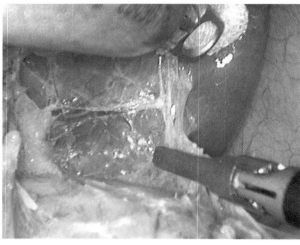

Fig. 17.**1**   Freeing of posterior attachments using UltraCision shears. The spleen is elevated with a swab. *S* spleen, *C* colon (left flexure), *UC* 5 mm LCS shears, *SW* swab.

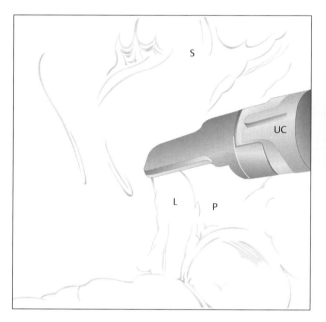

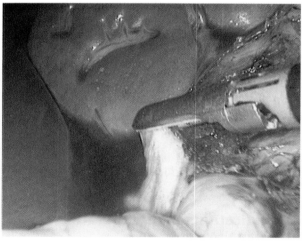

Fig. 17.**2**   Division of gastrosplenic ligament and short gastric vessels using UltraCision dissection. *S* spleen, *L* gastrosplenic ligament, *P* pancreas, *UC* 5 mm LCS shears.

Editor's tip: With five seconds of activation, the lateral spread of thermal injury is 1 mm with the UltraCision scalpel, as opposed to 5 mm with electrocoagulation and the same time of activation.

The spleen is mobilized and freed of all attachments, with the exception of the remaining ligaments attached to the upper pole ("hanging spleen"). The gastrosplenic ligaments, together with the short gastric vessels overlaying the hilum, are then divided (Fig. 17.**2**). This is carried out stepwise and safely using

UltraCision and clips are rarely required. When the lower pole of the spleen is elevated, the vessels in the hilum are put under tension and then exposed using a curved forceps. The tail of the pancreas, which is usually visualized during this procedure, is resected by performing the further dissection close to the spleen. For safety reasons, the large vessels in the hilum, or their branches, are divided with the aid of the vascular linear stapler. When placing the stapler, injury to the pancreas must be avoided. The spleen is placed in a cell-tight and water-tight recovery bag, in which it can be morcellated. For this purpose, the opening of the bag is brought out through a trocar incision enlarged to 2 cm, and the spleen is then fragmented with the finger or an instrument and recovered.

Summary of laparoscopic splenectomy:
- Division of the colosplenic, splenorenal, and, in part, the phrenicosplenic ligaments,
- Division of the gastrosplenic ligament and the short gastric vessels,
- Division of the hilar vessels or their branches using the linear stapler,
- Recovery of the spleen in a bag.

⚠ Hints and Pitfalls

- Overlooked accessory spleens are considered to be responsible for the recurrence of ITP (2). In series of open splenectomies, accessory spleens have been reported in 11–18% of the cases (12). In a review of the literature (4) reporting an incidence of 13%, however, these accessory spleens are also detected during laparoscopy and can be removed. The most common location of such accessory spleens is the hilum of the organ, the tail of the pancreas, the greater omentum, the greater curvature of the stomach, and the mesentery of the small and large bowels. A possible solution to the problem posed by accessory spleens might be preoperative scintigraphy using ^{99m}Tc (12) and the recommended CT scan.
- The lateral patient position described herein facilitates the exposure of the spleen, since the small and large bowels, together with the stomach, drop under the force of gravity to expose the operating area, thereby putting traction on the ligamentous attachment of the spleen. In the case of a very large spleen weighing more than 1.5 kg, which cannot readily be elevated with a swab, the supine position may be more favorable.

> Editor's tip: To achieve tension on the gastrosplenic fat in the supine position, the stomach is retracted to the patient's right with an atraumatic grasp and the spleen to the right with a swab. A dissection division of the short gastric vessels is performed entirely with the UltraCision shears. To diminish the risk of injury to the underlying hilum vessels, the inactive blade is turned downwards during activation.
> In such a case, however, the indication for a laparoscopic procedure should be carefully and critically considered.

- An indispensable instrument is the linear stapler for the control of the hilar vessels. Since, however, an occasional malfunctioning of the stapler cannot be excluded with absolute certainty, accurate prior visualization of the hilar vessels should always be attempted, in order to be able to control any hemorrhage that might occur (9). At the latest when,

during the operation, the need for blood transfusion becomes apparent, conversion to an open procedure should be considered.

🦉 Personal Experience

Since the introduction of UltraCision, we have carried out ten consecutive laparoscopic splenectomies with this instrument, as compared with the former use of titanium clips. The average operating time was about 2.5 hours, and the blood loss was negligible. A single splenectomy had to be converted to an open procedure since, after dividing all the splenic ligaments and with the patient in the lateral position, the large spleen (approximately 1000 g) could not be elevated for reliable control of the hilum. On the basis of this experience, we now leave the phrenicosplenic ligament attached to the upper pole of the spleen, thus leaving the organ "hanging" as it were, in order to ensure that the structures in the hilum are put under traction.

Discussion

The main complication associated with laparoscopic splenectomy is intraoperative bleeding. This is due to the numerous vascular connections and the delicate capsule of the organ that make manipulation with instruments a problem and which represents the main reason for a conversion. The mean conversion rate is roughly 10%, and increases to 25% with increasing size of the spleen (4). Bleeding in the surgical field not only endangers the patient, but also represents a stressful situation for the surgeon, since an unobstructed view, so necessary for specific management of the large vessels, is lost. Thus, some series report a blood loss of more than 250 ml (5). A possible solution to this problem is the use of UltraCision. In more recent studies it has been shown that the introduction of UltraCision has at least halved the intraoperative blood loss, and in many cases, has rendered it insignificant (6, 11). The use of the UltraCision scalpel avoids the formerly demanding divisioning of the short gastric vessels and the use of clips, and shortens the operating time. As in the case of mobilization of the greater curvature of the stomach during laparoscopic fundoplication, this is the greatest advantage of using UltraCision. Minimal mobilization of the individual vessels is required, and the risk of clips coming off is obviated. Not least due to the use of the UltraCision shears, the operating times in the current series have virtually been halved in comparison with earlier series (6, 11). Also reduced is the need for frequent changing of instruments, since grasping, cutting, and coagulation are all possible with a single instrument. The danger of injuring neighboring structures by electric current, as might occur to the colon during coagulation of the lower splenic pole, is obviated. In most cases, electrocoagulation can be avoided completely. In obese patients with excessive intra-abdominal fat, however, it has proved to be of advantage to coagulate and divide minor vessels, for example, those feeding the splenic poles, even without complete dissection, which would not be possible when using clips.

 References

1. Ballaux KEW, Himpens JM, Leman G, VandeBossche MRP. Hand-assisted splenectomy for hydatid cyst. Surg Endosc 1997; 11: 942–3.
2. Cadiere GB, Verroken R, Himpens J. Operative strategy in laparoscopic splenectomy. J Am Coll Surg 1994; 179: 668–72.
3. Carrol BJ, Phillips EH, Semel CJ, Fallas M, Morgenstern L. Laparoscopic splenectomy. Surg Endosc 1992; 6: 183–5.
4. Decker G, Millat B, Guillon F, Atger JA, Linon M. Laparoscopic Splenectomy for Benign and Malignant Hematologic Diseases: 35 Consecutive Cases. World J Surg 1998; 22: 62–8.
5. Flowers JL, Lefor AT, Steers J, Heyman M, Graham SM, Imbembo AL. Laparoscopic splenectomy in patients with hematologic diseases. Ann Surg 1996; 224: 19–28.
6. Gossot D, Fritsch S, Celerier M. Laparoscopic splenectomy. Optimal vascular control using the lateral approach and ultrasonic dissection. Surg Endosc 1999; 13: 21–5.
7. Marassi A, Vignali A, Zuliani W, Biguzzi E, Bergamo C, Gianotti L, Di Carlo V. Splenectomy for idiopathic thrombocytopenic purpura. Comparison of laparoscopic and conventional surgery. Surg Endosc 1999; 13: 17–20.
8. Park A, Gagner M, Pomp . The lateral approach to laparoscopic splenectomy. Am J Surg 1997; 173: 126–30.
9. Poulin EC, Thibault C, Mamazza J. Laparoscopic splenectomy. Surg Endosc 1995; 9: 172–7.
10. Reck T, Koeckerling F, Scheuerlein F, Hohenberger W. Laparoskopische Splenektomie. Zentralbl Chir 1998; 123: 295–300.
11. Rothenberg SS. Laparoscopic splenectomy using the harmonic scalpel. J Laparoend Surg 1996; 6(Suppl 1): 61–3.
12. Rudowski WJ. Accessory spleens: clinical significance with particular reference to the recurrence of idiopathic thrombocytopenic purpura. World J Surg 1985; 9: 422–30.

18 Laparoscopic Splenectomy with the 10 mm UltraCision Shears (LCS 15 Pistol Grip or LCS 6S Needle-Holder Grip) with Rotating Blade

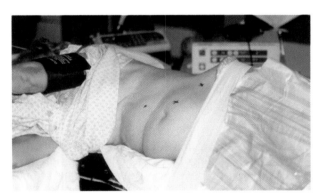

C. M. S. Royston, D. Zacharoulis, P. C. Sedman

The introduction of the UltraCision scalpel has transformed the operation of laparoscopic splenectomy. Prior to its introduction, splenectomy had been performed laparoscopically in only a few centers (beginning in 1991), and during these operations small- to medium-sized vessels had to be either ligated or clipped. This resulted in long operating times because ligation is time consuming and tedious and, since clipping is less secure, bleeding was a more significant problem. The benefits of splenectomy performed laparoscopically (as with cholecystectomy before it) are impressive with rapid mobilization and fewer post-operative general complications. The laparoscopic procedure has now become the "gold standard" for most elective splenectomies.

Indication and Preoperative Management

The common indications for splenectomy are listed in Table 18.1. Laparoscopic surgery is reserved for elective procedures especially where the spleen is of small size (up to 1 kg). In conditions where there is massive splenomegaly the open approach is preferred, not only for ease of dissection but also because splenic retrieval is a major problem. The most common indications are idiopathic thrombocytopenic purpura and spherocytosis. Caution is advised in patients with hypersplenism in association with portal hypertension. Previous upper abdominal surgery is not a contraindication. We suggest that when in doubt, patients should undergo ultrasound to assess the size of the spleen. As a general rule, impalpable spleens are suitable for the laparoscopic approach. Patients should be vaccinated against pneumococcus, meningococcus, and hemophilus and prophylactic antibiotics are also advised. Clotting should be checked and in cases of ITP the platelet count should be optimized with steroids or transfusion. Two units of blood are cross-matched. The arguments in favor of preoperative splenic artery embolization have become largely irrelevant with the introduction of the UltraCision scalpel and this is not now recommended.

Table 18.1 Common indications for elective splenectomy

- Treatment of hematological disease
- Anemias (e.g., hereditary spherocytosis)
- Thrombocytopenias (e.g., ITP)
- Myeloproliferative disorders
- Neoplasms
- Diagnosis/staging
- Lymphoma
- Metabolic/miscellaneous
- Cysts
- Aneurysms

Fig. 18.1 Position of patient on operating table and position of ports (X).

Operation

Position on the table Patients are placed in the half lateral position (Fig. 18.1), the left side of the body being elevated 45° and lying flat. In obese patients, breaking the table is helpful.

Introduction of trocars Pneumoperitoneum is established with a Veress needle or Hasson technique just above the umbilicus. A 12 mm trocar is inserted and a 30° telescope is introduced into the abdominal cavity. A 12 mm trocar is introduced in the left lumbar region and a 5 mm trocar in the epigastric region (Fig. 18.1). It

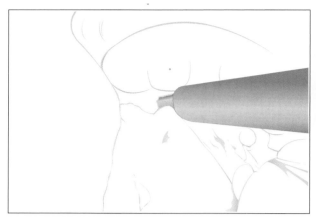
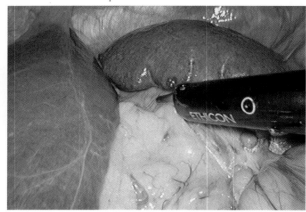

Fig. 18.**2**   Division of short gastric vessels using the UltraCision scalpel.

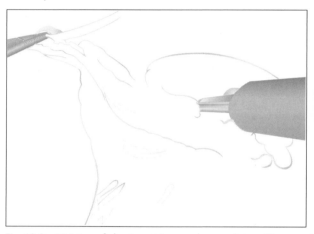
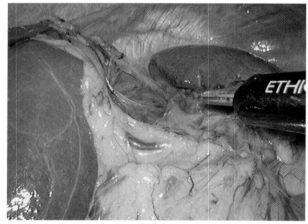

Fig. 18.**3**   Division of short gastric vessels complete with separation of greater curvature of stomach from the spleen.

is often useful to introduce a further 5 mm trocar in the left hypochondrium immediately below the left ribs for splenic retraction. There are often adhesions between the lower pole of the spleen and the splenic flexure of the colon. If these are present, they need to be dissected free and this dissection is started with the UltraCision scalpel from the lumbar port. These adhesions are completely removed to free the colon from the lower pole of the spleen.

Procedure The sequence of steps recommended is as follows:
1. Mobilization of the splenic flexure of the colon
2. Division of short gastric vessels and division of gastrosplenic ligament
3. Ligation of the splenic artery
4. Division of the splenic hilum
5. Removal of specimen

The short gastric vessels are divided and the lesser sac entered by introducing a retractor through the 5 mm subcostal trocar and gently pushing the spleen laterally. Movement of the spleen may be further aided by tilting the table right-side down, allowing the spleen to

fall posteriorly, away from the greater curve of the stomach and thus opening the gastrosplenic ligament. Once the lesser sac is entered, the stomach may be retracted medially, further displaying the short gastric vessels which are divided individually with the UltraCision scalpel in coagulation mode (Fig. 18.**2**).

> Editor's tip: Using the 10 mm LCS, the short gastric vessels are divided with the blunt side at level 3; using the 5 mm shears with the fixed blade, level 2 is recommended for reliable hemostasis.

The dissection of the gastrosplenic ligament continues inferiorly until the stomach is completely freed from the spleen. During this dissection, accessory spleens will become apparent in 10–20% of patients and these should be resected The tail of the pancreas is readily visualized in the lesser sac and the splenic artery usually seen running in the superior aspect of the pancreatic tail to the splenic hilum. With gentle dissection, an instrument (Petelin forceps or Delaitre) can be tunneled beneath and around the splenic artery via the lumbar port (Fig. 18.**3**). Once the splenic artery has

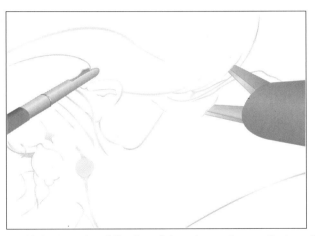 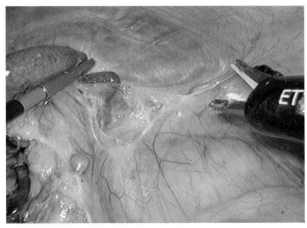

Fig. 18.**4** Lateral mobilization of the spleen using gravity to assist retraction medially.

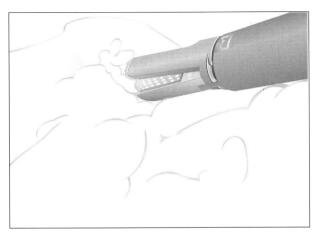 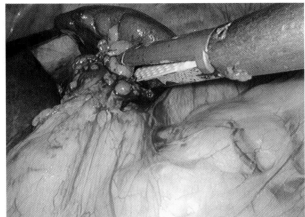

Fig. 18.**5** Transection of splenic hilum with an endoscopic linear stapling device.

been dissected from below, it is possible to pass a "0" vicryl suture around the artery and ligate it in continuity using needle holders to fashion the knot.

While splenic artery anatomy may be variable and it may have divided into several feeding arteries at this point, a splenic artery identified in this way is still dominant in 75% of people and can be confirmed by observing the spleen turning blue/black moments after ligation of the vessel. Retention of the pink color at either splenic pole will alert the surgeon to the presence of a further arterial supply, usually from small vessels. In obese patients, splenic artery ligation can be difficult and may be forgone, but some advantages of devascularization are then lost, namely a safer dissection in a devascularized organ and an easier dissection of a decongested splenic vein.

Dissection again turns to the inferior pole of the spleen. The inferior pole is mobilized, freeing the posterior surface of the spleen from the paracolic gutter. The peritoneum at this level is divided using the UltraCision scalpel. This proceeds until the spleen is completely mobilized posteriorly and inferiorly and

the splenic hilum is isolated (Fig. 18.**4**). The splenic hilum may now be secured, either by the use of a linear stapling and cutting device (TSW 45 Vascular endostapler) which is introduced from the lumbar port, or by ligation of the splenic vein in a similar fashion to the ligation of the splenic artery (Figs. 18.**5**, 18.**6**). If the latter method is preferred, careful dissection is performed using a combination of the UltraCision scalpel to remove the loose tissue around the splenic vein and dissecting forceps to get behind the vein. The vein is then tied in a similar fashion to the splenic artery using 2/0 vicryl sutures; at least two sutures are applied. A clip can be placed on the splenic side of the vein to control any back-bleeding.

If the endostapler is used to take the splenic pedicle, it is important to ensure that the whole of the splenic vein is placed into the jaws of the instrument. Two or three firings of the endostapler may be necessary to completely divide the pedicle. It is important to ensure that any loose, fatty tissue is removed. If it is too bulky, the splenic pedicle will not fit satisfactorily into the jaws of the endostapler. The pancreatic tail abuts the

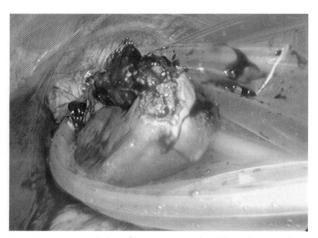

Fig. 18.**6** Splenic delivery into an impermeable endoscopic bag for morcellation and retrieval.

splenic hilum in up to 30% of patients. Care must be taken to avoid damaging it.

When the splenic pedicle has been divided, the final step to completely free the spleen is to divide the adhesions between the spleen and the left dome of the diaphragm. There may be a posterior vein or artery supplying the superior pole of the spleen which, if encountered, will need to be either clipped or ligated. When the spleen has been completely freed, the distal aspect of the pancreas is carefully checked. Any blood is removed by a sucker and the whole area irrigated. The telescope is removed from the supraumbilical trocar and inserted into the lumbar trocar.

The 10/12 mm trocar is changed for either a 15 mm or an 18 mm trocar and the retrieval bag is placed through this port. Two retrieval bags are recommended: either the large 15 mm Endocatch (AutoSuture), which opens spontaneously as soon as it is inserted into the abdominal cavity, or the larger Espiner (Espiner Medical Products) retrieval bag. For the smaller spleens (ITP, spherocytosis) either bag is satisfactory. For the larger spleens approaching l kg the Espiner bag is preferable as it is larger and considerably stronger. The retrieval bag is inserted via the 15 or 18 mm trocar at the umbilicus to lie immediately below the spleen, the spleen being in its original position in the left hypochondrium. The bag is opened (with the Endocatch this happens spontaneously). The lower part of the bag is placed below the inferior aspect of the spleen and with pressure on its superior pole, the spleen is forced into the bag.

As soon as the organ is completely inside the bag the tapes are pulled to disconnect the bag from the insertion mechanism. It is then pulled out of the abdominal cavity, the tapes are pulled tightly, and the mouth of the bag is brought on to the surface of the abdomen. If a 15 mm trocar has been used, it may be necessary to slightly enlarge the incision just above the umbilicus to allow a finger to be inserted into the retrieval bag to finger fracture the spleen.

The spleen is fractured, and tension is put on to the bag to push the fractured segments of the spleen through the abdominal wall where they can be removed using sponge-holding forceps. The sequence of finger fracturing the spleen, traction on bag to force the fractured particle into the mouth of the bag, and removal by the sponge-holding forceps is continued until the whole of the spleen is removed. This produces large chunks of spleen which are adequate for histology.

If the Espiner bag is used, an 18 mm trocar is necessary. The bag is introduced via the trocar. The posterior part of the bag, with the removal tape attached, is placed posterior to the spleen. The pouch of the bag is opened and, with downward traction on its superior aspect, the spleen is pushed into the bag. The tapes are then tightened around the bag to complete the capture of the spleen. The spleen is finally removed as described above. The Espiner bag is made of parachute material and is much stronger than the Endocatch which is made of plastic; much more tension can be applied to the former bag as there is no fear of it bursting.

When the spleen has been removed, the supraumbilical trocar site is closed with PDS and with fine, subcuticular PDS to skin. The abdomen is then reinsufflated to check the area of the splenic bed. This is done using a telescope in the lumbar port. Any remaining blood can be aspirated with a sucker and, if necessary, a redivac drain can be inserted via the 5 mm subcostal trocar. The remaining trocar sites are closed with PDS and fine PDS for skin closure. Postoperatively, oral fluids can commence as soon as the patient is comfortable.

⚠ Hints and Pitfalls

- The use of a 30° telescope is essential. A 0° telescope will not give satisfactory visualization of the inferior aspects of the dissection.
- In very large patients, it may be necessary to change the position of the primary trocar from just above the umbilicus, further up towards the left costal margin. The telescope may not be long enough to get good visualization, particularly in dissection of the superior pole of the spleen under these circumstances.
- If the patient has a very large left heptic lobe that obscures the upper part of the stomach and part of the spleen, it may be necessary to insert a retractor to elevate the liver. The stomach and spleen can thus be exposed in order to dissect the upper short gastric vessels and mobilize the superior pole of the spleen. This is best done using a Nathansen retractor which fixes the retraction to an external clamp and will keep the liver retracted for the duration of the procedure.
- The tip of the UltraCision scalpel becomes very hot with use and care should be taken to prevent the tip

from coming into contact with the stomach wall as this may lead to a perforation.

> Editor's tip: By turning the inactive blade towards sensible structures, the risk of injuries from the active blade might be diminished.

- The final mobilization of spleen tissue from the diaphragm may be facilitated by employing a left-side down tilt as described by Richardson et al. in the so-called "hanging spleen" position.
- At all stages during dissection it is most important not to traumatize the splenic capsule as splenunculi may result from spilled healthy splenocytes.

 ## Personal Experience

We have performed laparoscopic splenectomies in 27 patients over the last 18 months. There have been no deaths or intraoperative conversions but two significant complications have required delayed laparotomy for short gastric vessel bleeding (one patient) and for a late greater curve perforation on the third day (one patient).

This latter complication is thought to have been caused by inadvertently incorporating the greater curve in the jaws of the UltraCision scalpel during activation and a delayed thermal injury ensued. The remaining 25 operations were uncomplicated. The median operative time was 110 minutes, but it decreased during the learning curve in keeping with the experience of others. Now, for non-enlarged spleens, it takes only little longer than for open splenectomy. The median length of hospital stay was four days. Our finding of three splenunculi in this series corresponds closely with the reported incidence of splenunculi of 10–15% in autopsy series. To date we are not aware of any instance of persistent splenic tissue function postoperatively. This latter problem has been raised as being peculiar to the laparoscopic approach where it is perceived that there is a higher incidence of splenic capsular tears, splenic tissue spillage, and a higher potential for missing accessory spleens. Meticulous attention to avoid intraoperative splenic damage is required and attention paid to the efficient removal of the spleen from the abdomen either via the retrieval bags, which are still improving in design, or by separate incision. In our experience removal of the specimen can often be the most troublesome part of the procedure.

> Editor's tip: The large skin incision for safe retrieval of the specimen is a minor problem compared to splenic tissue spillage.

 ## Discussion

Laparoscopy is now the procedure of choice for performing elective splenectomy. The postoperative benefits enjoyed by the patient through avoiding an uncomfortable upper abdominal scar are hugely gratifying. The UltraCision scalpel has been largely responsible for its acceptance on a wide scale. Numerous, sizeable series of patients are reported, all attesting to the benefits of laparoscopic splenectomy over open splenectomy. Large spleens are still problematic for this approach. Improvements in the techniques of specimen retrieval will no doubt solve this problem. Complications do occur but can be minimized by attention to surgical detail.

 ## Suggested Reading

Cadiere GB, Verroken R, Himpens J, Bruyns J, Efira M, De Wit S. Operative strategy in laparoscopic splenectomy, J Am Coll Surg 1994; 179: 668–72.

Emmerman A, Zornig C, Peiper M, et al. Laparoscopic splenectomy: technique and results in a series of 27 cases. Surg Endosc 1995; 9: 924–7.

Poulin EC, Thibault C, Mamazza J. Laparoscopic splenectomy. Surg Endosc 1995; 9: 172–7.

Hyatt JR, Phillips EH, Morgenstern L. Surgical Diseases of the Spleen. Heidelberg, Berlin: Springer Verlag; 1997.

Taragona EM, Espert JJ, Cerdan G, Belague C, Piulachs J, Sugranes G, Atrigas V, Trias M. Effect of spleen size on splenectomy outcome. A comparison of open and laparoscopic surgery. Surg Endosc 1999; 13: 559–62.

Gigot JF, Lengele B, Gianello P, Etienne J, Claeys N. Present status of laparoscopic splenectomy for haematologic diseases: Certitudes and unresolved issues. Sem Laparosc Surg 1998; 5: 147–67.

Richardson WS, Smith CD, Branum CD, Hunter JG. Leaning spleen: A new approach to laparoscopic splenectomy. J Am Coll Surg 1997; 185: 412–5.

Targarona EM, Espert J-J, Balague C, Surgranes G, Ayuso C, Lomena F, Bosch F, Trias M. Residual splenic function after laparoscopic splenectomy: A clinical concern. Arch Surg 1998; 133: 56–60.

Gigot J-F, Jamar F. Ferrant A, van Beers BE, Lengele B, Pauwels S, Pringot J, Kerstens P-J, Gianello P, Detry R. Inadequate detection of accessory spleens and splenosis with laparoscopic splenectomy. Surg Endosc 1998; 12: 101–6.

Friedman RL, Hiatt JR, Korman JL, Facklis K, Cymerman J, Phillips EH. Laparoscopic or open splenectomy for hematologic disease: which approach is superior? J Am Coll Surg 1997; 185: 49–54.

Katkhouda N, Hurwitz MB, Rivea RT, Chandra M, Waldrep DJ, Gugenheim J, Mouiel J. Laparoscopic splenectomy. Outcome and efficacy in 103 consecutive patients. Ann Surg 1998; 228: 568–73.

Szold A, Sagi B, Klausner JM. Optimizing laparoscopic splenectomy. Technical details and experience in 59 patients, Surg Endosc 1998; 12: 1078–81.

Decker G, Millat B, Guillon F, Atger J, Linon M. Laparoscopic splenectomy for benign and malignant diseases: 35 consecutive cases. World J Surg 1998; 22: 62–8.

Trias M, Targarona EM, Espert JJ, Balague C. Laparoscopic surgery for splenic disorders. Lessons learned from a series of 64 cases. Surg Endosc 1998; 12: 66–72.

19 Pancreatic Resection with the 10 mm UltraCision.Shears for Open (CS 6S) and Laparoscopic Surgery (LCS 15)

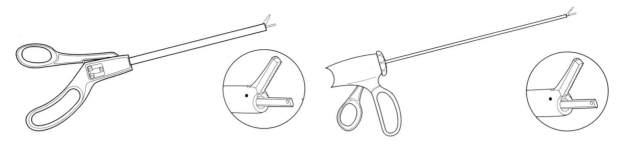

P. C. Giulianotti

Throughout the 1970s duodenopancreatectomy (DP) carried a hospital mortality rate in the range of 25%; some believed that the operation should be abandoned (6, 12). During the 1980s, however, this changed dramatically, with many centers reporting hospital mortality rates of less than 5%. The reason for this improvement involves several factors: better anesthesia, intensive care support, and perhaps specialization within surgery have all played important roles (5, 7, 28).

Familiarity with anatomy, reduction of operative time, and lower operative blood loss, as well as better anticipation and management of postoperative complications have been major factors. But improvements in technology, materials, combined with the lessons learned from minimally invasive surgery, minimal tissue trauma, minimal losses, and perfect anatomical dissection, have also provided a major benefit.

Today, virtually any patient who is acceptable for general anesthesia can undergo duodenopancreatectomy with little risk of hospital mortality. Since the operation can be performed with low risk, the indications for resection have greatly expanded (5, 19).

The introduction of the UltraCision scalpel is one of the most important technological improvements of recent years. It allows a delicate and effective hemostasis, avoiding the risk of electric and thermal injury (1, 16).

The operative blood and lymphatic losses that were one of the main causes of morbidity have been dramatically reduced by the use of the UltraCision scalpel. This technology may be used both in open and laparoscopic surgery, where previously impracticable operations have been made routinely feasible (14, 22).

Two standard operations will be presented here: right pancreatectomy which is still essentially an open procedure, and left pancreatectomy, which is becoming a laparoscopic standard.

Indication and Preoperative Management

The indications for pancreatic resections are a variety of neoplasms of the pancreas, duodenum, ampulla of Vater and distal common bile duct, and certain complications of chronic pancreatitis and trauma (2, 19, 27, 30).

Surgical resection of pancreatic cancer still remains the best therapeutic option, even though few patients are cured (30). There have been some encouraging results in survival, and further improvements are expected from combining adjuvant chemotherapy and radiation therapy (2).

The diagnostic evaluation of patients with suspected cancer comprises ultrasound (US), spiral computed tomography (CT), upper gastrointestinal endoscopy, and baseline serum markers. Angiography, endoscopic retrograde cholangiopancreatography (ERCP), nuclear magnetic resonance (NMR), fine needle aspiration cytology (FNAC), endoscopic US (EUS), and staging laparoscopy are indicated in selected cases (15, 19, 22).

Most patients with cancer have significant weight loss and various durations of jaundice. Preoperative endoscopic stenting may result in cholangitis; this is avoided if the laparotomy is planned (19). The jaundiced patient is given parenteral vitamin K preoperatively and the prothrombin level is monitored; fresh frozen plasma may be required intraoperatively.

Preoperative preparation should address those clinical profiles that are usually tested for any individual undergoing general anesthesia and major abdominal procedures (2). Preparation of the patient for surgery includes bowel cleansing the day before operation. Prior to arrival in the operating theater an initial dose of broad-spectrum antibiotic is administered intravenously and antiembolism cuffs are applied. A urinary Foley catheter and nasogastric tube are inserted. A central venous line is prepared.

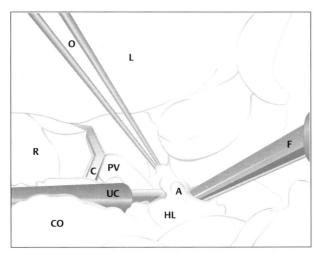

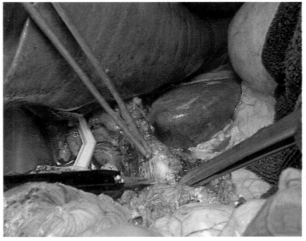

Fig. 19.**1** Resection of the hepatoduodenal ligament. The inactive side of the UltraCision shears gently slides over the hepatic artery. *UC* UltraCision, *HL* hepatoduodenal ligament, *O* operator forceps, *F* first assistant forceps, *A* hepatic artery, *C* clamp on the bile duct, *PV* portal vein, *L* liver, *CO* colon (right flexure), *R* retractor.

 Operation

Right Pancreatectomy

For the open DP procedure patients are positioned supine, the chest and abdomen are shaved and draped, including the femoral and cervical regions for vascular access.

The instruments required are those for general abdominal operation with the integration of a vascular kit, the UltraCision 10 mm shears for open surgery (needle holder hand grip CS6S) and a linear cutter.

The usual approach is a bilateral subcostal incision. The first step is an accurate inspection of the entire peritoneal cavity for evidence of metastatic disease, especially in the liver, omentum, peritoneal surface, and periaortic nodes.

Peritoneal washing cytology and intraoperative US are an integral part of the preliminary assessment.

The sharp side of the rotating active blade of the 10 mm shears is used to divide the lateral peritoneum along the hepatic flexure of the colon, which is mobilized medially and inferiorly away from the duodenum. Next, the blunt or flat side is used to incise the thickened the often vascularized peritoneum lateral to the duodenal loop.

> Editor's tip: When the UltraCision shears are open, more of the effect is transmitted from the active blade to the tissues.

A generous Kocher maneuver is performed, elevating the head of the pancreas containing the tumor and palpating the superior mesenteric artery and vein to ensure that these vessels are not encased by a tumor extending from the uncinate process.

The gastrocolic ligament is opened starting from the left side where the lesser cavity may be more easily entered. This step is very efficiently done with UltraCision using the flat side of the active blade (level 5).

The gastroepiploic vessels along the greater curvature are preserved if a pylorus-sparing procedure (PPDP) is to be performed.

Through the gastrocolic space, the anterior surface of the pancreas can be examined. The greater omentum is easily detached from the right half of the colon using the sharp side of the shears.

> Editor's tip: While the assistant holds the greater omentum firmly and steadily, the surgeon can adjust the tension in the tissues by varying the traction of the transverse colon. More tension means faster cutting.

The gallbladder is grasped at the fundus and detached from its hepatic bed in a subserous, avascular plane that is easily found by pricking the serosa with the active tip of the instrument. Any oozing from the hepatic bed is controlled with the flat side of the shears. The cystic artery is divided in the same way.

The entire dissection of the hepatoduodenal ligament is performed with the blunt side (level 5), starting from the hilum and gently sliding down the vascular and biliary structures performing a complete lymphadenectomy (Fig. 19.**1**).

In order to facilitate skeletonization, the hepatic artery and common bile duct are encircled with umbilical tape.

The hepatic duct is divided with normal scissors (to avoid any tissue trauma for the anastomosis) just proximal to the cystic duct. A cross-section of the duct is excised for frozen section. The distal bile duct and gallbladder are pulled down, leaving a clean portal vein

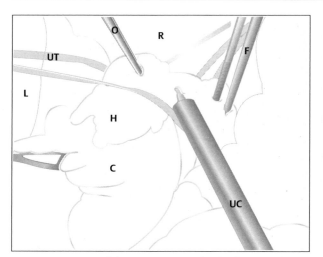
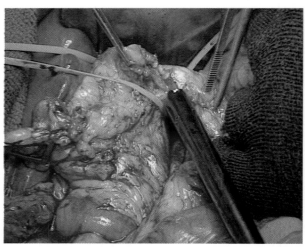

Fig. 19.**2**   Section of the pancreatic neck. The flat side of the UltraCision shears used at level 3. *UC* UltraCision, *UT* umbilical tape under the neck, *H* head of the pancreas, *L* liver, *O* operator forceps, *F* first assistant forceps, *R* retractor.

and hepatic artery. The small right gastric artery is divided with the flat side of the UltraCision blade; the larger gastroduodenal artery is cautiously sectioned between ligatures.

> Editor's tip: To enhance fluent progress of the intervention, the vessel between the ligatures and the threads of the ligatures can easily be divided with the UltraCision shears or even the active blade alone.

The dissection of the hepatic artery is continued right up to the celiac axis.

The next step in the classical Whipple procedure is the gastric division, which allows a better exposure of the anterior surface of the pancreas. The stomach is transected through the mid-body above the incisura (hemigastrectomy).

The gastroepiploic arcade is divided with the flat side of the UltraCision shears; the left gastric artery and vein are sectioned in the same way (the artery may be ligated) near the gastric wall to permit cleaning of the periaortic lymph nodes at the origin of these vessels.

> Editor's tip: The left gastric artery should be ligated because most of the time this vessel is larger than 3 mm and with too much traction in the vessel the hemostasis will fail.

For an ampullary or small pancreatic tumor a pylorus-preserving resection is possible; in this case the duodenum is transected below the pylorus, leaving about 1.5–2 cm of duodenum. The right gastroepiploic artery is divided in PPDP near the pylorus, as is the right gastric artery, so that the proximal portion of the artery remains attached to the pancreatic specimen, allowing the removal of the retropyloric nodes. The incision of the peritoneum of the transverse mesocolon

with the sharp blade along the inferior border of the gland allows the exposition of the superior mesenteric vein at the splenomesenteric confluence.

With the help of two hanging stitches, the neck of the pancreas is lifted and may be transected with the flat side (level 3) (Fig. 19.**2**). There are usually two small arteries in the cut surface of the gland which are controlled with the UltraCision scalpel; sometimes they need a few 4/0 prolene suture ligatures.

The division of the pancreas exposes the portal vein. The main pancreatic duct is identified on the caudal side of the transection. Identification of Wirsung's duct may occasionally be uncertain if the gland is soft and the duct small (the duct may be occluded by the UltraCision scalpel, but the occlusion may be transient and may cause juice leakage).

> Editor's tip: In distal pancreatectomy, ultrasonic division significantly reduced the incidence of pancreatic fistulas compared with conventional techniques in a randomised trial (25). In both arms, the pancreatic duct was ligated.

The head of the pancreas is rotated to the patient's right and the dissection is extended to completely free the superior mesenteric vein from the uncinate lobe.

Holding the specimen in the left hand and making traction towards the right facilitates the dissection. This phase may be performed entirely with the flat side of the blade (level 3), dividing the small branches of the superior mesenteric artery and the venous tributaries to the superior mesenteric vein.

Occasionally, bleeding from small tears of the mesenteric vein may be controlled with finger pressure followed by repair with 6/0 prolene. The superior mesenteric artery and vein can be completely skeletonized. The jejunum distal to the ligament of Treitz (about 15 cm) is divided with a linear stapler and its tributary vessels (quite short) are controlled close to

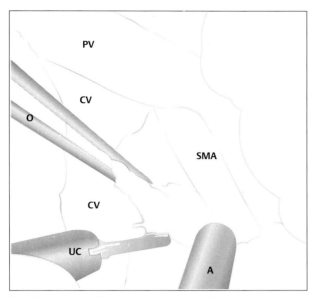

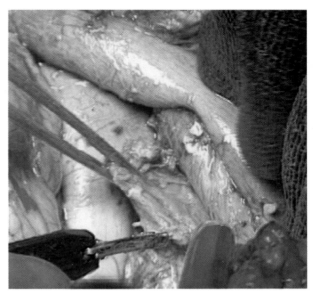

Fig. 19.**3** Lymphadenectomy is completed by clearing the tissues around the superior mesenteric artery with the blunt side of the UltraCision shears at level 5. *UC* UltraCision, *O* operator forceps, *A* aspiration, *CV* caval vein, *PV* portal vein, *SMA* superior mesenteric artery.

the wall of the bowel (flat side, level 3), taking account of the position of the SMA.

Upon completion of the dissection, the jejunum may be rotated and brought behind the superior mesenteric vessels so that the entire specimen may be resected. In cases of cancer, the resection may be completed by extending the field of lymphatic and soft tissue clearance (Fig. 19.**3**). The pancreatic stump is mobilized to allow a further resection of 3–5 cm towards the tail and all lymph nodes of the periaortic area may be removed (extended lymphadenectomy).

This phase of the operation may be performed entirely by alternating the blunt and the flat side of the shears, UltraCision, level 3–5. Reconstruction can then proceed in the preferred way.

Laparoscopic Left Pancreatectomy

Preoperative preparation The operation is performed under general anesthesia with endotracheal intubation. A nasogastric tube is inserted to keep the stomach deflated and the patient's urinary bladder is catheterized.

The supine position used in the earlier experience with laparoscopic splenectomy is replaced by a right lateral decubitus position with the left side up at a 60° angle to allow gravity to retract the organs in a modified Delaitre-Gagner position (11) (Fig. 19.**4a, b**).

The table is broken slightly to open the flank space between the ribs and the iliac crest. Reverse Trendelenburg is added and the patient is rotated slightly to the anterior side. The patient is secured safety to the operating table to permit changes in gravitational retraction.

The following choice of instruments is recommended:

- 3 × 10 mm ports (camera, UltraCision, Babcock, suction/irrigation)
- 2 × 5 mm ports (assistant complementary retraction, suction/irrigation)
- UltraCision 10 mm shears (LCS15)
- Babcock grasper
- 2 × 5 mm grasping instruments
- One needle holder
- 3/0 prolene sutures
- One Endolinear cutter (vascular stitches)
- One Endobag
- Suction-irrigation device
- 30° optical scope
- US laparoscopic probe

The pneumoperitoneum is created by an open or closed technique. The abdomen is insufflated with CO_2 and the intra-abdominal pressure is maintained between 12 and 14 mmHg.

Port sites are: 10 mm umbilical port for laparoscope, 10 mm lateral left subcostal for surgeon's right hand (UC, stapler), 10 mm right subcostal for surgeon's left hand (Babcock), 5 mm lateral right subcostal for first assistant (retraction, suction, irrigation), 5 mm lateral left for second assistant (complementary retraction) (Fig. 19.**4**).

After full exploration of the abdominal cavity to check for metastatic lesions or other incidental pathologies, the other ports are inserted with minimal adjustment according to the patient's anatomy.

Endolaparoscopic echography is performed before starting the dissection to evaluate the liver, to clear the pancreatic vascular anatomy, and localize the tumor (20). The preparation is started with the blunt side of the UltraCision shears (level 3) opening the

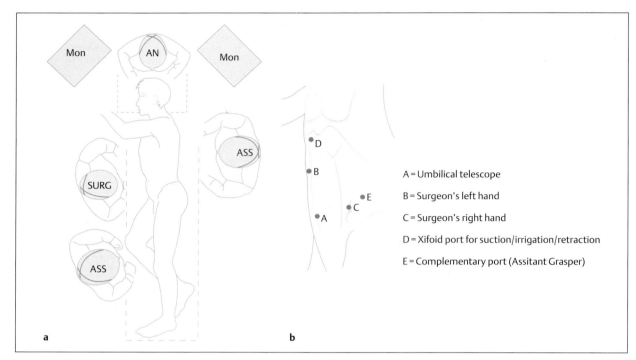

Fig. 19.**4 a, b**   Patient and port positioning for laparoscopic left pancreatectomy.

lesser sac while preserving the gastroepiploic arcade vessels.

The gastrocolic omentum is divided with the blunt side of the UltraCision shears (level 3), using the active tip to open the avascular fat and then picking up the vessels between the blades.

The short gastric vessels are divided with the flat side of the shears (level 3), exposing the entire anterior surface of the pancreas and spleen. The splenic artery is easily identified at the superior border of the gland, and isolated from surrounding tissue near its origin from the celiac axis. A blunt right-angle dissector is helpful. The artery is sectioned with a vascular Endolinear cutter.

Making a downward retraction of the left colonic flexure with the Babcock, the phrenocolic and splenocolic ligaments are completely detached with the sharp blade (level 5) exposing all the inferior border of the pancreatic body.

The ligament of Treitz is divided, preserving the inferior mesenteric vein. (Sometimes it is necessary to allow a wide mobilization of the body up to the neck over the portal vein, and to divide the inferior mesenteric vein between clips.)

The spleen is mobilized from the diaphragm at the end (the hanging spleen simplifies the earlier steps of the procedure) by incision of its lateral peritoneal attachments, allowing medial and inferior rotation of the spleen and tail of the pancreas (Fig. 19.**5**). The body is then bluntly dissected from the retroperitoneum and Gerota's fascia through an avascular plane.

A site, 2–3 cm proximal to the tumor, is identified where the pancreas can be transected. The splenic vein

may be gently isolated from the posterior aspect of the pancreatic body (blunt, level 3). But, if there is some difficulty or bleeding, the vein may be stapled along with the pancreas. If the gland is soft, a linear stapling device may be used; if it has become hard due to chronic pancreatitis, it may be transected by UltraCision (level 3) (see previous editor's tip) (Fig. 19.**6**).

A closed suction drain is placed near the stump of the pancreas and brought out through a side port.

 Hints and Pitfalls

Right Pancreatectomy

- During the dissection of the hepatoduodenal ligament, and when skeletonizing the vessels, be careful with the active tip of shears and work with gentle movements, sliding on the structures and turning away from them while in action.

  Editor's tip: When turning the inactive blade towards the vessels and the common bile duct during activation of the instrument, the risk of injury is diminished.

- An aberrant, right hepatic artery originates from the superior mesenteric artery in 20% of cases and is usually situated on the right side of the portal vein and common bile duct. It must be detected and preserved, as it is sometimes necessary to resect and re-implant it (3).

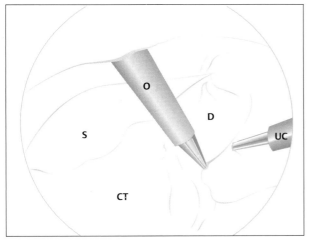
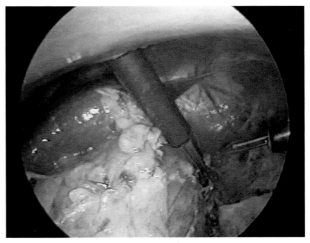

Fig. 19.**5**   Medial and inferior rotation of the spleen and tail of the pancreas after the spleen is mobilized from the diaphragm. *S* spleen, *CT* cystic tumor, *UC* UltraCision, *D* diaphragm, *O* operator forceps.

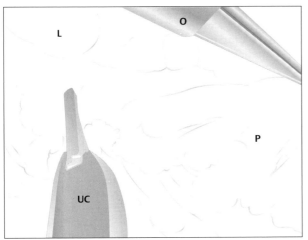
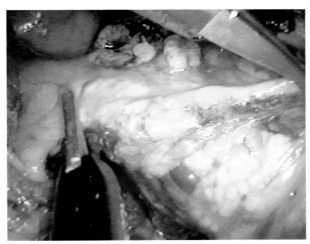

Fig. 19.**6**   Ultracision transection of the pancreatic body during a laparoscopic splenopancreatectomy. *P* pancreas, *UC* UltraCision, *L* liver, *O* operator forceps.

- If a pancreatojejunal anastomosis is to be performed, take care in performing hemostasis on the pancreatic stump to avoid involuntary occlusion of the duct of Wirsung, picked between bites of tissue.
- Before starting the dissection of the uncinate process, it is worthwhile to prepare and expose the SMA on the left of the superior mesenteric vein. This provides a reference point for working more expeditiously with the UltraCision shears.
- Bleeding from small tears in the mesenteric vein can usually be controlled with finger pressure, followed by repair with 6–0 vascular sutures.

Laparoscopic Left Pancreatectomy

- If the lesion is bulky and hampers the preliminary isolation of the splenic artery, it is advisable not to insist on preparing the vessels at the beginning of the procedure but to mobilize the whole splenopancreatic block first and then to handle the artery from behind (Fig. 19.**7**).
- The most common postoperative complication after laparoscopic pancreatic resection and enucleation is pancreatic fistula. The incidence of this complication may be reduced by suture-closure of the transected pancreatic duct and application of fibrin glue (9).

Editor's tip: Suture closure of the pancreatic duct is always recommended to diminish the frequency of pancreatic fistulas. The UltraCision shears seems to be the most reliable intraoperative tool for pancreatic division and can be combined with octreotide administration and fibrin glue sealing.

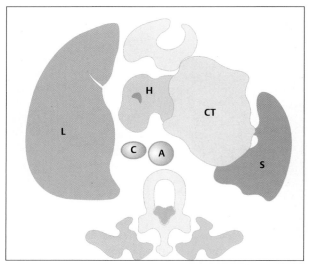 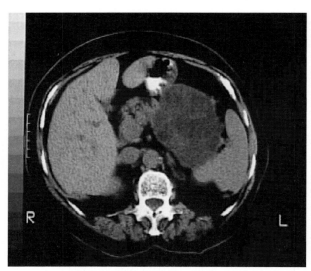

Fig. 19.**7**   Computed tomography scan showing the large cystic tumor of the tail of the pancreas. *L* liver, *S* spleen, *CT* cystic tumor, *A* aorta, *C* caval vein, *H* head of pancreas.

If there is some technical trouble, the procedure may be hand-assisted utilizing a small, muscle-splitting right lower quadrant incision. This allows for palpation of the peritoneal cavity and for safe and expeditious pancreatectomy (18).

● During the dissection of the short gastric vessels, it is advisable not to work close to the gastric wall, but to stay at a little distance, so that if there is some bleeding it easier to pick the vascular stump again with the blunt side (level 3).

● In handling the spleen, particular care is necessary to avoid capsular tears during splenic mobilization. In case of bleeding do not try to coagulate on the capsula, but use a sponge to apply compression though the assistant's port.

 Personal Experience

In the last three years we can report 71 consecutive cases of pancreatic resections (open and laparoscopic surgery). The patients were divided in two groups: Group A, containing 26 patients operated with the Ul-traCision scalpel; Group B, containing 45 patients submitted to traditional surgery.

In Group A, 16 patients received a pancreatoduo-denectomy (DP) and 10 patients a splenopancreat-ectomy (SP) (seven of which laparoscopically); in Group B, 36 had DP and nine had SP; 19 vascular resections were associated (four in Group A and 15 in Group B).

Mean intraoperative blood loss was 273.1 ± 211.2 ml (Group A) and 563.1 ± 334.1 ml (Group B), respectively.

The mean length of the operation was statistically similar in the two groups (350.0 ± 97.5 minutes to 368.6 ± 110.8 minutes).

There were five postoperative deaths: two in Group A (cardiac failure and stump necrotizing pancreatitis)

and three in Group B (leukemic recurrence, pneumonia, and progression of a metastatic disease).

Five patients in Group A and nine in Group B had a low-output pancreatic fistula (13 DP with stump sclerosis and one SP).

Morbidity was 23.1 % in Group A and 24.4 % in Group B. The mean hospital stay for the patients without complications was similar (about 15 days).

Discussion

Ultrasonic dissection may contribute to a further lowering of the postoperative morbidity in pancreatic resections. In open surgery it reduces blood and lymphatic losses, does not increase operating times, and, on the whole, clinically improves the quality of the postoperative course. Blood loss and the need for transfusion seem to correlate with the oncological prognosis (4).

Lymphatic losses may contribute to the immunological impairment of patients submitted to surgery.

The "gold standard" of DP is still the open procedure (8, 21, 23). No benefits seem to be derived, at the moment, from the use of a complete laparoscopic Whipple operation, which still remains an experimental matter (9, 13, 29). In a series of ten patients, Gagner reported a rate of conversion to an open procedure of 40 % and complications were seen in the non-converted group. The average operating time was 8.5 hours and the hospital stay was 22.3 days (13).

On the other hand, acquiring experience with the use of ultrasonic dissection in open surgery gives the operator the skill and confidence to also work in laparoscopic surgery and it may constitute an optimal procedural training.

Laparoscopic distal pancreatectomy, with or without splenectomy and enucleation, is technically easier to perform and seems to greatly benefit patients by improving morbidity and shortening hospital stay (9, 17, 24). Careful patient selection is important. These operations should be only be attempted by surgeons who have experience in open pancreatic surgery and who have acquired the necessary advanced laparoscopic skills (8, 9, 10, 23, 24, 25, 26, 29).

Acknowledgements

I want to express my consideration and gratitude to Doctor Tommaso Balestracci and Doctor Giuseppe Caravaglios for their valuable assistance.

References

1. Amaral JF. Ultrasonic dissection. Endosc Surg Allied Technol 1994; 2: 181–5.
2. Bearly RM. Pancreatic cancer. In: McKenna RJ, Murphy GP. editors. Cancer Surgery. New York: Lippincott Company; 1994. pp. 105–18.
3. Branum G, Skandalakis LJ. Pancreas and duodenum. In: Wood WC, Skandalakis JE. editors. Anatomic basis of Tumor Surgery. St. Louis: Quality Medical Publishing; 1999. pp. 600–43.
4. Cameron JL, Crist DW, Sitzmann JV, Hruban RH, Boitnott JK, Seidler AJ, et al. Factors influencing survival following pancreatoduodenectomy for pancreatic cancer. Am J Surg 1991; 161: 120–4.
5. Cameron JL, Henry AP, Charles JY, Keith D, Lillemoe HS, Kaufman S. One hundred and forty-five consecutive pancreaticoduodenectomies without mortality. Ann Surg 1993; 217: 430–8.
6. Crile G Jr. The advantages of bypass operations over pancreaticoduodenectomy in the treatment of pancreatic cancer. SG&O 1970; 130: 1049–53.
7. Crist DW, Sitzmann JV, Cameron JL. Improved hospital morbidity, mortality, and survival after the Whipple procedure. Ann Surg 1987; 206: 358–65.
8. Cuschieri A. Laparoscopy for pancreatic cancer: does it benefit the patient? Eur J Surg Oncol 1998; 14: 41–4.
9. Cuschieri SA, Jakimowicz JJ. Laparoscopic pancreatic resection. Semin Laparosc Surg 1998; 5: 168–79.
10. Cuschieri A, Jakimowicz JJ, van Spreeuwel J. Laparoscopic distal 70% pancreatectomy and splenectomy for chronic pancreatitis. Ann Surg 1996; 223: 280–5.
11. Delaitre B. Laparoscopic splenectomy: "the hanged spleen" technique. Surg End 1995; 9: 528–9.
12. Fingerhut A, Cudeville C. Laparoscopic bypass for inoperable disease of the pancreas. Semin Laparosc Surg 199; 3: 10–4.
13. Gagner M, Pomp A. Laparoscopic pancreatic resection: is it worthwhile? J Gastrointest Surg 1997; 1: 20–6.
14. Gill BS, MacFayden BV Jr. Ultrasonic dissectors and minimally invasive surgery. Semin Laparosc Surg 1999; 6: 229–34.
15. Gouma DJ, Nieveen van Dijkun EJ, De Wit LT, Obertop H. Laparoscopic staging of biliopancreatic malignancy. Ann Oncol 1999; 10 Suppl 4: 33–6.
16. Kanehira E, Kinoshita T, Omura K. Fundamental principles and pitfalls linked to the use of ultrasonic scissors. Ann Chir 2000; 125: 363–9.
17. Kimura W, Inoue T, Futakawa N, Shinkai H, Han I, Muto T. Spleen-preserving distal pancreatectomy with conservation of the splenic artery and vein. Surgery 1996; 120: 885–90.
18. Klingler PJ, Hinder RA, Menke DM, Smith SL. Hand-assisted laparoscopic distal pancreatectomy for pancreatic cystadenoma. Surg Laparosc Endosc 1998; 8: 180–4.
19. Howard JM. Pancreatoduodenectomy (Whipple resection) with skeletonization of vessels for cancers of the pancreas and adjacent organs. In: Ihse I, Prinz R, Idezuck Y. editors. Surgical Disease of the Pancreas. 3 rd edn., Baltimore: Williams and Wilkins; 1998.
20. Menak MJ, Arregui ME. Laparoscopic sonography of the biliary tree and pancreas. Surg Clin North Am 2000; 80: 1151–70.
21. Park A, Schwartz R, Tandan V, Anvari M. Laparoscopic pancreatic surgery. Am J Surg. 1999; 177: 158–63.
22. Rumstadt B, Schwab M, Schuster K, Hagmuller E, Trede M. The role of laparoscopy in the preoperative staging of pancreatic carcinoma. J Gastrointest Surg 1997; 1: 245–50.
23. Salky BA, Edye M. Laparoscopic pancreatectomy. Surg Clin North Am 1996; 76: 539–45.
24. Sugo H, Mikami Y, Matsumoto F, Tsumura H, Watanabe Y, Futagawa S. Distal pancreatectomy using the harmonic scalpel. Surgery 2000; 128: 490–1.
25. Suzuki Y, Fujino Y, Tanioka Y, Hori Y, Ueda T, Takeyama Y, Tominaga M, Ku Y, Yamamoto YM, Kuroda Y. Randomized clinical trial of ultrasonic dissector or conventional division in distal pancreatectomy for non-fibrotic pancreas. Br J Surg 1999; 86: 608–11.
26. Takao S, Shinchi H, Maemura K, Aikou T. Ultrasonically activated scalpel is an effective tool for cutting the pancreas in biliary-pancreatic surgery: experimental and clinical studies. J Hepatobiliary Pancreat Surg 2000; 7: 58–62.
27. Trede M. Technique of Whipple pancreatoduodenectomy. In: Trede M, Carter DC. editors. Surgery of the Pancreas. New York, NY: Churchill Livingstone; 1997. pp. 487–98.
28. Trede M, Chir B, Hon FRCS, Schwall G. The complications of pancreatectomy. Ann Surg 1988; 207: 39–47.
29. Underwood RA, Soper NJ: Current status of laparoscopic surgery of the pancreas. J Hepatobiliary Pancreat Surg 1999; 6: 154–64.
30. Wanebo HJ, Koness RJ. Pancreatic Cancer: Surgical Approach. In: James D, Ahlgren JS, MacDonald JB. editors. Gastrointestinal Oncology. Philadelphia: Lippincott Company; 1992. pp. 209–14.

20 Laparoscopic Adrenalectomy with the 10 mm UltraCision Shears (LCS 15 Pistol Hand Grip or LCS 6S Needle Hand Grip)

C. Haglund, J. Sirén

Surgical handling of patients with adrenal tumors depends on the endocrine function of the tumor and on which method the surgeon is familiar with. Adrenal tumors are often small and benign. Therefore, they are well suited for mini-invasive surgery. The first report of laparoscopic adrenalectomy was published in 1992 (9). Like many other mini-invasive operations, laparoscopic adrenalectomy has, in a short period of time, gained great popularity, and numerous reports on early experience of the method have been published (5, 15, 17, 18, 19). Prospective randomized studies to compare open and laparoscopic adrenalectomy have not been performed, but in many hospitals throughout the world laparoscopic adrenalectomy has become the new "gold standard" in adrenal surgery. Laparoscopic adrenalectomy has proven to be a convenient and safe technique. It is associated with less postoperative pain and shorter hospital stay compared to the open method (3), and it has shown to be cost-effective.

Indication and Preoperative Management

The indications for adrenalectomy are clear: hormone-producing tumors, large tumors (>4 cm), suspected or verified malignancy, tumors that grow during follow-up, and symptomatic tumors. Hormone-producing tumors may be cortical tumors producing aldosterone (Conn's syndrome) or cortisol (Cushing's adenoma) or medullary tumors, pheochromocytomas, producing catecholamines. In rare cases, bilateral adrenalectomy is recommended because of cortical hyperplasia (Cushing's disease) (2).

An increasing number of adrenal tumors today are found by coincidence during ultrasound, CT scan, or MRI performed as diagnostic procedures for reasons other than suspicion of adrenal tumor. These tumors are called "incidentalomas." The advantage of laparoscopic adrenalectomy over open surgery should not change the policy in handling incidentalomas. Some incidentalomas are hormonally active. Therefore, all incidentaloma patients should be screened for hormonal overproduction. Hormonally inactive tumors smaller than 4 cm (some authors advocate 6 cm) in diameter, which show no tendency to grow during 3–6 months follow-up should not be operated on. For large tumors, surgery is recommended because of an increased risk of a malignancy.

Laparoscopic adrenalectomy is well suited for operation of most types of adrenal tumors. If malignancy is suspected, based on the size of the tumor or rapid growth, open operation should be considered. Laparoscopic operation of tumors larger than 10 cm is associated with an increased number of technical problems. Therefore, open surgery should be considered. In laparoscopic cholecystectomies of gallbladder carcinomas not known before operation and in laparoscopic surgery of colonic cancer, port site metastases have been described. There is limited data on the possible risks if malignant adrenal tumors are operated on laparoscopically.

It is extremely important to optimize the preoperative pharmacological adrenergic blockade treatment of patients with pheochromocytoma in order to avoid intraoperative problems with blood pressure control and cardiac arrhythmia.

Operation

The following choice of instruments is recommended:
- 30° laparoscope
- 3, 4, or 5 × 5–10 mm ports
- UltraCision 5 mm/10 mm shears
- 2 × 5 mm grasping instruments
- Liver retractor (in right-sided operations)
- Instrument holder for the liver retractor
- Suction device
- 1 × plastic bag (10 mm)

The following instruments may be used additionally or alternatively:

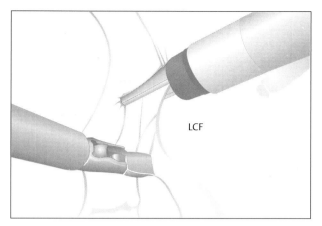 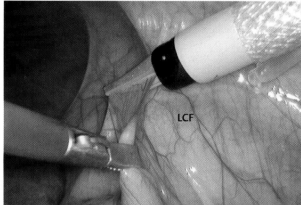

Fig. 20.**1** The peritoneal attachments of the splenic flexure of the colon are incised with the UltraCision shears. *LCF* left colonic flexure.

- 2 × needle holders (in case of bleedings that have to be sealed by suturing)
- 5/0 or 6/0 unresorbable monofilament sutures

There are four principal techniques to perform videoscopic adrenalectomy: anterior transabdominal, lateral transabdominal, lateral extraperitoneal, and posterior extraperitoneal. Most surgeons prefer the lateral transabdominal approach described by Gagner et al. (10, 12). There also are several reports on the extraperitoneal approach. The anterior transabdominal technique has mainly been used for bilateral adrenalectomy.

Lateral Transabdominal Laparoscopic Adrenalectomy

The patient is positioned in a lateral decubitus position with the side to be operated on up. The upper arm should be extended and suspended. The operating table should be extended at the waist to increase the space between the costal margin and the iliac crest. A 10–20° reverse Trendelenburg position is favorable. The surgeon and assistant stand on the anterior side of the patient. The monitor is placed on the opposite side behind the patient's shoulder. The assisting nurse stands on the opposite side to the surgeon. After establishing a 12 mmHg carbon dioxide pneumoperitoneum a 10 mm port for the camera is inserted between the costal margin and the umbilicus. One working port is inserted in the ventral axillary line and another in the dorsal axillary line. One to two additional 10 mm trocars are inserted below the costal margin when necessary. One trocar should be a traditional 10–12 mm trocar to allow enlargement of the port site when removing the specimen. The other ports can be trocars not requiring closure of the fascial layer. The 10 mm 30° laparoscope and, when necessary, a grasping forceps are held by the assistant. In right-sided adrenalectomy, a liver retractor is used to hold the liver. The liver retrac-

tor is handled by the assistant or alternatively fixed to a holding system. Dissection is preferably carried out using the UltraCision shears. Electrocautery may be used, but coagulation is more precise and secure with the UltraCision shears.

> Editor's Tip: When the UltraCision shears are activated for five seconds, it gives 1 mm lateral spread of thermal injury in the tissues compared to 5 mm with electrocautery.

The tissue effect of the UltraCision shears can be adjusted by the power setting of the generator, the pressure applied to the shears, and the shape of the blade.

Operation of the left adrenal The preparation is started with the sharp and/or blunt side of the UltraCision shears, which can also be used as a grasping and holding tool. The peritoneal attachments of the splenic flexure of the colon are incised (Fig. 20.**1**), when necessary, to expose the space between the spleen and the upper pole of the kidney. The peritoneum, i.e., splenorenal ligament, between spleen and kidney is incised beginning from the medial border of the spleen and continuing laterally towards the diaphragm (Fig. 20.**2**). A small cuff of peritoneum is left towards the spleen. The spleen does not have to be mobilized, although incision of the lower part of the splenophrenic ligament may help in many patients. The spleen may be lifted with the shaft of a grasper or if preferred with a liver retractor. At this point the adrenal gland may be identified superior and medial to the kidney by its typical bright yellow color. In many patients, retroperitoneal fat has to be dissected between the upper pole of the kidney and the spleen to expose the gland. When dissecting the superior and inferior borders of the adrenal, tissues are divided using the UltraCision shears (Fig. 20.**3**). The shears securely seal small arterial and venous branches. Care has to be taken not to injure the tail of the pancreas, which even

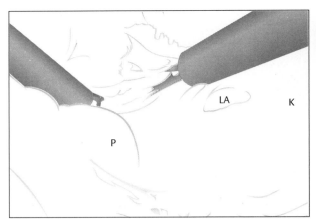
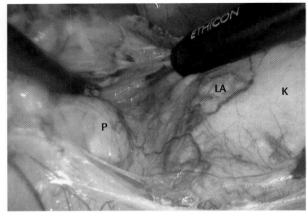

Fig. 20.**2**   The upper border of the left spleen is dissected using the UltraCision shears. *P* pancreatic tail, *K* kidney, *LA* left adrenal.

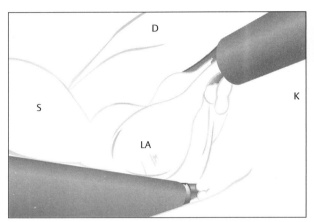
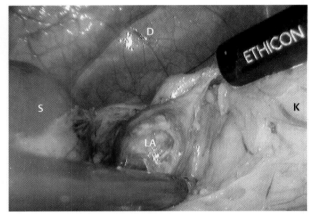

Fig. 20.**3**   The inferior border of the left spleen is dissected using the UltraCision shears. *LA* left adrenal, *S* spleen, *D* diaphragm, *K* kidney.

might be mistaken for the adrenal. During dissection grasping the adrenal gland should be avoided.

> Editor's Tip: A small tear in the adrenal gland can result in a severe bleeding impossible to deal with laparoscopically; therefore, keep away from the adrenal gland by using a grasper.

Preferably, the perinephric fat should be grasped or the gland should be lifted or pushed with a blunt grasper. If the gland has to be grasped, an atraumatic bowel grasper should be used. The adrenal vein should be divided early in the operation, when pheochromocytomas are operated on. In other types of lesions, it might be easier to divide it at a later stage of the operation after mobilization of the gland. The adrenal vein is located at the inferior medial corner of the gland and is usually the only structure that has to be divided between clips (Fig. 20.**4**). Occasionally, an accessory vein at the inferior border of the gland may be found and is divided between clips when necessary. All other dissections are performed with the UltraCision shears, which reliably transect all small vessels to the adrenal. Once the gland

is free, a plastic bag is introduced through a trocar of traditional model and the specimen is removed in one piece via the trocar site by spreading the muscle layer with a finger or by enlarging the incision when necessary, depending on the size of the tumor. Postoperative drainage of the operation site is not needed.

Operation of the right side   The right lobe of the liver is lifted with a retractor, which can be held by the assistant or alternatively fixed to a holding system. Mobilization of the right colonic flexure is seldom necessary. The triangular ligament is divided exposing the adrenal gland and the caval vein. The dissection can be started from the inferior or superior border of the adrenal. The medial border is freed next along the lateral edge of the caval vein and the adrenal vein is identified and clipped. An accessory adrenal vein is sometimes found at the upper border of the gland and must be searched for and divided between clips if encountered. All other vessels can be coagulated by the UltraCision shears.

Bilateral adrenalectomy   For bilateral operations an anterior transabdominal approach with the patient in

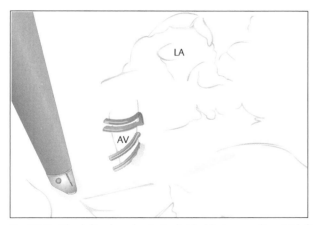 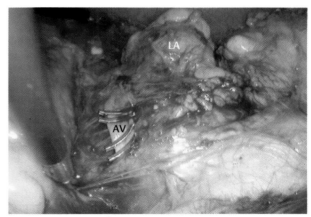

Fig. 20.**4** The left adrenal vein is divided between clips. *LA* left adrenal, *AV* adrenal vein.

a supine position can be used. However, this technique requires more dissection and retraction of adjacent organs than the lateral transabdominal approach (8). We find it easier to use the lateral approach and to reposition and redrape the patient between the two operations.

Lateral Extraperitoneal Videoscopic Adrenalectomy

The lateral extraperitoneal videoscopic adrenalectomy is performed on the patient in a semilateral position with the side of the tumor elevated. The retroperitoneal space is entered through an incision about 5 cm below the costal margin at the dorsal axillary line, and first dissected with a finger. A balloon trocar is then inserted and inflated, and then after a few minutes replaced with a blunt trocar. The space is maintained with carbon dioxide insufflation. An additional three trocars are inserted: one at the dorsal, one at the ventral border of the created space, and one below the costal margin along the dorsal axillary line. Gerota's capsule is opened and the superior pole of the kidney is identified. The gland is dissected free as in transabdominal procedures (16).

Posterior Extraperitoneal Videoscopic Adrenalectomy

The posterior extraperitoneal operation is performed on the patient in a prone semi-jack-knife position. The retroperitoneal space is entered 2–3 cm lateral to the 12th rib, and a balloon catheter is inserted aiming toward the costal-vertebral angle. After creation of a pneumoretroperitoneum as described above, three additional trocars are inserted, one medial just below the 12th rib, another 1 cm lateral to the 11th rib, and the third between the 9th and 10th ribs. The kidney is retracted downward from the medial trocar, and dissection takes place from the two lateral trocars, the camera being positioned at the first trocar. The dissec-

tion is started from the superior and anterior aspects of the gland at both sides. Retraction of the liver or spleen is not necessary. The gland is dissected free as in other procedures (15).

Summary of the laparoscopic adrenalectomy:
- Mobilization of the colonic flexure,
- Incision of the retroperitoneum,
- Dissection of the superior/inferior border of the adrenal,
- Dissection of the medial border and identification of the adrenal vein,
- Division of the adrenal vein between clips,
- Completion of dissection of the gland,
- Enlargement of one of the port sites, when necessary,
- Removal of the gland in a plastic bag.

⚠ Hints and Pitfalls

- The position of the trocars depends on the individual anatomy of the patient, mainly the distance between umbilicus and costal margin. Also, the number of trocars needed varies according the anatomy of the patient. When retraction of adjacent organs is needed during dissection of the adrenal, additional trocars may be used for the instruments.
- For retraction of the right liver lobe, a retractor is needed. The retractor is handled by the assistant or is preferably fixed to a holding-system. In patients with a clearly enlarged liver, retraction of the organ may be difficult, thus limiting the working space and sometimes making it difficult to reach the upper border of the gland.
- Sometimes there may be problems with fragile venous side branches of the caval vein or the renal vein. Bleedings from these veins can be difficult to seal in laparoscopic operations. When possible, suturing with 6–0 polypropylene sutures will handle the bleeding properly.

- Although the lateral spread of heat when using the UltraCision shears is minimal, it still is recommended to be careful when dissecting close to large veins.

> Editor's Tip: Turning the inactive blade towards the vessels when activating the shears will diminish the risk of unpleasant bleedings.

- In left side operations, the pancreatic tail might be mistaken for the adrenal gland.
- Closure of the fascial layer when using traditional trocars close to the costal margin may cause nerve entrapment. The use of trocars which do not require closure of the fascia probably reduces the risk of nerve injury.

 ## Personal Experience

The authors have no personal experience of the retroperitoneal technique. It seems to be popular among surgeons who are used to the retroperitoneal approach in open surgery as well (1, 13). The space obtained retroperitoneally is limited. Therefore, only rather small tumors seem convenient to operate with this technique. The authors have experience with 65 lateral transabdominal laparoscopic adrenalectomies.

The first 40 adrenalectomies in 38 patients have been analyzed for a report. The following indications for surgery were suspected: aldosterone-producing adenoma ($n = 20$), pheochromocytoma ($n = 9$), Cushing's adenoma ($n = 3$), Cushing's disease ($n = 1$; bilateral), adrenocortical hyperplasia with hypercortisolism caused by ectopic ACTH production ($n = 1$; bilateral), and incidentally discovered hormonally inactive adrenal tumor ($n = 4$). Two of the Conn's adenomas had been detected as incidentalomas. One of the suspected Cushing's adenomas turned out to be a low-grade cortical carcinoma. One suspected pheochromocytoma turned out to be a hematoma. (The four hormonally inactive incidentalomas were: one hematoma, one cyst, one inactive cortical hyperplasia, and one inactive cortical adenoma.) The mean size of the tumors was 2.6 cm. Sixteen lesions were on the right side, 24 on the left side; in two patients both adrenals were removed. The mean weight of the patients was 81 kg (range 27–121 kg) and the BMI was on average 28 kg/m² (range 17–31 kg/m²).

The mean operating time was 121 minutes (range 53–360 minutes). The size of the tumor, BMI, or side of the tumor did not have a significant effect on the operative time. The mean operating time for the last 20 operations (112 minutes) was shorter than for the first 20 operations (131 minutes), but the difference was not significant. The estimated intraoperative bleeding was on average 80 ml.

Conversion to laparotomy was done in one case (2.4%), an obese woman (BMI 35 kg/m²) with hypercortisolism caused by bilateral adrenocortical hyperplasia due to ectopic ACTH syndrome. (She had undergone right hemicolectomy for a colon carcinoma.) The left adrenal was successfully removed laparoscopically, but the right-sided procedure was not possible because of an extremely enlarged liver and postoperative adhesions.

The median postoperative hospital stay was three days. All patients were able to start oral intake during the first postoperative day. The patients needed narcotic analgesics on average 1.8 days postoperatively. The median postoperative sick leave was 17 days. There was no mortality or reoperations. Seven patients had postoperative complications (18%). The patient converted to laparotomy had transient postoperative dyspnea caused by a small pulmonary embolus. One patient developed a pneumothorax (treated with pleural suction for 4 days). Two postoperative bleedings at the operative site required red blood cell transfusions. Two patients had prolonged pain at a trocar wound. One patient had a urinary tract infection.

Discussion

A large number of studies on laparoscopic adrenalectomy have been published, but in most studies the number of patients has been small and the results of laparoscopic adrenalectomy have been retrospectively compared with those of conventional operations. In spite of this lack of adequate randomized trials, it is apparent that the laparoscopic method has advantages for the patient compared with open surgery. Laparoscopic adrenalectomy is associated with shorter postoperative recovery than open surgery. This is true both for comparisons between laparoscopic and open abdominal operations (14, 17) and for comparisons between videoscopic and open posterior approaches (1).

Most reports describe a transabdominal laparoscopic technique. There are, however, some potential advantages when using the retroperitoneal route. The abdominal cavity is not entered and the need for dissection and retraction of adjacent organs is limited. In the posterior extraperitoneal approach, both adrenals can be operated on without having to change the patient's position. On the other hand, in the extraperitoneal approaches the working space is limited, and the anatomical landmarks for the location of the adrenal gland may be more difficult to identify. In conventional open surgery one must consider small risks associated with laparotomies, like the risk of postoperative adhesions and the risk of incisional hernias. These complications are, however, rare after laparoscopic surgery.

In comparisons between transabdominal and posterior videoscopic operations no clear differences in postoperative recovery or in sick leave have been found (6). In both groups the hospital stay is 3–4 days and sick leave 12–13 days. The operation time varies in different reports between 100 and 180 minutes. Like in other laparoscopic operations the operation time decreases with increased experience. The morbidity in larger collectives is about 10% and the mortality almost zero (12).

Introduction of the UltraCision shears and scalpel for open and laparoscopic surgery has, to a high degree, enhanced the development of the laparoscopic adrenalectomy technique. Transection in laparoscopic adrenalectomy can be performed with traditional electrocautery, but in our experience the use of the UltraCision shears improves hemostatic control and, although studies comparing these methods are lacking, it is obvious that operation time and bleeding are decreased.

Laparoscopic adrenalectomy is today to be considered the "gold standard" for operation of most types of benign adrenal lesions, including pheochromocytomas. However, the surgeon and anesthesiologist should always show respect for pheochromocytomas and the difficult hemodynamic changes which may be caused by manipulation of the tumor. It has been shown that the problems are not larger than in open surgery, but rather smaller. The adrenal gland is manipulated less than in open surgery (4, 7, 20). Therefore, the laparoscopic approach is well suited for operation of benign pheochromocytomas. The operation time is usually somewhat longer than for other adrenal tumors and the postoperative hospital stay is longer (11). In the postoperative period, there is a risk of hypotension. These patients should preferably be followed up in an intensive care unit for 1–2 days postoperatively.

Who should perform laparoscopic adrenalectomies? The surgeon should be familiar with advanced laparoscopic techniques and also experienced in endocrine surgery. These operations should be centralized in hospitals with a large enough yearly number of adrenal operations to ensure that the surgeons will gain experience with both laparoscopic and open techniques.

References

1. Baba S, Miyajima A, Uchida A, Asanuma H, Miyakawa A, Murai M. A posterior lumbar approach for retroperitoneoscopic adrenalectomy: assessment of surgical efficacy. Urology 1997; 50: 19.
2. Bax TW, Marcus DR, Galloway GQ, Swanstrom LL, Sheppard BC. Laparoscopic bilateral adrenalectomy following failed hypophysectomy. Surg Endosc 1996; 10: 1150.
3. Brunt LM, Doherty GM, Norton JA, Soper NJ, Quasebarth MA, Moley JF. Laparoscopic adrenalectomy compared to open adrenalectomy for benign adrenal neoplasms [see comments]. J Am Coll Surg 1996; 183: 1.
4. Col V, de Cannieri L, Collard E, Michel L, Donckier J. Laparoscopic adrenalectomy for pheochromocytoma: endocrinological and surgical aspects of a new therapeutic approach. Clin Endocrinol (Oxf) 1999; 50: 121.
5. Duh QY, Siperstein AE, Clark OH, Schecter WP, Horn JK, Harrison MR, et al. Laparoscopic adrenalectomy. Comparison of the lateral and posterior approaches. Arch Surg 1996; 131: 870.
6. Fernandez-Cruz L, Saenz A, Benarroch G, Astudillo E, Taura P, Sabater L. Laparoscopic unilateral and bilateral adrenalectomy for Cushing's syndrome. Transperitoneal and retroperitoneal approaches. Ann Surg 1996; 224: 727.
7. Fernandez-Cruz L, Taura P, Saenz A, Benarroch G, Sabater L. Laparoscopic approach to pheochromocytoma: hemodynamic changes and catecholamine secretion. World J Surg 1996; 20: 762.
8. Fernandez-Cruz L, Saenz A, Benarroch G, Sabater L, Taura P. Total bilateral laparoscopic adrenalectomy in patients with Cushing's syndrome and multiple endocrine neoplasia (IIa). Surg Endosc 1997; 11: 103.
9. Gagner M, Lacroix A, Bolte E. Laparoscopic adrenalectomy in Cushing's syndrome and pheochromocytoma [letter]. N Engl J Med 1992; 327: 1033.
10. Gagner M, Lacroix A, Prinz RA, Bolte E, Albala D, Potvin C, Hamet P, Kuchel O, Qurin S, Pomp A. Early experience with laparoscopic approach for adrenalectomy. Surgery 1993; 114: 1120.
11. Gagner M, Breton G, Pharand D, Pomp A. Is laparoscopic adrenalectomy indicated for pheochromocytomas? Surgery 1996; 120: 1076.
12. Gagner M, Pomp A, Heniford BT, Pharand D, Lacroix A. Laparoscopic adrenalectomy: lessons learned from 100 consecutive procedures. Ann Surg 1997; 226: 238.
13. Gasman D, Droupy S, Koutani A, Salomon L, Antiphon P, Chassagnon J, et al. Laparoscopic adrenalectomy: the retroperitoneal approach. J Urol 1998; 159: 1816.
14. Jacobs JK, Goldstein RE, Geer RJ. Laparoscopic adrenalectomy. A new standard of care. Ann Surg 1997; 225(5): 495–501; discussion. Mercan S, Seven R, Ozarmagan S, Tezelman S. Endoscopic retroperitoneal adrenalectomy. Surgery 1995; 118: 1071.
15. Mercan S, Seven R, Ozarmagan S, Tezelman S. Endoscopic retroperitoneal adrenalectomy. Surgery 1995; 118: 1071.
16. Parilla P, Lijan AJ, Rodriguez JM, Robles R, Illana J. Initial experience with endoscopic retroperitoneal adrenalectomy. Br J Cancer 1996; 83: 987.
17. Prinz RA. A comparison of laparoscopic and open adrenalectomies. Arch Surg 1995; 130: 489.
18. Rutherford JC, Stowasser M, Tunny TJ, Klemm SA, Gordon RD. Laparoscopic adrenalectomy. World J Surg 1996; 20: 758.
19. Shichman SJ, Herndon CD, Sosa RE, Whalen GF, MacGillivray DC, Malchoff CD, Vaughan ED. Lateral transperitoneal laparoscopic adrenalectomy. World J Urol 1999; 17: 48.
20. Sprung J, O'Hara JF, Gill IS, Abdelmalak B, Sarnaik A, Bravo EL. Anesthetic aspects of laparoscopic and open adrenalectomy for pheochromocytoma. Urology 2000; 55: 339.

21 Thyroid Surgery with the UltraCision Blade

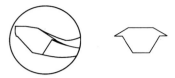

W. Feil

Austria, especially the Alpine regions, is a country with a long history of endemic goiter. The problem has been reduced by the addition of iodine to cooking salt. It was not until recently that the iodine concentration in salt had to be elevated because of the overall dietary sodium reduction in food. However, thyroid surgery is number six in the frequency ranking of all surgical operations. In Austria (population 8 million), about 9000 thyroid resections are performed per year.

Indication and Preoperative Management

Preoperative assessment and indication to operation follow the international standardized criteria: intraoperative frozen section analysis is mandatory in all cases. In cases with cold nodules, unilateral hemithyroidectomy is performed. Separated parathyroid glands are treated "as if it was the last gland" and autotransplanted in the ipsilateral sternocleid muscle.

For local logistic reasons, patients enter the hospital the day before surgery. Outpatient thyroid surgery is not performed.

Operation

For thyroid resection, the patients are brought into a modified beach-chair position with the neck slightly extended.

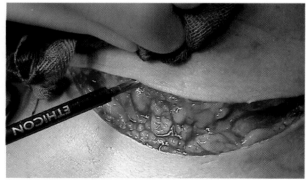

Fig. 21.1 Coagulation of dermal bleeders in the corium with the HC blade avoids burn marks to the skin.

The following choice of instruments is recommended:
- UltraCision generator and hand piece
- 5 mm HC blade, or
- 5 mm HF blade, or
- 5 mm SH or DH blade (10 cm long), or
- Reusable HS2 blade, and if available
- Hand activation for generator 300

Editor's tip: Practical use has shown that the HC blade is the most convenient for thyroid surgery. Excellent results can also be achieved with the HF blade, but this blade is very sharp. Presumably, the sickle-like blades will disappear from the OR in the course of time.

The skin incision following the surgical rules by Kocher is performed with a regular steel scalpel, as UltraCision is not intended for skin incisions. Thereafter, all surgical preparation, dissection and most of coagulation procedures are done with the selected blade.

Coaptation/coagulation of small bleeders in the subcutaneous tissue is easily performed with the blade (Fig. 21.1). In contrast to electrosurgery, the tissue is not grasped with a forceps and a burn mark produced, rather the bleeder is distinctly localized. For this, the skin can be everted, the bleeding vessel is compressed and energy activated for a short moment (less than 0.5 seconds). The vessel walls are welded and bleeding stops without collateral damage and skin burn. Following the subcutaneous tissue, the platysma is transected (Fig. 21.2). The residue of coagulation is a distinct area of tissue alteration visible as grayish-red colored tissue (Fig. 21.3). A cranial skin-platysma lobe is prepared (Fig. 21.4) with the blade. Even thicker veins in the subplatysmal region can be treated sufficiently with the activated blade (Fig. 21.5). The tissue is loaded on the flat side of the blade; energy is activated and the sufficiently welded tissue is transected.

A custom-made retractor is inserted and the deeper muscle layer is medially incised with the blade (Fig. 21.6). Thereafter, the thyroid gland is peeled out. The tissues layer can be separated bluntly (Fig. 21.7) and by dissection with the activated blade (Fig. 21.8). Even thicker veins (Fig. 21.9) can be controlled with UltraCision. In the next step, the isthmus is transected (Fig. 21.10) and the anterior parts of the thyroid lobes are dissected from the trachea (Fig. 21.11). In the following stages, the surgical procedure depends on the necessity and extent of resection. In cases where a

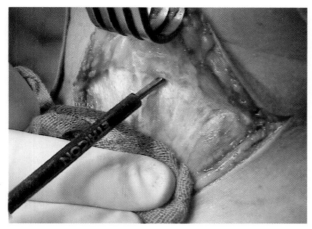

Fig. 21.**2**   Transection of the subcutaneous tissue. Prestretching enhances quick cutting.

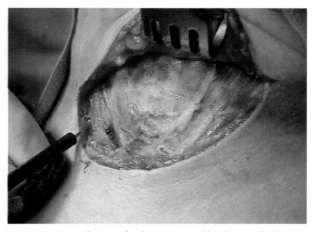

Fig. 21.**3**   Coagulation of subcutaneous bleeders with the HC blade by compression and application of energy.

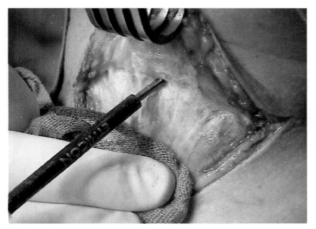

Fig. 21.**4**   Preparation of the cranial skin-platysma lobe. Prestretching enhances quick cutting.

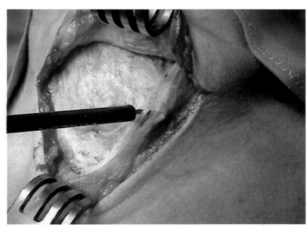

Fig. 21. **5**   Thicker veins are loaded on the blade and coagulated under direct visualization.

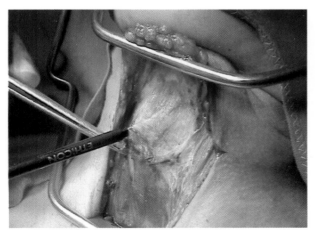

Fig. 21.**6**   Median splitting of the muscle layer.

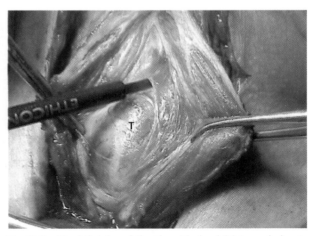

Fig. 21.**7**   The left lobe of the thyroid gland (*T*) is peeled out. Separation of the layers can be performed bluntly.

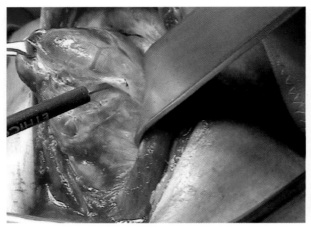

Fig. 21.**8** Preparation of the left lobe. Connective tissue is transected with the activated blade.

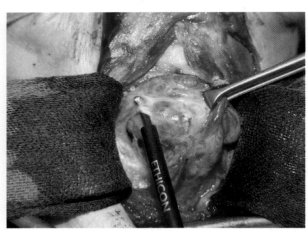

Fig. 21.**9** Thicker veins are loaded on the blade, carefully coagulated and thereafter transected without any bleeding.

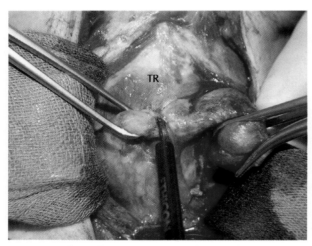

Fig. 21.**10** The isthmus is transected with the HC blade. Bleeders can be controlled by simultaneous compression and application of energy. *TR* trachea.

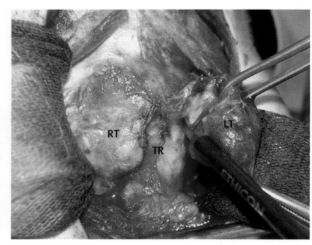

Fig. 21.**11** Dissection of the left lobe from the trachea. Punctual bleeders on the tracheal wall (*TR*) can be controlled easily. *LT* left thyroid lobe, *RT* right thyroid lobe.

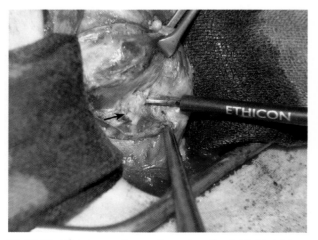

Fig. 21.**12** The recurrent nerve (*arrow*) on the right side is identified. Care must be taken with the nerve, which must not be touched with the activated blade.

hemithyroidectomy is indicated, the recurrent nerve (Fig. 21.**12**) and the parathyroid glands (Fig. 21.**13**) are identified.

> Editor's tip: When the parathyroid gland and the recurrent nerve are identified and separated it may be useful to use gentle clamps for the surrounding small vessels in order to be sure that absolutely no thermal injury is produced. The hot blade cools down immediately when not activated, but residual heat could be harmful to the nerve. Thus, it is recommended not to touch the nerve directly with the blade.

A neuromonitoring equipment was not available for this study, but is highly recommended, especially in cases of surgery for recurrent disease.

The superior and inferior thyroid vessels are identified and transected, if indicated. In certain situations it is possible to load smaller arterial vessels on the blade, then coagulate and transect them with the activated blade (Figs. 21.**14**, 21.**15**). If there is too much tension on these structures—and this is frequently the case—it is recommended to use clamps for the pole arteries in order to avoid the slipping back of an incompletely welded vessel that subsequently starts bleeding.

> Editor's tip: The superior and inferior pole vessels should generally be transected between clamps when a blade is used for thyroid surgery in order to play it safe. When the 5 mm C14 shears are used, all vessels can be safely controlled and transected in thyroid surgery.

In many cases, it is possible to perform the resection or hemithyroidectomy closest to the capsule of the gland. Thus, it is not necessary to ligate the trunks of, e.g., the inferior artery, but it is possible to control the vessels as they diverge in the capsule. The structures can be loaded on the blade (Fig. 21.**16**), coagulated (Fig. 21.**17**) and dissected thereafter (Fig. 21.**18**).

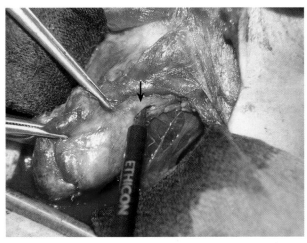

Fig. 21.**13**　The left superior parathyroid (*arrow*) gland is identified and carefully separated from the thyroid gland. Care has to be taken not to compromise the parathyroid gland's blood supply. However, blade dissection can go close to the gland without compromising vitality and function.

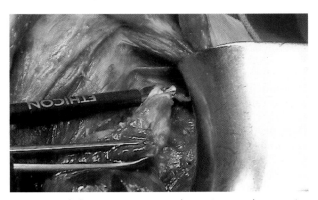

Fig. 21.**14**　If there is not too much tension on the superior pole, vessels they can be carefully loaded on the blade and coagulated.

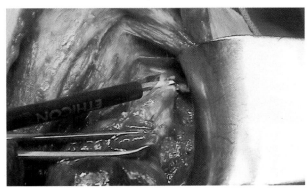

Fig. 21.**15**　If there is not too much tension on the superior pole, vessels they can be transected after coagulation with the blade.

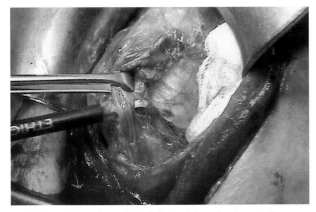

Fig. 21.**16**　Dissection of the inferior left pole close to the capsule. The diverted pole vessels can be loaded up on the blade.

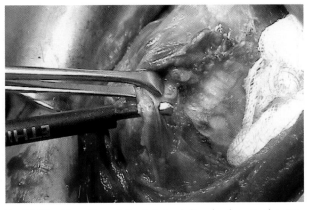

Fig. 21.**17**　Dissection of the inferior left pole close to the capsule. The loaded branches of the pole vessels can be coagulated with the activated blade.

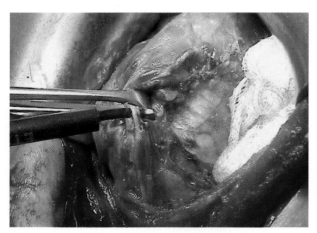

Fig. 21.**18** The coagulated vessels are transected with the blade rotated to the sharper edge.

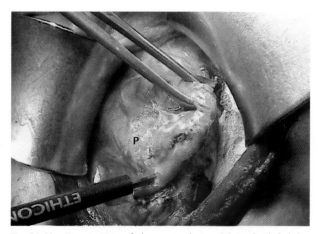

Fig. 21.**19** Transection of the parenchyma (*P*) in the left lobe with the activated HC blade.

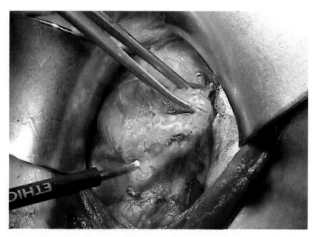

Fig. 21.**20** Bleeders in the parenchyma can be controlled by compression and application of energy.

Editor's tip: Preparation, coagulation and dissection can be performed with one instrument. Thus, the surgical focus is maintained on the operative field and frequent instrument changes are avoided. The benefit of this procedure is obvious.

When a partial resection or enucleation or subtotal resection is performed, the parenchyma can be transected with the blade (Fig. 21.**19**). Residual bleeders can be controlled by compression and activation of the blade (Fig. 21.**20**).

In countries where a reusable HS2 blade is available, thyroid resection can be easily performed with that blade (Fig. 21.**21 a–c**).

Editor's tip: Parenchyma dissection with the blade may be unsatisfactory in cases of thyroiditis, Hashimoto's disease or severe hyperthyrosis. Bleeding may occur and additional sutures may be necessary.

⚠ Hints and Pitfalls

- Even the thicker veins (e.g., under the platysma) can be coagulated and dissected with the blade. Thereafter, some tension is applied to the skin lobes with the retractor. Hence, it may happen that properly sealed vessels are mechanically reopened by tissue tension and bleed. In this situation, ligatures are the means of choice. The same may occur with thicker veins (e.g., Kocher's vein) on the gland itself.
- Bleeding may also occur when the parenchyma is dissected in certain cases of Hashimoto's disease or hyperthyroidism. Most of the time, bleeding control can be achieved by local pressure and energy application, but in some cases sutures are necessary anyway.
- Care has to be taken around the recurrent nerve. The nerve must not be touched with the activated blade. In spite of the problem of local tissue temperature, it is still unclear if close contact with the vibrating blade may cause permanent or temporary lesions to the nerve induced by the strong ultrasound waves alone.
- Care has to be taken with the parathyroid glands. It is also unclear if the ultrasound wave itself may be harmful to the gland function postoperatively. It is also recommended to stay away from the gland with the activated blade in order to avoid thermal lesions.
- Drainage is unnecessary because there is no bleeding during the operation and nothing rebleeds.

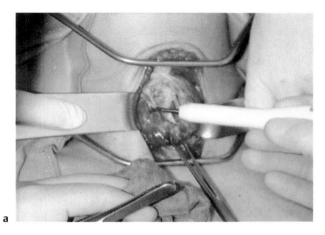

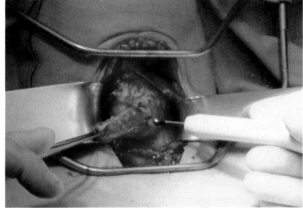

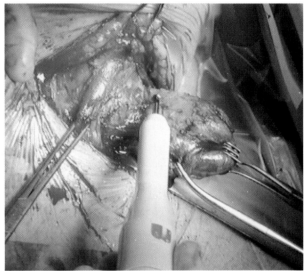

Fig. 21.**21 a** Thyroid surgery can also be performed with a reusable HS2 blade (if available). Dissection of the right lobe. **b** Dissection of the thyroid gland's parenchyma with a reusable HS2 blade. **c** Parenchyma transection of the left lobe with a reusable HS2 blade.

Personal Experience

In a personal series, 215 consecutive unselected patients underwent thyroid surgery with UltraCision between 1997 and 2002. In 175 cases an UltraCision blade (HS2, SH, HC, HF) and in 40 recent cases the 5 mm C14 shears were used. In no case was it necessary to use another energy modality (HF surgery). The operations performed were subtotal (uni- and bilateral) resection, hemithyroidectomies, total thyroidectomies, and modified neck dissections for thyroid cancer. In one patient a parathyroid gland was detached from the resected specimen and retransplanted; in two patients a gland was deprived from local blood supply and also retransplanted.

The suction device was used in only a few cases with gigantic intrathoracal goiters or cases of severe thyroiditis, where minimal bleeding was unavoidable. In "regular" thyroid surgery, the suction device was never used and blood loss was negligible. One patient had subsequent bleeding on the OR table. The reason was an injury to a vein by the trocar for the suction drainage. The wound was reopened and the bleeder controlled. After that incident (case 112), no drainage has been introduced. There were no other bleeding complications before that and thereafter.

Thirteen patients (all after total thyroidectomy, none of them autotransplanted) had temporary malfunction of the parathyroid glands and had to be substituted with calcium for up to 10 days. All patients recovered completely and are free from substitution thereafter.

Perioperative lethality was zero. Patients were discharged after 2–3 days postoperatively.

All patients underwent control for recurrent nerve function the day before as well as one or two days after surgery. There was one patient with a complete unilateral lesion of the recurrent nerve after resection of a T4N2 papillary cancer. There were no other permanent lesions. In 11 patients partial lesions were detected after surgery phonetically, they all had recovered after 6–8 weeks.

Discussion

Thyroid surgery follows standardized rules, valid not only for the surgical procedure, but also for preoperative measurements and postoperative therapy. The introduction of UltraCision does not influence the surgical standards, but may ameliorate surgical performance, reduce OR time and the frequency of postoperative complications.

In this study, comparisons are only possible to historic control groups or to the other patients operated at the same institution at the same time period. Both methods have a methodological bias, but there are no other data available reflecting a prospective clinical trial.

It is evident from personal experience that the operation times are significantly reduced by the use of UltraCision. Most of the preparation and dissection is performed with one instrument and the surgical focus is maintained on the operative field. Following a subjective estimation, OP time can be reduced by at least one third. It will be the task of cost-controlling institutions to calculate the savings in OR time and put them into relation to the costs of disposable instruments.

It is also evident from personal experience that blood loss is significantly reduced. The benefit for the patient can only be estimated, as blood substitution occurs very infrequently in thyroid surgery and was never needed during this study.

In the "control group" of the other patients from the same institution, cases of rebleeding on the ward postoperatively, that made surgical intervention necessary, were reported. The clear benefit of UltraCision is the argument that there were no rebleeders in the UltraCision group. The dictum "what does not bleed at the end of the operation does not rebleed" can be interpreted dogmatically in this context. It is a clear benefit for the patients having surgery with UltraCision that rebleeding does not occur.

The argument that the only bleeding complication in this series was due to a trocar for the drainage led to the conclusion that drainage is no longer inserted. Another argument is the personal experience that in all known cases of rebleeding on the ward in the "control group" the drainage reservoir was empty, the line clotted and the neck of the suffocating patient extremely swollen by the local hematoma.

There are no significant data for hospital stay or cosmetic result in respect to the use of UltraCision. There is a strong feeling that patients who underwent thyroid surgery with UltraCision recover more quickly and perform better, but this argument cannot be reflected in significant data. The frequency of complications (bleeding) in the control group is too low to influence the data and the overall hospital stay for both groups is too short to be statistically valuable. The rate of permanent and/or temporary lesions of the recurrent nerve is equal in both groups.

The only prospective study was performed by Meurisse et al. and showed a significant reduction of OR time, blood loss, analgesics consumption and incidence of temporary hyoparathyroidism when the UltraCision hook was used for thyroid surgery.

These data also support the arguments that surgery is facilitated from the technical point of view, OR time is reduced and bleeding complications are diminished when UltraCision is used. This is a clear vote for the implementation of UltraCision.

Suggested Reading

Dralle H, Lorenz K, Nguyen-Thanh P. Minimally invasive video-assisted parathyroidectomy—selective approach to localized single gland adenoma. Langenbecks Arch Surg 1999 Dec; 384(6): 556–62.

Hermann M, Alk G, Roka R, Glaser K, Freissmuth M. Laryngeal recurrent nerve injury in surgery for benign thyroid diseases: effect of nerve dissection and impact of individual surgeon in more than 27,000 nerves at risk. Ann Surg 2002 Feb; 235(2): 261–8.

Meurisse M, Defechereux T, Maweja S, Degauque C, Vandelaer M, Hamoir E. Evaluation of the UltraCision ultrasonic dissector in thyroid surgery. Prospective randomized study. Ann Chir 2000; 125: 468–472.

Mourad M, Saab N, Malaise J, Ngongang C, Fournier B, Daumerie C, Squifflet JP. Minimally invasive video-assisted approach for partial and total thyroidectomy. Surg Endosc 2001 Oct; 15(10): 1108–11.

Prager G, Czerny C, Kurtaran A, Passler C, Scheuba C, Bieglmayer C, Niederle B. Minimally invasive open parathyroidectomy in an endemic goiter area: a prospective study. Arch Surg 2001 Jul; 136(7): 810–6.

Roeher HD, Simon D, Witte J, Goretzki PE. Principals of limited or radical surgery for differentiated thyroid cancer. Thyroidology 1993 Dec; 5(3): 93–6.

Runkel N, Riede E, Mann B, Buhr HJ. Surgical training and vocal-cord paralysis in benign thyroid disease. Langenbecks Arch Surg 1998 Aug; 383(3–4):240–2.

Schwartz AE, Friedman EW. Preservation of the parathyroid glands in total thyroidectomy. Surg Gynecol Obstet 1987; 165: 327–32.

Steurer M, Passler C, Denk DM, Schneider B, Niederle B, Bigenzahn W. Advantages of recurrent laryngeal nerve identification in thyroidectomy and parathyroidectomy and the importance of preoperative and postoperative laryngoscopic examination in more than 1,000 nerves at risk. Laryngoscope 2002; 112): 124–33.

Udelsman R, Chen H. The current management of thyroid cancer. Adv Surg 1999; 33: 1–27.

22 Minimally Invasive Thyroid Surgery with the UltraCision Shears (CS 14C)

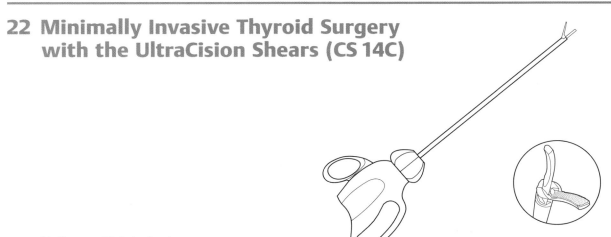

M. Gagner, W. B. Inabnet

In the late nineteenth century, Theodor Kocher developed the technique of thyroidectomy, an operation that required a transverse cervical incision and the creation of myocutaneous flaps to gain access to the thyroid. Although conventional thyroidectomy can be performed safely with little morbidity, this approach leaves an undesirable scar on the anterior surface of the neck. Until recently, there had been few major refinements in the surgical approach to the thyroid gland. However, with the advent of laparoscopic surgery in the latter part of the twentieth century, endoscopic techniques have been developed for surgery of the neck (1, 2, 3, 4, 5). We have developed the technique of endoscopic thyroidectomy, a minimally invasive technique which permits thyroid excision without the unfavorable cosmetic results associated with conventional thyroidectomy.

Indication and Preoperative Management

Multiple factors play a role in patient selection for endoscopic thyroidectomy, including the type of pathology, thyroid size, and body habitus. The presence of a solitary thyroid nodule with indeterminate cytology is an excellent indication for endoscopic thyroidectomy. Accordingly, the preoperative evaluation should include a thorough history and physical examination, indirect laryngoscopy, thyroid function tests, and fine needle aspiration. Ultrasonography is used as an extension of the physical examination, providing useful information on the size and location of the pathology and permitting evaluation of the contralateral thyroid lobe. Other indications for endoscopic thyroidectomy include a solitary toxic nodule, recurrent thyroid cysts, and small multinodular goiters.

Since the neck offers a limited working space, endoscopic thyroidectomy should not be performed in patients with thyroid nodules great than 4 cm. Other relative contraindications include a large multinodular goiter, Graves' disease, a history of prior neck surgery, and morbid obesity as a short, wide neck will limit maneuverability. Until more data are available, endoscopic thyroidectomy should not be performed for thyroid carcinoma.

Operation

After inducing general endotracheal anesthesia, the patient is placed on the operating table in the supine position with the neck slightly extended. Anatomical landmarks are outlined with a marking pen, including the sternal notch, the midline, the anterior border of the sternoclediomastoid muscle (SCM), and the external jugular veins. The head is slightly rotated to maximize access to the ipsilateral neck.

A 0.5 cm incision is made at the sternal notch and the cervical fascia is opened under direct vision. The subplatsymal space is developed along the anterior border of the ipsilateral SCM. A purse-string suture is placed in the subcutaneous tissue and a 5 mm trocar is inserted. Carbon dioxide is insufflated to a pressure of 12 mmHg, but once an adequate working space has been developed, the insufflation pressures are decreased to 8–10 mmHg for the remainder of the procedure. A 0°, 5 mm endoscope is used to perform the initial dissection. This maneuver is performed by gently advancing the endoscope along the avascular space of the anteromedial border of the ipsilateral sternocleidomastoid muscle.

Once an adequate working space has been developed, a 30°, 5 mm endoscope is used for the remainder of the procedure. Additional trocars are inserted under direct vision including a 2 mm trocar at the midline, a 2 mm trocar at the mid-portion of the ispilateral SCM, and a 5–1 mm trocar superolaterally along the anterior border of the SCM. The latter trocar site, which is located in a cosmetically favorable location, may be used to extract the specimen at the conclusion of the operation.

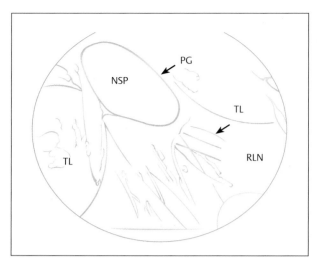
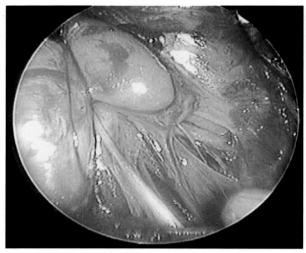

Fig. 22.**1**   Identification of the superior parathyroid gland (*PG*) and the recurrent laryngeal (*RLN*). *TL* thyroid lobe, *NSP* normal superior parathyroid gland.

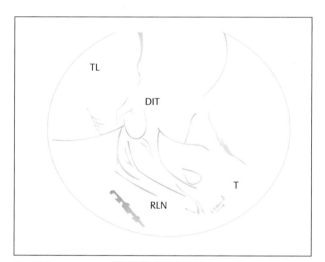
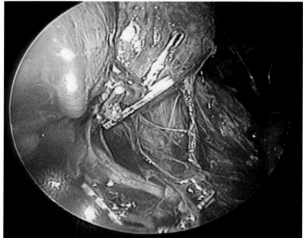

Fig. 22.**2**   Division of the inferior thyroid artery. *TL* thyroid lobe, *DIT* divided inferior thyroid artery, *RLN* recurrent laryngeal nerve, *T* trachea.

The carotid artery is identified and the space between the lateral border of the strap muscles and the medial edge of the carotid artery is developed. The strap muscles are not divided but rather retracted anteromedially. The thyroid lobe is visualized and mobilized using a combination of sharp and blunt dissection. The use of cautery is to be avoided, especially in the deeper tissue planes. The middle thyroid vein is ligated using 5 mm clips or the 5 mm UltraCision shears. Using blunt dissection, the recurrent laryngeal nerve and parathyroid glands are identified and carefully dissected free of their attachments to the thyroid gland (Fig. 22.1). The inferior thyroid artery is mobilized at its junction with the recurrent laryngeal nerve and ligated with the 5 mm clip applier. With the recurrent laryngeal nerve in full view, the inferior thyroid artery is divided (Fig. 22.**2**).

The superior pole vessels are isolated, clipped, and divided. The superior laryngeal nerve is identified and protected during this maneuver. In a similar manner, the inferior pole vessels are clipped and divided. Alternatively, the UltraCision shears can be used to divide the inferior thyroid vasculature. After releasing the anteriomedial attachments of the recurrent laryngeal nerve by blunt dissection, the UltraCision shears are used to divide the ligament of Berry. The recurrent laryngeal nerve must be in full view during this maneuver. Finally, the isthmus is divided with the UltraCision shears.

A small sac is constructed by removing the thumb portion of a surgical glove and a purse-string suture is fashioned. The specimen is placed in the sac and extracted through the superolateral trocar site, which may need to be slightly enlarged to accommodate the specimen. Steri strips are used to close the incisions.

Hints and Pitfalls

- Proper patient selection plays an important role in endoscopic thyroidectomy. Patients with a long, narrow neck provide more space for endoscopic maneuvering.
- Carbon dioxide may leak around the 2 mm trocars thereby compromising exposure; however, small towel clips or purse string sutures may be applied to the skin to minimize CO_2 leakage.
- Typically, a 30° endoscope provides adequate endoscopic visualization, but occasionally a 45° endoscope can improve visualization, especially if the thyroid gland is large.
- The use of an energy source (i.e., cautery, UltraCision shears) is to be avoided in the deeper tissue planes, especially in proximity to the recurrent laryngeal nerve.

> Editor's tip: The recommendation of avoiding energy sources in dissecting deeper tissue planes in minimal invasive thyroid surgery is easy to accept when the distances between sensible structures, the carotid artery, the recurrent laryngeal nerve and the inferior thyroid artery, sometimes are less than 1 mm, which is the lateral spread of thermal injuries for ultrasonic instruments. For cautery it is 5 mm at the same time of activation, i.e., 5 seconds.

- If the surgeon does not unequivocally identify the recurrent laryngeal nerve and parathyroid glands, the operation should be converted to an open, conventional approach.
- We routinely submit the specimen for frozen section analysis. If a diagnosis of thyroid carcinoma is established, an open completion thyroidectomy is performed.

Personal Experience

Sixteen patients with a solitary thyroid nodule have undergone endoscopic thyroidectomy at our institution. Exclusion criteria included patients with nodules greater than 4 cm, multinodular goiter, Graves' disease, or a high index of suspicion of thyroid malignancy. There were 14 females and two males with a mean age of 43 years (17–66 years). Indications for surgery included indeterminate cytology ($n = 6$), follicular neoplasm ($n = 6$), recurrent thyroid cyst ($n = 2$), Hürthle cell neoplasm ($n = 1$), and toxic thyroid nodule ($n = 1$) (Fig. 22.**3**). The mean nodule diameter was 2.8 cm (0.6–7 cm). Analgesic requirement, return to normal activity, and cosmetic results were compared to those for 16 consecutive patients who had conventional thyroidectomy.

Operative procedures included left thyroid lobectomy ($n = 7$), left subtotal thyroidectomy ($n = 2$), right thyroid lobectomy ($n = 2$), right subtotal thyroidectomy ($n = 2$), and isthmusectomy ($n = 3$) (Fig. 22.**4**). Fifteen of 16 cases were successfully completed endoscopically. In one patient with a large 7 cm cyst, the procedure was completed through a small ipsilateral incision. The mean operating time was 220 minutes (120–330 minutes). There were no major complications, but two patients developed mild hypercarbia and one patient had an incidental parathyroidectomy. Final pathology yielded a diagnosis of follicular adenoma ($n = 9$), Hürthle cell adenoma ($n = 1$), oncocytic adenoma ($n = 1$), thyroid cyst ($n = 2$), multinodular goiter ($n = 1$), and papillary thyroid carcinoma ($n = 2$). One of the patients with papillary carcinoma underwent open completion thyroidectomy without evidence of residual neoplasia. When compared to conventional thyroidectomy, patients undergoing endoscopic thyroidectomy had a significantly superior cosmetic result ($p < 0.005$) and a quicker return to normal activity ($p < 0.05$).

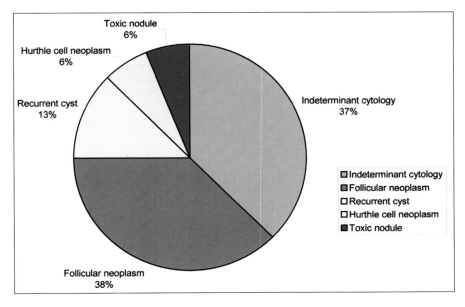

Fig. 22.**3** Indications for thyroidectomy.

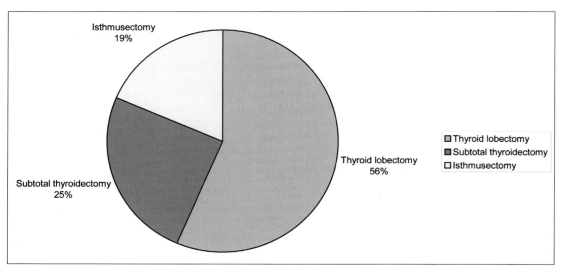

Fig. 22.**4**   Endoscopic thyroidectomy.

 Discussion

Endoscopic thyroidectomy is one of the most significant new advances in thyroid surgery. Although conventional open thyroidectomy can be performed with few complications, this approach leaves a visible scar on the anterior surface of the neck in a cosmetically unfavorable location. The endoscopic approach undoubtedly provides a superior cosmetic result when compared to conventional thyroidectomy and results in a quicker return to normal activity. Endoscopic thyroidectomy provides fantastic magnification of thyroid anatomy, including the recurrent laryngeal nerve, superior laryngeal nerve, and the parathyroid glands.

> Editor's tip: The extraordinary good imaging is perhaps the greatest advantage with minimal invasive thyroid surgery in comparison with conventional thyroidectomy.

In addition, since muscle is not divided during endoscopic thyroidectomy, there is less tissue trauma, resulting in a quicker return to normal activity. The longer duration of surgery is the primary disadvantage of endoscopic thyroidectomy; however, this should decrease as additional experience is gained. In addition, CO_2 insufflation may not be tolerated in the elderly or in patients with comorbid medical problems. Careful patient selection is paramount.

The results of our series of patients demonstrate that endoscopic thyroidectomy can be performed safely with minimal morbidity. As our experience grows, it may be possible to broaden the indications for this new minimally invasive technique for thyroid excision.

 References

1. Gagner M. Endoscopic subtotal parathyroidectomy in patients with primary hyperparathyroidism. Br J Surg 1996; 83: 875.
2. Hüscher CSG, Chiodini S, Napolitano C, Recher A. Endoscopic right thyroid lobectomy. Surg Endosc 1997; 11: 877.
3. Yeung GHC. Endoscopic surgery of the neck. Surg Laparosc Endosc 1998; 8: 227–32.
4. Bellantone R, Lombardi CP, Raffaelli M, et al. Minimally invasive, totally gasless video-assisted thyroid lobectomy. Am J Surg 1999; 177: 342–3.
5. Shimizu K, Akira S, Jasmi AY, et al. Video-assisted neck surgery: endoscopic resection of thyroid tumors with a very minimal neck wound. J Am Coll Surg 1999; 188: 697–703.

23 Thyroid Surgery with the 10 mm UltraCision Shears (CS 150 Pistol Grip or CS 6S Needle-Holder Hand Grip) for Open Surgery

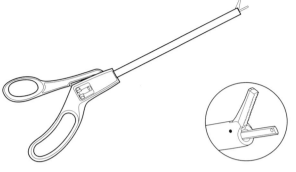

C. Haglund, P. Voutilainen

The thyroid gland has a rich blood supply. In conventional thyroidectomies, a great number of vessels have to be clamped, divided, and tied which takes a considerable part of the operating time. Many surgeons prefer clips instead of sutures, others use bipolar diathermy. Recently, a major development in the use of energy for cutting and hemostasis in surgery was achieved by introduction of UltraCision's ultrasonically activated surgical devices, including shears and blades that cut and coagulate at the same time. These instruments cause a lateral thermal injury of only 1–3 mm in width, which is about half of that caused by bipolar systems (4).

Following an initial learning phase of our own and of others, where we used UltraCision in open abdominal and laparoscopic surgery (5, 7), we began to use the device in thyroid surgery. The impression in a masked, match-paired study was positive, and a randomized trial comparing the UltraCision technique with a conservative operation technique routinely used in our department was performed (9, 10). Both studies showed reductions in operation time, without increase in complication rate.

Indication and Preoperative Management

The main indication for thyroidectomy today is a thyroid nodule, in which malignancy cannot be excluded without performing a lobectomy of the side of the tumor. Surgery for goiter is indicated in patients, in whom the goiter is enlarged sufficiently to cause symptoms due to compression of the trachea or esophagus, or when the goiter is associated with hyperthyroidism. Removal of goiters exclusively for cosmetic reasons is seldom indicated.

The optimal treatment of papillary thyroid carcinoma has been debated. The extent of thyroid resection, and the question of prophylactic neck dissection, and in case of lymph node metastases of modified ver-

sus conventional neck dissection have been points of debate. In follicular carcinoma, the mode of spreading is via the blood stream. Neck dissection is practically never indicated because lymph node spread is so rare. Medullary carcinomas, on the other hand, have an early potential for lymphatic spread and high incidence of multicentricity. The standard practice in our department is to treat all of these carcinomas by total thyroidectomy. In medullary carcinomas, central neck dissection is recommended; in papillary carcinomas, a modfied neck dissection is done in patients with suspected or verified lymph node metastases. All patients with papillary and follicular carcinoma are routinely given postoperative radioiodine therapy.

Operation

Total Lobectomy and Thyroid ectomy

The patient should be positioned with the neck extended to its fullest extent. The horizontal line of incision is marked on the skin by pressure with a suture thread approximately two fingers above the sternal notch. The skin and subcutaneous tissues are incised down to the platysma, which is divided in the line of the incision to expose the underlying deep fascia of the neck and the anterior jugular veins. The upper edge of the incision is raised and the areolar layer subjacent to the platysma is dissected up to the prominence of the thyroid cartilage using a combination of sharp and blunt dissection. The lower skin edge is freed in a similar manner down to the suprasternal notch. The wound edges are spread with a self-retaining retractor.

The fascia is incised in the midline, from the thyroid cartilage to the sternal notch using UltraCision (Fig. 23.**1**). The incision does not always exactly define the gap in the strap muscles. By using UltraCision, the risk of small bleedings can be avoided. The sternohyoid muscles are now retracted away from the midline to expose the underlying thyroid gland, partially over-

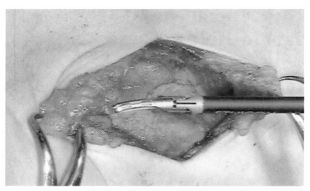

Fig. 23.**1**   The deep fascia of the neck is incised in the midline using the UltraCision shears.

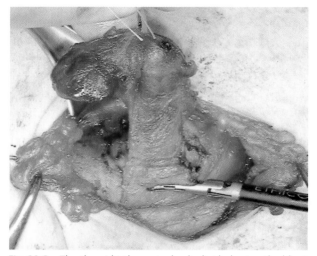

Fig. 23.**2**   The thyroid isthmus is slowly divided using the blunt part of the blade of the UltraCision shears.

lapped by the sternothyroid strap muscles. Cervical muscles should be cut only when necessary. The UltraCision shears cut muscle tissue with good hemostasis. The muscles are freed from the thyroid by dissecting their medial areolar attachments to the capsule of the gland. With a sweeping movement of the index finger between the thyroid gland and the strap muscles, the thyroid lobe is freed from its lateral attachments.

The isthmus of the gland is pushed upward and the inferior thyroid veins are divided by the UltraCision shears. Large vessels might first be coagulated with the flat part of the blade and then divided with the blunt part. For most vessels, the blunt part only can be used.

> Editor's tip: For division of vessels given names and up to 3 mm in size, level 3 and the blunt side of the active blade are recommended when using the 10 mm shears.

The pyramidal lobe, where present, together with the associated pretracheal blood vessels, are stripped down off the anterior surface of the trachea and the vessels are divided with the shears.

The thyroid lobe is then grasped with the help of stay sutures and rotated medially. The middle thyroid veins are divided. The areolar planes adjacent to the thyroid, trachea, and esophagus are carefully dissected. The inferior thyroid artery and its intersection with the recurrent laryngeal nerve are identified. The inferior parathyroid gland is often found close to the intersection of the artery and nerve. Some surgeons ligate the inferior thyroid artery at this level. The authors prefer to divide the arterial branches close to the surface of the gland using the UltraCision shears.

> Editor's tip: The lateral spread of thermal injury of 1 mm at 5 seconds of activation is especially noteworthy when dissecting close to sensible structures.

With the recurrent laryngeal nerve and one or both parathyroid glands identified, the thyroid lobe may be freed and removed. The thyroid isthmus is dissected free from the underlying trachea by blunt dissection with a clamp. It is slowly divided close to the opposite lobe using the blunt part of the blade (Fig. 23.**2**).

> Editor's tip: A complete hemostasis is achieved with a minimal risk of injury to the trachea when using level 3 with the blunt side of the active blade. The inactive blade is placed towards the trachea with no tension on the tissues.

The raw surface of the divided isthmus may be oversewn where needed with running 4–0 resorbable suture. Alternatively, the isthmus may be divided after freeing the lobe completely.

By dislocating the lobe forward and medially, the posterior attachments are put on stretch. The thyroid can now be mobilized upward by dividing its fascial attachments to the trachea and by dividing the secondary branches of the inferior thyroid artery. The recurrent laryngeal nerve is kept in view at all times. The parathyroid glands are carefully dissected from the thyroid capsule, taking care to preserve their blood supply. Bleedings close to the parathyroid glands are clamped and tied with absorbable sutures. The use of the UltraCision shears close to the parathyroids should be avoided. The lobe is then pulled laterally and downwards away from the site of the larynx, permitting division of the superior thyroid vascular pedicle without injuring the external laryngeal nerve (Fig. 23.**3**). The vessels are divided at the same point as they would be if ligatures were being used in the conventional method.

Using the UltraCision shears, the lobe is freed posteriorly by dividing the ligament of Berry, the dense vascular connective tissue, which binds the thyroid to the first and second tracheal rings. Division of this ligament releases the lobe. At this level, the recurrent nerve is vulnerable and the course of the nerve must be clearly identified. The shears should not be used close to the nerve, but all structures should be clamped, divided and tied with absorbable sutures.

> Editor's tip: All form of energy source dissectors are to be avoided in the absolute vicinity of the recurrent laryngeal nerve.

In total a thyroidectomy, a similar procedure is performed on the opposite site.

The authors always use fine suction drains, that are lead out laterally at the end of the incision. Some surgeons do not use drains if the operating field is dry. If the strap muscles have been divided, they are reapproximated with interrupted absorbable mattress sutures. The midline cervical fascia is approximated with interrupted or running 3–0 resorbable sutures. The platysma is closed with interrupted or running 4–0 resorbable sutures. The skin is normally closed with clips, or alternatively with interrupted 5–0 monofilament, nonresorbable sutures or a running subcuticular stitch.

⚠ Hints and Pitfalls

- There are three different positions of the blade when using the 10 mm coagulating shears (CS 150 and CS 6S): sharp for cutting, flat for coagulation, and blunt for a combination of these effects. The speed of cutting and the amount of coagulation can be adjusted by the power setting of the generator and the pressure applied on the shears. When dividing thyroid blood vessels, the UltraCision shears were used with the power setting mainly at level 3 to achieve optimal balance between cutting power and hemostasis.
- To obtain a better coagulation effect before dividing large vessels, the flat part of the blade may be used before dividing with the blunt part. The authors often use a technique, where the vessel is coagulated with the blunt part of the blade using light pressure. The UltraCision shears are then moved a few millimeters closer to the gland, and the vessel is coagulated and divided. Thus, a larger area of coagulation is achieved.
- For excision of the glands from the trachea, the "knife effect" of the shears can be used.

> Editor's tip: To optimize the effect of the active blade of the shears, the instrument should be opened and the tip of the blade should be used.

- The relationships to the thyroid of the recurrent and superior laryngeal nerves are of great importance in thyroidectomy. The lateral thermal effect of the UltraCision shears is minimal. Still care has to be taken not to use them close to the nerves.
- The parathyroids are situated in close relationship to the posterior and lateral aspects of the thyroid.

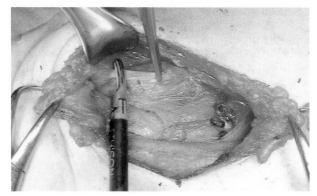

Fig. 23.**3** The superior thyroid vascular pedicle is divided with the UltraCision shears.

The parathyroid glands may be inadvertently damaged or removed during thyroidectomy. The UltraCision shears should not be used close to the parathyroids, in order to avoid thermal injury.

🦉 Personal Experience

In a masked, match-pair study, we evaluated our impression of the UltraCision shears in thyroidectomies (9). We observed a clinically and economically significant reduction in operating time without any increase in the complication rate. Later, a randomized, controlled trial was performed to confirm the initial expression and results (10). Patients were recruited from the Division of Endocrine Surgery, Helsinki University Central Hospital, from August 1997 to January 1999. Patients, destined to undergo total thyroidectomy or lobectomy because of toxic goiter, suspicion of differentiated thyroid carcinoma or follicular adenoma were included in the study. The main outcome measure was the operating time. Additional outcome measures were intraoperative bleeding, postoperative bleeding, injury to parathyroid glands, and postoperative palsy of the recurrent laryngeal nerve. Injury of parathyroid glands was estimated by calculating the ratio between serum calcium level on first postoperative morning and before surgery.

The mean operating time with the UltraCision shears was 99.1 minutes, (range 63–157 minutes). The mean operating time with the conventional method 134.9 minutes (range 86–286 minutes). The average savings in operating time when using UltraCision was 35.8 minutes ($p = 0.013$). The mean amount of intraoperative bleeding was 128 ml in the UltraCision group and 268 ml in the conventional group. The difference was not statistically significant ($p = 0.16$) because of the high variation in the amount of bleeding caused by the tendency of some patients with toxic goiter to bleed a great deal. The mean postoperative drainage until the next morning was 67.2 ml in the UltraCision group and 51.8 ml in the conventional group ($p = 0.36$). The mean serum calcium level on the first postoperative morning was 86.9 % of the preoperative level in the UltraCision group, and 88.4 % in the conventional group ($p = 0.60$). The median hospital stay was 2.5 days in the UltraCision group, and 3.0 days in the conventional group ($p = 0.41$).

Since 1997, UltraCision has routinely been used at our department for thyroid operations, except for the patients included in the conventional group of our trial.

Discussion

In a randomized trial, when the UltraCision shears were used in thyroid surgery, operating time was reduced by 23.2 % over the conventional method (10). Intraoperative bleeding tended to be less with UltraCision, but the difference was not statistically significant. There were no remarkable differences between study groups in the complication rates. Complications with long-term consequences in thyroid surgery are hypocalcemia and recurrent laryngeal nerve injury, and the complication rate increases in direct relation to the extent of thyroid resection (3). So far, we have not used the UltraCision shears close to the recurrent laryngeal nerve or the parathyroid glands; rather, we have used resorbable ligatures.

In our cost/benefit analysis of the randomized trial, we examined the costs of the device and the savings in operating time. In our hospital, the calculated price of the use of the impulse generator and the shears was equal to the calculated savings in operating time.

We have also used UltraCision for partial lobectomy and subtotal thyroidectomy with good results (unpublished data). In some patients the UltraCision has been used for resections.

In conclusion, UltraCision is a suitable tool for use in total thyroidectomies and lobectomies, and compared with the conventional method it saves operating time.

Editor's tip: The timesaving effect is also true for laparoscopic Nissen fundoplication and explained by the shortened time for division of the short gastric vessels (see Chapter 5). The superior sealing effect with ultrasonic instruments is demonstrated in pancreatic surgery (Suzuki Y, Fujino Y, Tanjoka Y, et al. Randomized clinical trial of ultrasonic dissector or conventional division in distal pancreatectomy for non-fibrotic pancreas. Br J Surg 1999; 86: 608–611).

However, to obtain full benefit of the device, approximately 10 hours of experience with it is required. In spite of minimal lateral thermal effect of the device, it can still not be recommended to be used close to the nerves or parathyroids.

References

1. Amaral JF. The experimental development of an ultrasonically activated scalpel for laparoscopic use. Surg Laparosc Endosc 1994; 4: 92–99.
2. Amaral JF. Laparoscopic cholecystectomy in 200 consecutive patients using an ultrasonically activated scalpel. Surg Laparosc Endosc 1995; 5: 255–262.
3. Flynn MB, Lyons KJ, Tarter JW, Ragsdale TL. Local complications after surgical resection for thyroid carcinoma. Am J Surg 1994; 168: 404–407.
4. Hoenig DM, Chrostek CA, Amaral JF. Laparosonic coagulating shears: alternative method of hemostatic control of unsupported tissue. J Endourol 1996; 10: 431–433.
5. Laycock WS, Trus TL, Hunter JG. New technology for the division of short gastric vessels during laparoscopic Nissen fundoplication. A prospective randomized trial. Surg Endosc 1996; 10: 71–73.
6. Psacioglu H, Atay Y, Cetindag B, Saribulbul O, Buket S, Hamulu A. Easy harvesting of radial artery with ultrasonically RK, Haglund CH. Ultrasonically activated shears in thyroid surgery. Am J Surg 1998; 175: 491 activated scalpel. Ann Thorac Surg 1998; 65: 984–985.
7. Swanstrom LL, Pennings JL. Laparoscopic control of short gastric vessels. J Am Coll Surg 1995; 181: 347–351.
8. Takami H, Ikeda Y, Niimi M. Ultrasonically activated scalpel for subtotal thyroidectomy in Graves' disease. Letter. Am J Surg 1999; 178: 433.
9. Voutilainen PE, Haapiainen RK, Haglund CH. Ultrasonically activated shears in thyroid surgery. Am J Surg 1998; 175: 491–493.
10. Voutilainen PE, and Haglund CH. Ultrasonically activated shears in thyroidectomies. A randomized trial. Ann Surg 2000; 231: 322–328.

24 Laparoscopic Hysterectomy: with or without Ophorectomy

M. Kauko

Since the first laparoscopic hysterectomy by Harry Reich in 1989 (1) the topic has been under constant surveillance within the gynecological surgical community. All possible hemostatic and cutting methods have been introduced, but electrosurgery, especially with bipolar forceps, and endostaplers has been most widely accepted (1, 2). The UltraCision harmonic scalpel with its novel qualities both in coagulation and cutting has proved to be an effective tool in hysterectomy and has earned its place among the laparoscopic instrumentation.

This chapter will deal with the special features of the UltraCision scalpel in laparoscopic hysterectomy. Laparoscopic hysterectomy is defined as a hysterectomy in which the uterine arteries are sealed laparoscopically. The supporting ligaments of the uterus are, in most cases, cut laparoscopically as well as the colpotomy. Finally, the uterus is removed and the vaginal cuff is sutured vaginally. These steps follow the definitions proposed by Garry and Reich in 1993 (3). Basic knowledge about operative laparoscopy is not covered in this context; there are several textbooks available for this purpose.

Indication and Preoperative Management

The UltraCision scalpel with the laparosonic coagulating shears (LCS) is a multifunctional instrument. Whether 10 mm or 5 mm in diameter it grasps, dissects, coagulates, and cuts the tissue. The multifunctionality cannot be overemphasized, because this simplifies the procedure and potentially allows the surgeon to reduce the number of operating ports down to two, the first for the optic and the other for the LCS. A strong uterine manipulator with different axes to move the uterus is obligatory. Of the conventional laparoscopic instrumentation, only a suction-irrigation device is usually needed, but instruments like graspers, scissors, and even a bipolar electrosurgery device should be available and might be useful depending on the case.

The simplicity offered by the UltraCision scalpel should, however, never lead to compromising visibility of the surgical field and thereby compromising the safety of the procedure. The procedure can be started with the intention of using only the UltraCision scalpel, but during the course of the operation more instruments may be needed; they have to be at hand, and the surgeon has to know how to use them. He/she has to be open-minded enough to change to them if necessary (Table 24.1).

Table 24.1 Instrumentation for laparoscopic hysterectomy with UltraCision

Instrument	Obligatory	Depending on the case
Trocars (2–4)	+	
LCS (5 mm/10 mm)	+	
Uterine manipulator	+	
Suction-irrigation	+	
Grasper (1–2)		+
Bipolar forceps		+
Scissors		+
Needle holders		+
Clip applicator		+

Editor's tip: When using one operating port only, the port should have an insufflating channel which can be kept open to remove the mist produced by the UltraCision scalpel during coagulation.

Extensive descriptions of the ultrasonic energy used for coagulation and cutting as well as the differences from other energy modalities are given in the first two chapters of this book. However, some features will be noted here, because of the novelties ultrasonic energy has brought to the traditional gynecological surgical thinking.

Coagulation and cutting with UltraCision are basically dependent on four interconnected features: power level, tissue tension, blade sharpness, grip force/pressure. Obviously, activation time is important and is linearly correlated to the tissue destruction (4). In hysterectomy, a delicate balance between the tension in the target tissue and the grip force in the hand piece of the instrument is important. A rule of thumb is that the target tissue should not be under tension while coagulating; otherwise, it will be cut too fast before adequate coagulation is achieved and the vessels will not be sealed. This is very different from conventional surgical techniques in open and laparoscopic approaches in which the tissue to be severed is first grasped then stretched. In most cases, the tension created by mobilizing the uterus with a manipulator is enough. If gaspers are used to enhance visibility, the surgeon must pay attention to not stretching the tissue under coagulation, because that will lead to hemostatic problems in highly vascular areas.

Adequate coagulation also requires a delicate adjustment in the grip force of the hand piece. During the learning curve for the method, adjustment of the grip

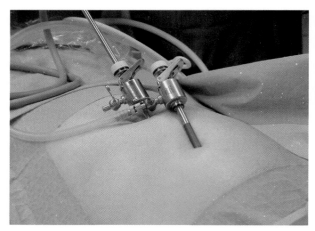

Fig. 24.**1** Position of ports.

force becomes more automatic and the force varies according to the vascularity, tissue thickness, and desired speed for coagulation and cutting. The selected power level and the blade shape are equally important in balancing the coagulation and cutting, but they can be predetermined while the tissue tension and grip force are determined by the surgeon's hand.

![] Operation

The patient is positioned in the lithotomy position. If the surgeon intends to mobilize the uterus him/herself, the legs should be low enough for the surgeon to be able to reach the manipulator without effort with one hand while operating with the UltraCision scalpel in the other hand. The degree of Trendelenburg position depends on the anatomic situation within the pelvis. Sometimes good visibility requires tilting by as much as 20–30°, in which case shoulder braces are needed to support the patient steadily on the table. Patient positioning does not differ from the standard position for the gynecologic laparoscopic approach but, if the advantage provided by UltraCision is fully appreciated, the surgeon should have an easy access to the uterine manipulator him/herself.

After standard preparations including cleansing the abdomen and the vagina and wrapping the patient, the Foley catheter and the uterine manipulator are inserted. When using a manipulator with different choices of uterine tips, the largest possible tip to fit into the cavity should be selected. This will enhance the maximal movements of the uterus with the manipulator, thereby minimizing the possibility for needing graspers and extra ports for them.

After insufflating the abdominal cavity, a trocar for the optic is inserted through the belly. After checking the abdominal cavity and the pelvis, a second 5 mm trocar is inserted in the midline, cranial to the uterus. There is no rule of thumb for the height of the positioning of the operating trocar, but when operating with

one port only, the surgeon has to be able to reach the uterine sides tangentially with the UltraCision scalpel from above (Fig. 24.**1**).

> Editor's tip: The author currently uses a 5 mm, 0° optic, which gives as good an image as a 10 mm one, although the tolerance for diminishing light is narrow.

When preserving the ovaries, the procedure starts by grasping the utero-ovarian ligament or the fallopian tube with the shears. There is no guideline for the sequence of severing the structures; the individual anatomic situation guides the decision. Every bite of tissue between the blades is coagulated and cut using power level 3. Depending on the thickness of the tissue bundle, this has to be done in several steps (Fig. 24.**2**). The capacity of the blades to grip is 10 mm in length. Coagulation is highly dependent on the tissues type, i.e., penetration of the ultrasound energy to the tissue. The energy will be transmitted to the tissue parallel to the applied force, so only the tissue between the blades in which the force is applied will be affected. It is important to keep the uterus under maximal tension and pushed upwards with the manipulator to let the adnexa hang freely alongside. This will create just enough tissue tension for the UltraCision scalpel to achieve adequate coagulation before the tissue is cut. The gripping force should be only moderate—just enough to keep the tissue bundle between the blades.

> Editor's tip: By carefully rotating the tip of the instrument while coagulating the effect is enhanced.

If the dissection plane is too close to the uterus, annoying back-bleeding from the uterus may occur. Large fundal myomas tend to retract the adnexa very close to the uterine body, leaving little room for an adequate pedicle on the uterine side. For diffuse back-bleeding, pushing the active blade tangentially against the bleeding area while utilizing power level 3 is usually satisfactory. Visible bleeders are grasped and coagulated. In any case, the back-bleeding in this step of the procedure should be stopped because several steps are still to be done before the uterine blood supply is cut completely.

The procedure is continued by grasping, coagulating, and cutting the round ligaments. Depending on the thickness of the ligament, several bites may be needed. Power level 5 will give adequate hemostasis in this relatively avascular tissue. The bladder flap is cut by using the instrument as a knife, either keeping the blades open and using the active blade only or using the posterior, free edge or the active blade. Starting from the severed round ligament, the bladder peritoneum is lifted upwards with the active blade. Proceeding medially towards the contralateral round ligament while stretching the cervix with the manipulator, the uterovesical junction can easily be identified and the bladder peritoneum opened at the proper level,

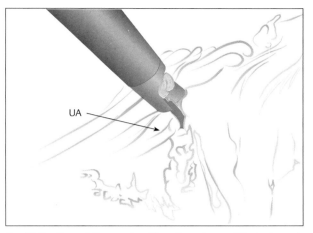

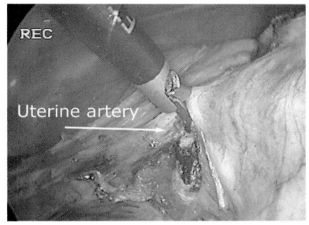

Fig. 24.**2**   Coagulation and cutting the adnexa. *UA* uterine artery.

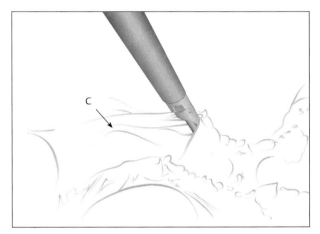

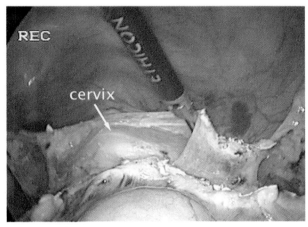

Fig. 24.**3**   Opening the bladder flap. *C* cervix.

which will *per se* retract the bladder side of the peritoneum downwards and hence visualize the cervical fascia (Fig. 24.**3**). This step is fast and usually almost bloodless with power level 5. The cavitational effect of UltraCision will promote separation of the tissue planes and dissection of the bladder from the cervix. Then, the bladder pillars can be coagulated and cut, but being more vascular, more hemostatic effect is needed and power level 3 is advised. The bladder itself can be gently pushed further down along the cervix with the tip of the instrument against the cervix, not against the bladder, since that might cause perforation of the bladder.

If the patient has had previous caesarean sections, the uterovesical junction may be adherent, and sharp dissection is required to free the bladder. The UltraCision scalpel is a very delicate and safe instrument for sharp dissection because the thermal destruction zone is narrow and predictable, i.e., linearly correlated to the activation time. The risk of thermal damage to the bladder wall is decreased in comparison to electrosurgery (4, 5). However adherent the bladder peritoneum might be, UltraCision alone is usually sufficient, thus demonstrating the multifunctionality of the instrument.

After opening the posterior leaf of the broad ligament, the uterine vessels are dissected free from the surrounding connective tissue by using the instrument as a normal blunt dissector. The uterus is pushed maximally upwards and contralaterally to visualize the vessels and stretch the cervix, against which the vessels are grasped, coagulated, and cut using power level 3. It is important to apply as little grip force as possible, just enough to keep the vessel bundle between the blades, which is facilitated by pushing the tip of the instrument against the cervix, leaving no room for the escape for any of the vessels. The instrument should be left to do its work, as it will, if enough time is allowed for coagulation (Fig. 24.**4**). If the artery seems to recover, a second application with UltraCision is needed. The cervix has to be stretched all the time to keep the coagulation zone far from the ureter.

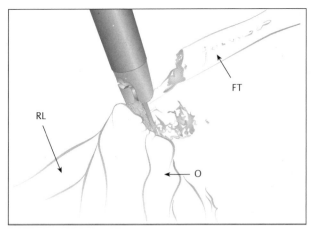
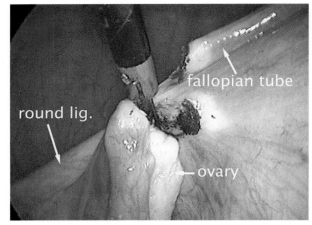

Fig. 24.**4**   Coagulation and cutting the uterine vessels. *RL* round ligament, *FT* fallopian tube, *O* ovary.

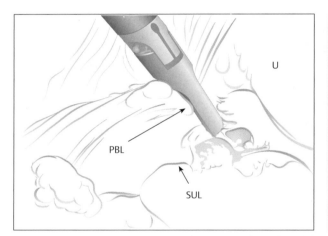
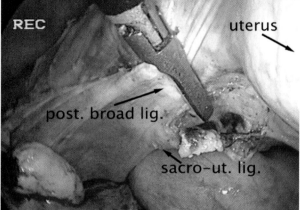

Fig. 24.**5**   Cutting the parametria, colpotomy. *PBL* post broad ligament, *U* uterus, *SUL* sacro-uterin ligament.

Editor's tip: As with any other hemostatic method, coagulating and cutting too close to the uterine wall with the UltraCision scalpel tends to cause back-bleeding from the myometrium. This might be extremely difficult to stop and a good tip is to seal the vessels on the contralateral side, which will eventually stop the uterine blood supply and, obviously, the back-bleeding.

Whether the parametria should be cut from above or below depends on the supportive status of the pelvic floor. If any descensus is present, the supporting ligaments should be cut vaginally, followed by the standard steps for the vaginal pelvic floor support. If the pelvic supportive status is normal, the lateral and posterior parametria are coagulated and cut laparoscopically with the UltraCision scalpel using power level 3 or 5. This is, again, enhanced by pushing the uterus strongly upwards and adjusting the angle of anteflexion of the cervix to give the best access to the target tissue. An intrafascial technique is preferred and easy to manage with UltraCision. The precervical fascia

should be penetrated by using the instrument as a knife and the fascia is pushed downwards, simultaneously coagulating the small vessels (Fig. 24.5). After the anterior fornix has been reached it will be opened by the UltraCision scalpel against any instrument lifting up the anterior fornix from the vagina. If special instruments for sealing the vagina airtight are used, the colpotomy can easily be done circularly with UltraCision. Otherwise, the procedure continues vaginally by completing the colpotomy and suturing any of the possibly remaining supporting ligaments from below. The vaginal vault is closed from below with a running suture. The author uses 2–0 polypropylene suture.

Editor's tip: A good, practical suggestion is to cut the sacrouterine ligaments close to their insertion to the uterus at the very beginning of the procedure. This will give an excellent landmark at the end of the procedure, as to how far down one should attempt to go.

It is important to check the hemostasis laparoscopically after the vagina has been closed. The vault is lifted up with a sponge, to visualize any possible small bleeders. The time gap between coagulating the uterine vessels and rechecking the hemostasis after the vaginal phase seems to be long enough for any recoveries of the uterine arteries to show up. If any bleeding in the pedicle is encountered, recoagulating with UltraCision is usually enough.

If the operation has thus far proceeded with one instrument only, a grasper will sometimes be needed at this point to remove the bowel loops and enhance visibility. Recovery of the uterine arteries after coagulation is rare but potentially hazardous and the possibility should be totally excluded.

If one or both ovaries are to be removed, the procedure starts from the infundipulo-pelvic ligaments (I-P ligament). The conduit of the ureter (when crossing the iliac vessels and descending to the pelvis) has to be verified before any further steps are taken. If there is any question about the conduit of the ureters, they should be dissected and visualized retroperitoneally. In difficult anatomic situations, it saves time and trouble to insert a ureteral stent via a cystoscope to be able to orientate correctly. Even though the UltraCision scalpel acts as a grasper, its grasping capacity might not be enough to retract the ligament medially from the pelvic side-wall. A grasper is needed to hold the ovary while coagulating and cutting the I-P ligament with the instrument. Again, it is necessary to leave the tissue under coagulation loose enough to achieve adequate coagulation before it is cut. For coagulation and cutting the I-P ligament, power level 3 is appropriate.

> Editor's tip: If the surgeon does not want to use an extra grasper but rather only the UltraCision scalpel for grasping and coagulation, it is advisable to open the peritoneum around the I-P ligament in order to create a rougher tissue surface, which the instrument can hold better.

After sealing the vessels in the I-P ligament, the mesovarium and mesosalpinx down to the round ligament are severed by using power level 3 or 5 depending on the vascularity. The posterior leaf of the broad ligament is opened just by lifting the peritoneum up with the active blade and cutting it with power level 5 to the insertion of the sacro-uterine ligament. Often the uterine vessels are clearly visibly by now and the procedure can continue by further dissecting them or by opening the bladder peritoneum as described above. The hysterectomy described above will then follow.

 Hints and Pitfalls

- In the 10 mm UltraCision scalpel, the active blade rotates and offers three different blade shapes for coagulation and cutting. The flat surface of the blade has excellent coagulation capability. It can be used to coagulate the more vascular areas before turning the blade for cutting. On the other hand, the wider shaft decreases the visual field when working tangentially with the optical axis. The tip of the instrument can be partly hidden behind the shaft. The author's choice is the 5 mm instrument, with which the tip can always be seen, even though the choice for the different blades is lost.
- If adhesions impair the operation field, UltraCision is a safe and effective instrument for excision. In difficult anatomic situations the ports (as many as are needed) should be placed according to the operative requirements to be able to reach the adhesions safely. Do not forget to check the umbilical region from another port if there are any suspicions for bowel adhesions in that region.
- After a final check of the hemostasis, it is sometimes necessary to leave a drainage in the pouch of Douglas to drain the possible venous oozing and to avoid hematomas in the vault. The drain can be placed via a 5 mm port.
- Morcellation of large uterine myomas can be extremely tedious work. If the uterine blood supply is cut, morcellation from above with an electric device may save time. The uterus can be shaped for more easy vaginal extraction. If an electric morcellator is not available, the procedure has to be done vaginally (Table 24.**2**).

 Personal Experience

The total number of laparoscopic hysterectomies performed with UltraCision in our department exceeds 250. The series of the first 50 patients operated with this technique was thoroughly followed. The indications for hysterectomy were: uterine myomas (68 %), endometriosis (12 %), ovarian tumors (5 %), and miscellaneous (10 %). In 35 % of the cases, concomitant ophorectomy was done. The mean uterine weight was 190 g (115–430 g), mean operation time 60 minutes (35–90 minutes) and the mean blood loss 170 ml (50–600 ml). Eighty-five percent of the patients left the hospital on the first postoperative day. No major complications were encountered. One patient required hemotransfusion because of operative bleeding of 600 ml. Two patients developed a minor pelvic floor infection and were treated by oral antibiotics. These complications are comparable to the larger series reported in laparoscopic hysterectomies (6, 7). After this series using UltraCision as a hemostatic and cutting device, use of the instrument as the operating tool has

Table 24.**2**   Steps of hysterectomy with UltraCision, including technical advice

Step	LCS/power level	LCS/blade shape	Other optional instruments*
Infundibulopelvic ligament	3	Shears	Grasper
Utero-ovarian ligament	3	Shears	Grasper
Round ligament	5	Shears	
Bladder flap	5	Knife	
Posterior peritoneum	5	Knife/shears	
Uterine vessels	3	Shears	
Ligaments	3	Shears	
Colpotomy	3	Knife	Vaginal instrument to lift the fornix
Morcellation			Electric morcellator, vaginal instruments
Vaginal closure			Vaginal instruments for closure
Checking hemostasis	3 (on demand)	Shears (on demand)	Grasper, clip applicator (on demand)

* A suction-irrigation device must always be at hand, to regain visibility if bleeding is encountered

become routine for laparoscopic hysterectomy in our department. The operating time is shorter in comparison to electrosurgery after the personal learning curves for UltraCision have been completed. The learning curve is dependent on the overall experience in major laparoscopic surgery. After experience with other hemostatic methods, about 10 cases will give a sufficient learning curve for UltraCision.

Discussion

Ultrasound energy and the UltraCision harmonic scalpel with its multifunctionality have brought simplicity to the instrumentation of laparoscopic hysterectomy. The approach and the procedure can become very minimalistic, in which the steps are easy to follow and learn. It is not only simplicity, but also the increased safety in comparison to electrosurgery, which should promote the idea of using ultrasound energy more widely in the laparoscopic approach (8, 9). The preliminary concern of UltraCision being slow in action is counteracted by the fact that the surgeon does not need to change instruments for coagulation and cutting. Because no tissue is cut before it is coagulated, the operation field tends to remain very dry with excellent visibility.

References

1. Reich H, DeCaprio J, Mc Glynn F. Laparoscopic hysterectomy. J Gynecol Surg 1989; 5: 213–6.
2. Reich H, McGlynn F, Sekel L. Total laparoscopic hysterectomy, Gynaecol Laparosc 1993; 2: 59–63.
3. Garry R, Reich H. Laparoscopic hysterectomy. In: Garry R, Reich H. editors. Laparoscopic Hysterectomy, 1st edn. Oxford: Blackwell Scientific Publications; 1993. pp. 79–117.
4. Amaral JF, Chrostek C. Depth of thermal injury: ultrasonically activated scalpel vs. electrosurgery. Surg Endosc 1995; 9: 226.
5. Amaral JF. Laparoscopic cholecystectomy in 200 consecutive patients using ultrasonically activated scalpel. Surg Laparosc Endosc 1995; 4: 255–62.
6. Härkki-Siren P, Sjöberg J, Mäkinen J, Heinonen PK, Kauko M, Tomas E, Laatikainen T. Finnish national register of laparoscopic hysterectomies: A review and complications of 1165 operations. Am J Obstet Gynecol 1997; 176: 118–22.
7. Olsson JH, Ellström M, Hahlin M. A randomised prospective trial comparing laparoscopic hysterectomy and abdominal hysterectomy. Br J Obstet Gynecol 1996; 103: 345–50.
8. Amaral JF, Chrostek CA. Experimental comparison of the ultrasonically activated scalpel to electrosurgery and laser surgery for laparoscopic use. Min Invas Ther & Allied Technol 1997; 6: 324–31.
9. McCarus SD. Physiologic mechanism of the ultrasonically activated scalpel. J Am Assoc Gynecol Laparosc 1996; 3: 601–8.

25 Laparoscopic Myomectomy

M. Degueldre, J. Vandromme

Uterine leiomyomas are found in 20 to 30% of women over 30 years of age and in 75% of hysterectomy specimens (1, 2). Although few patients are symptomatic, this pathology is the major indication for hysterectomy in premenopausal women (3, 4). A clonal aberration, commonly on chromosomes 7 and 12, is associated with these benign tumors (5). Estrogen and progesterone receptors play an important role in the growth of the leiomyoma (6). Clinical results with hormonal competition or suppression of sex steroid secretion show only temporary relief of symptoms or reduction in size (7). Delayed childbearing age, body image, and symptomatology will determine the indications for conservative surgery. Besides the standard open surgery, interest is increasingly shown for minimally invasive surgical techniques in the management of myomas.

This article will focus on the laparoscopic treatment of intramural/subserosal myomas.

Indication and Preoperative Management

Leiomyomas are associated with menstrual abnormalities, menometrorrhagia, pelvic pain or pressure, reproductive disorders, urinary and G. I. tract symptoms in one third of the patients (8). Localization, size, number, and tumor growth will determine whether a medical and/or surgical approach is chosen. Submucosal fibroids bulging in the uterine cavity and pedunculated intracavitary fibroids are treated through the hysteroscopic route. Intramural, subserosal, and pedunculated fibroids are treated abdominally (9). Rapid tumor growth, confirmed by echography and vascular Doppler flow, for symptomatic or intramyometrial fibroids of over 4 cm in diameter are indications, in premenopausal women, for laparoscopic conservative surgery. A well-trained endoscopic surgical team can operate any fibroid. In our experience, as well as that reflected by the literature, a consensus is gradually emerging that a maximal size of 8–10 cm and a total number of four fibroids should not be exceeded (10).

Ultrasonography

Ultrasonography is the most accurate method to determine the number, size, localization and, combined with a Doppler flow-meter, vascularization. Both transvaginal and transabdominal scanning are important, because large pedunculated fibroids on the fundus may be overlooked with the transvaginal scan. As stated above, the number and size will determine the intended approach for surgery. Preoperative localization is important regarding the relation to the endometrial cavity and the spatial orientation in some forms of intramural situation. Doppler flow measurement is a good indicator for rapid growth but is of little practical interest for the operation as such.

Medical Therapy

GnRH agonist treatment before myomectomy aims to reduce the size of the myoma and restore the patient's hemoglobin in cases of severe anemia. Optimal reduction of myoma size (32–84%, mean 51%) is obtained after three months of therapy (11).

Although according to the calculation of a sphere, a volume reduction of 50% will only reduce the size of a fibroid of 8 cm to 6.5 cm, this small reduction of the diameter will have important implications as to the length of myometrial incision, dissection, and morcellation time.

Amenorrhea induced in the majority of cases after 2–3 months of GnRH agonist therapy increases hemoglobin levels, avoiding unnecessary perioperative blood transfusions. Some authors have demonstrated significantly less operative blood loss after GnRH agonist treatment in open as well as in laparoscopic myomectomy procedures (12).

Operation

The patient is placed in a dorsal lithotomy position, legs flexed, with shoulder straps fixed, to allow a maximal Trendelenburg position. After vesical catheterization, a strong uterine manipulator is placed in order to mobilize and rotate the uterus.

The following choice of instruments is recommended:
- 2 × 10 mm ports (camera and grasper)
- 1 × 12 mm port (UltraCision with curved blade, morcellator)
- UltraCision curved blade (HC 325)
- UltraCision coagulation ball
- 1 × atraumatic dissecting forceps
- 1 × myoma grasper
- 2 × needle holders
- Resorbable sutures 1 (4 metric), 1/2, 27 mm, round tip needle (polygalactyn)
- Morcellator (Steiner, Karl Storz)

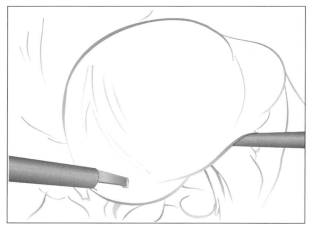

Fig. 25.**1**   Exposure of the myoma for incision.

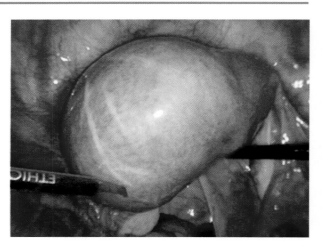

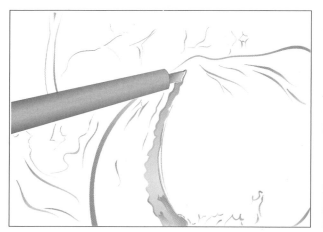

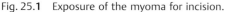

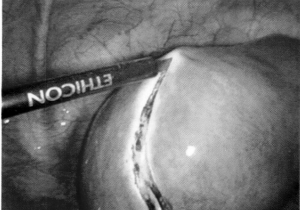

Fig. 25.**2**   Serosal incision using the cutting edge of the UltraCision blade.

After creation of a pneumoperitoneum and umbilical insertion of a 10 mm port for the laparoscope, two lateral ports are placed, high (approximately 2 cm under the umbilical line) and lateral (exterior to the epigastric artery and rectus muscle).

> Editor's tip: Port localization must allow instruments to work perpendicular on the main operation site. This is important for the dissection as well as for the suture.

The uterus is positioned in such a manner as to face the UltraCision curved blade at the site of incision (Fig. 25.**1**). Careful examination and comparison with echographic data will help determine the incision line with the least myometrial depth. The incision line resects the longitudinal axis of the uterus. This will, according to the vascularization, avoid unnecessary bleeding. The curved blade (level 3) progresses slowly through the myometrium with the sharp edge. Incision length must be approximately 2/3 of the diameter of the myoma (Fig. 25.**2**).

> Editor's tip: Start the incision at the lowest end and move upwards in order to avoid bleeding on the incision site.

While cutting, bleeding can be controlled by pushing the flat part of the blade against the myometrium on both sides of the incision (level 3). This procedure is continued until the white surface of the myoma is reached (Fig. 25.**3**). With the curved blade used as a smooth retractor and an atraumatic grasping forceps, margins are separated. The myoma is then stabilized with large tenaculum forceps.

From this moment on, it is essential to work on the surface of the myoma. While the tenaculum forceps exert a gentle traction, the curved blade is used as a dissector, a coagulation device, and a retractor. Dissection is carried out with the flat part of the blade (level 3) by sliding it over the surface of the myometrium. The myometrial fibers of the pseudocapsula are gradually disconnected and small vessels coagulated. The myoma is gradually extracted (Fig. 25.**4**). No bleeding will occur as long as the dissection remains

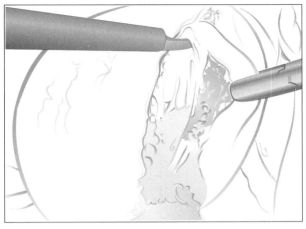

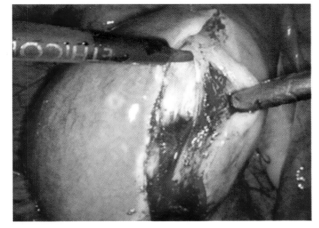

Fig. 25.**3** Myometrial incision on the surface of the myoma.

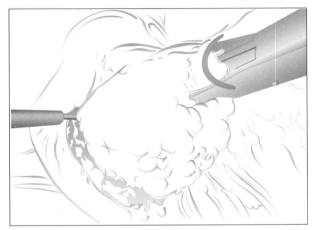

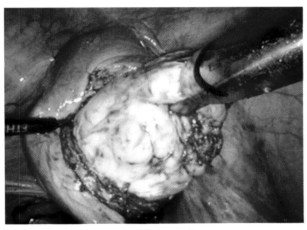

Fig. 25.**4** Gradual extraction of the myoma with large tenaculum forceps and the UltraCision blade used as a retractor.

under the pseudocapsula, leaving no myometrium on the surface of the myoma.

> Editor's tip: Coagulation, when needed, can be controlled with the UltraCision ball tip. The instrument is applied firmly on the myometrial surface at level 3. Rotation of the tip while applying energy will avoid "sticking" to the tissue.

Incision closure will then be performed in one layer with absorbable suture material (Vycril 1). This suture is a double-U with the needle passing through the entire mass of the dissected myometrial capsule with entry and exit through the intact serosal surface (Fig. 25.**5 a, b**). This stitch combines hemostasis, closure of the defect, and anatomical reconstruction simultaneously, leaving only intact serosa on the surface (Fig. 25.**6 a, b**). One stitch is needed for every 2 cm of myometrial incision. Suture and knotting are performed with two needle holders. The knot is tied intracorporeally to ensure optimal traction without a cutting effect on the muscle.

After completion of the suture, myomas are morcellated with an electromechanical morcellator. This part of the operation is time-consuming and accounts often for more than half of the total operating time.

After thorough rinsing of the abdominal cavity and control of the hemostasis, the fascia of the lateral ports is closed and the pneumoperitoneum is deflated.

⚠ Hints and Pitfalls

- As this operation addresses often voluminous intra-abdominal masses, it is important to position the trocars as lateral and as high as possible. When needed, a fourth 5 mm suprapubic port is inserted. The diameter of the lateral ports is determined by the size of the myoma grasper and the morcellator.
- A strong uterine manipulator is mandatory in order to mobilize heavy uterine masses.
- The use of dilute vasopressin (10–20 units in 100 ml saline) is often advocated for myometrial injection at the incision site. This product can be dangerous

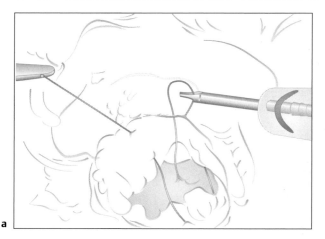

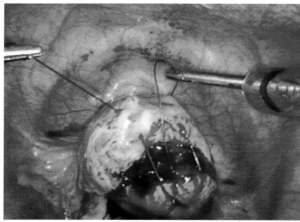

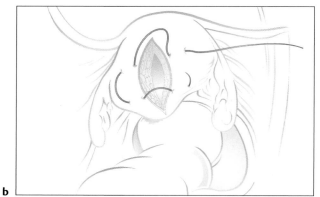

Fig. 25.**5 a, b** Double-U suture. The thread is passed 4 times through the serosa and the entire myometrial thickness.

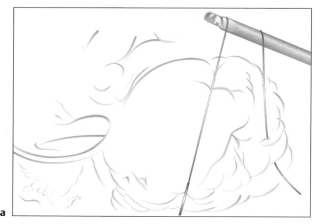

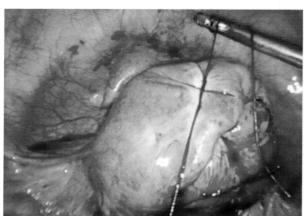

Fig. 25.**6 a, b** The knot is tied intracorporeally. Only intact serosa is left on the surface.

for the patient when injected in the blood vessels. In some countries legislation has banned its use.

- We do not advocate rinsing during the operation, but only aspiration of blood, as light absorption by hemoglobin is a major factor in reducing the visibility.
- The UltraCision blade finds its way slowly through the tissue. If the surgeon applies too much force on the instrument, the coagulation effect is suboptimal.
- The vycril thread does not slide easily. It is important to pull the thread through at every step of the myometrial suture. This will also avoid damage to the muscle when tying knots.

Discussion

Assuming that the indication for myomectomy has been correctly assessed (13), the operative technique and approach must be defined. Randomized studies comparing laparoscopy with laparotomy showed less postoperative pain, shorter recovery time, and less blood loss for laparoscopy (14, 15). In spite of this, laparoscopic myomectomy remains a controversial technique. The major criticisms for laparoscopic myomectomy are the inability to palpate the uterus, the loss of degrees of freedom inherent to the design of the instruments, and the difficulty of intracorporeal suturing and knotting. The decision whether to remove myomas by laparoscopy is very much influenced by surgical skill and experience (16).

As the ultimate goal is the restoration of the integrity of an organ, tissue trauma must be avoided. We therefore prefer ultrasonic dissection rather than the commonly used monopolar current. Monopolar current induces the risk for direct coupling, capacitative coupling, and high frequency leakage. Due to the high temperature, carbonization of the tissue is a common phenomenon and the thermal injury to the adjacent myometrium is important. This may hamper optimal tissue healing.

As stated by Topel: "Excessive thermal injury to the myometrium secondary to monopolar cautery use may be the cause of reported fistula formation, uterine dehiscence, and extensive postoperative adhesions" (17).

On the other hand, ultrasonic energy avoids the risks inherent to monopolar current. The energy source is extra-abdominal. The system operates at low temperature with minimal dispersion, reducing tissue damage (18). In contrast to the important smoke emission of monopolar current, ultrasonic energy emits only small water droplets.

The UltraCision blade is a multifunctional instrument, combining cutting, coagulation, and dissection. This improves the ergonomics of the operation as only two instruments are needed for the dissection of the myometrium. The unique shape of the curved blade has several advantages. The sharp sides are used for cutting (level 3) while simultaneously the flat part coagulates minor bleeders by pressure on the cut edges. For the dissection of the pseudocapsula from the myoma the blade glides under the tissue (level 5). The cavitation effect separates the capsula from the tumor.

Considering the large dissection surface and the need to reconstruct an organ while avoiding postoperative adhesions, the suture must be hemostatic, strong, and consistent with the power lines, leaving only intact serosa on the surface.

We have developed a double-U suture (Fig. 25.**5 a, b**), passing through the serosa, with the full thickness of the myometrium taken in. This suture meets the above-mentioned criteria. Uterine reconstruction is completed with only one layer of sutures.

Myometrial dissection, energy sources applied on the tissue and suture type are separately or together responsible for postoperative uterine ruptures during pregnancy (19). At this stage, there is no evidence-based approach to evaluate the risk for labor after myomectomy (laparotomy or laparoscopy) but one has to keep in mind that the risk for uterine rupture after a classical caesarean section is 12 % (20).

Laparoscopic myomectomy remains a difficult and delicate operation. The UltraCision blade proves to be ergonomic, efficient, and safe for the patient. This technique induces minimal tissue damage, allowing better wound healing.

References

1. Cramer SF, Patal A. The frequency of uterine leiyomyoma. Am J Clin Pathol 1990; 94: 435–8.
2. Cramer DW. Epidemiology of myomas. Semin Reprod Endocrinol 1992; 10: 320–4.
3. Bachman G. Hysterectomy: a critical review. J Reprod Med 1990; 35: 839–62.
4. Stewart EA. Uterine fibroids. Lancet 2001; 357: 293–8.
5. Pandis N, Heim S, Bardi G et al. Chromosome analysis of 96 leiomyomatas. Cancer Genet Cytogenet 1991; 55: 11–8.
6. Soules MR, McCarty KS. Leiomyomas: steroid receptor content. Am J Obstet Gynecol 1982; 143: 6–11.
7. Fedele L, Vercellini P, Bianchi S, Brioschi D, Dorta M. Treatment with GnRH agonists before myomectomy and the risk of short-term myoma recurrence. Br J Obstet Gynaecol 1990; 97: 393–6.
8. Buttram VC, Reiter RC. Uterine leiomyoma: etiology, symptomatology, and management. Fertil Steril 1981; 36: 433–45.
9. Tulandi T, Al-Took S. Endoscopic myomectomy. Obstet Gynecol Clin North Am 1999; 26: 135–48.
10. Dubuisson JB, Chapron C, Mouly M, Foulot H, Aubriot F. Laparoscopic myomectomy. Gynaecological Endoscopy 1993; 2: 171–3.
11. Campo S, Garcea N. Laparoscopic myomectomy in premenopausal women with and without preoperative treatment using gonadotrophin-releasing hormone analogue. Hum Reprod 1999; 14: 44–8.
12. Mais V, Ajossa S, Guerriero S et al. Laparoscopy versus abdominal myomectomy: A prospective randomized trial to evaluate benefits in early outcome. Am J Obstet Gynecol 1996; 174: 654–8.
13. Haney AF. Clinical decision making regarding leiomyomata: what we need the next millennium. Environ Health Perspect 2000; 108(Suppl 5): 835–9.
14. Stringer NH, Walker JC, Meyer PM. Comparison of 49 laparoscopic myomectomies with 49 open myomectomies. J Am Assoc Gynecol Laparosc 1999; 4: 457–64.

15. Baggish MS, Diamond MP, Nezhat C, Rock JA, SanFilippo JS. Overcoming complications of laparoscopic surgery. I. Contemp Ob Gyn 1994; 39: 92–106.
16. Landi S, Zaccoletti R, Ferrari L, Minelli L. Laparoscopic myomectomy: technique, complications, and ultrasound scan evaluation. J Am Assoc Laparosc 2001; 8: 231–40.
17. Topel HC. Laparoscopic myomectomy, In: Bieber EJ, Maclin VM. editors. Myomectomy. London: Blackwell Science; 1998. pp. 280–92.
18. Amaral JF. Depth of thermal injury: Ultrasonically activated scalpel vs. electrosurgery. Surg Endosc 1995; 9: 226.
19. Pelosi MA 3 rd, Pelosi MA. Spontaneous uterine rupture at thirty-three weeks subsequent to previous superficial laparoscopic myomectomy. Am J Obstet Gynecol 1997; 177: 1547–9.
20. McMahon MJ. Vaginal birth after cesarean. Clin Obstet Gynecol 1999; 41: 369–81.

26 Resection of Deep Infiltrating Endometriosis

W. Feil, J. Scholler

Endometriosis is described as a pathology that necessitates radical surgery. Its etiology is still unclear. This disease is defined morphologically as endometrial glands and stroma outside the uterine cavity. Patients present with severe pelvic pain, dysmenorrhea, deep dyspareunia and chronic pelvic pain. The association with infertility appears logical, but is not definitively proven. A few patients present with symptoms of chronic bowel obstruction.

As a consequence of the introduction of laparoscopy, the awareness that endometriosis is a very frequent disease has progressively increased. Laparoscopy showed that endometriosis does not only mean "chocolate cysts" and black, puckered lesions, but endometriosis can appear also as small white vesicles, red vesicles, flame-like lesions, polypoid lesions and brown lesions. The introduction of CO_2-laser excision techniques confirmed the observation that some lesions also infiltrate deeper than expected in the subperitoneal stroma. Endometriosis infiltrating deeper than 5 mm has been defined as deep endometriosis.

Indication and Preoperative Management

Endometriosis surgery is usually performed by a gynecological surgeon. The general surgeon takes part in the operation of deep infiltrating endometriosis from the beginning when bowel resection has to be assumed or is clearly necessary from preoperative investigations.

All patients with endometriosis undergo flexible sigmoidoscopy. In cases, where obstruction is present or where the endoscope has difficulty in surpassing the proximal rectum and when pushing up the scope is extremely painful to the patient, further investigation is inevitable. Sphincter manometry is performed when compromised function is assumed and stapler surgery may be risky for the sphincter.

The preoperative assessment includes:
- Gynecological examination including ultrasound examination of the pelvis
- CT of abdomen and pelvis
- Barium enema
- Colonoscopy
- Sphincter manometry (when indicated)
- Intravenous pyelography

The day before surgery the bowel is adequately prepared for colon surgery.

If an obstruction of a ureter (normally the left ureter) is suspected from preoperative examinations a double-

J catheter is brought into the ureter cystoscopically the day before surgery. When this procedure becomes necessary during laparoscopy, the double-J catheter is placed intraoperatively.

Operation

The operation of selected patients with severe and extensive endometriosis is planned and performed by an experienced surgeon and an experienced gynecologist. Surgery is performed under general anesthesia. The patient is brought into a modified Lloyd-Davies position. A Foley catheter is introduced into the bladder. The uterus is fixed with a Valtchev uterus manipulator that is introduced through the vagina. This device allows extreme anteflexion of the uterus to enhance the view to the deep pelvic region.

Figure 26.1 shows the fifth postoperative day after removal of postoperative drainage. The patient is discharged. The suture lines give the places of the ports

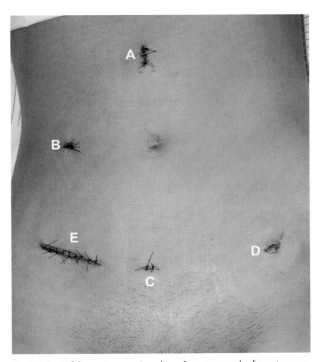

Fig. 26.1 Fifth postoperative day after removal of postoperative drainage. *A* 511 port for camera, *B* 355 port for Endo-Dissect, *C* 355 port for suction device, *D* 355 port for Endo-Babcock and postoperative drainage, *E* 355 port for UltraCision shears, changed to 512 port for Endo-Linear Cutter and extended for mini-laparotomy.

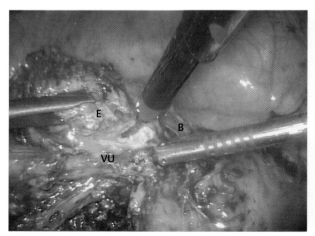

Fig. 26.**2**   Resection of deep infiltrating endometriosis (*E*) from the vesicouterine ligament (*VU*). *B* bladder.

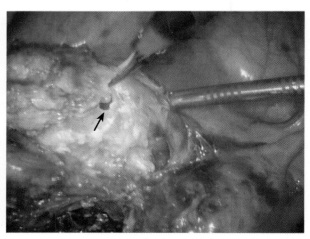

Fig. 26.**3**   During resection of a deep infiltrating endometriosis from the vesicouterine ligament the bladder (*arrow*) is opened.

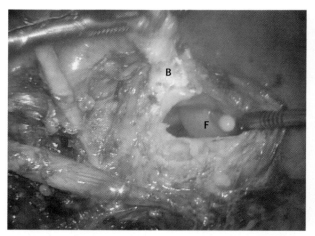

Fig. 26.**4**   During resection of a deep infiltrating endometriosis from the vesicouterine ligament the bladder wall (*B*) is resected and the Foley (*F*) catheter becomes visible.

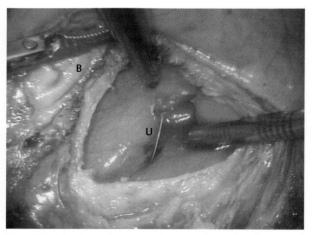

Fig. 26.**5**   Bladder wall (*B*) resection is performed under control of ureter splint (*U*), in order to prevent injury of the trigonum vesicae and its structures.

used for laparoscopic resection of endometriosis, low anterior rectum and sigmoid resection for deep infiltrating endometriosis, resection of the bladder wall, resection of the left ovary and laparoscopically assisted low anterior descendorectostomy with the ILS CDH 29 stapler. In this case the mini-laparotomy was performed in this untypical location, because a scar was present after previous appendectomy. The first port (511) is placed in the umbilicus or in the midline above the umbilicus. Three 5 mm 355 ports are placed in the left and right quadrant and in the median a few centimeters above the symphysis. If bowel resection is necessary, an additional 512 port is required.

Deep infiltrating endometriosis affects not only the posterior vaginal fornix but also the tissue around the ureter (mainly the left ureter), the uterine artery and the rectouterine, sacrouterine and vesicouterine ligaments.

The extent and type of endometriosis is explored and the extent of the resection is reevaluated. Deep in-

filtrating endometriosis of the sigmoid colon and/or rectum makes bowel resection necessary. In patients with extensive and/or recurrent endometriosis, preparation and/or desobliteration of the left ureter is a common surgical challenge. Preoperative splinting enhances preparation. Bladder affection can make wall resection inevitable.

Not infrequently endometriosis is found in the vesicouterine ligament (Fig. 26.**2**). During resection it may happen that the bladder is opened (Fig. 26.**3**) and excision of the bladder wall becomes necessary (Fig. 26.**4**). Resection is performed with the UltraCision shears easily and without bleeding. The position of the trigonum is identified by the location of the ureter splint (Fig. 26.**5**). After excision, the bladder wall is closed with 2/0 PDS sutures (Fig. 26.**6**) and checked for water-tightness by instillation of approx. 200 ml saline with 5 ml methylene blue through the Foley catheter.

Endometriosis may be found in the posterior vaginal fornix and make segmental resection of the anterior

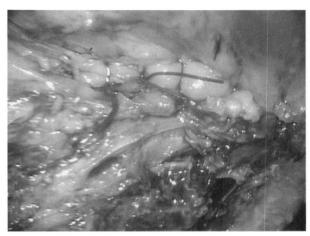

Fig. 26.**6** The bladder wall is closed with two layers of 2/0 PDS and 2/0 Vicryl. The water-tightness is proved by installation of 200 ml saline with 5 ml methylene blue.

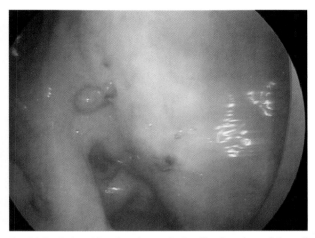

Fig. 26.**7** Polypoid red endometriosis affecting the pelvic wall and the rectum.

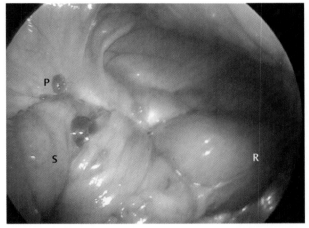

Fig. 26.**8** Superficial black and red polypoid endometriosis and deep infiltrating endometriosis affecting the sigmoid colon (*S*) and rectum (*R*) and pelvic wall (*P*). The leading symptom in this patient was bowel obstruction.

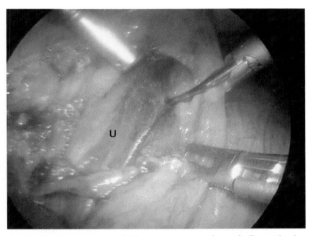

Fig. 26.**9** Transection of the mesosigmoid medially with the UltraCision 5 mm CS shears. The left ureter (*U*) is identified.

rectal wall necessary. The mobilized rectum is closed in these cases with 3/0 Vicryl sutures. Not infrequently endometriosis affects not only the outer parts of the rectal wall (Fig. 26.**7**) but also the sigmoid colon at the level of the promontory (Fig. 26.**8**). In these cases, the sigmoid colon may be fixed tightly with a double loop to the lateral pelvic entrance. Resection begins with the transection of the sigmoid mesentery at the height of the promontory. The left ureter is identified clearly (Fig. 26.**9**). Then the sigmoid colon can be dissected from the lateral pelvic wall (Fig. 26.**10**).

There may be a conglomerate of the lateral part of the sigmoid and the left ovary (Fig. 26.**11**), which has to be identified with its vessels. If the ovary has already been resected in a previous operation, the left horn of the uterus may be directly fixed to the left pelvic entrance close to the ureter (Fig. 26.**12**). These conglomerates can also be fixed to the uterus (Fig. 26.**13**) and make sharp dissection necessary in order to preserve the uterus (Fig. 26.**14**).

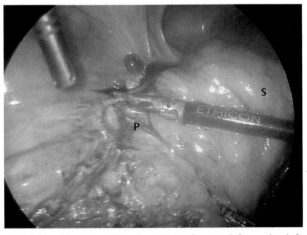

Fig. 26.**10** The sigmoid colon (*S*) is dissected from the left lateral pelvic entrance (*P*) en bloc with the endometriosis lesions.

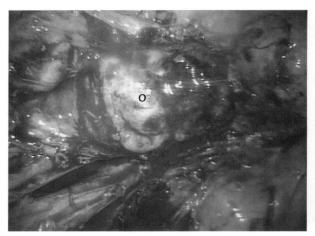

Fig. 26.**11**   After mobilization of the sigmoid colon, the left ovary (*O*) is identified.

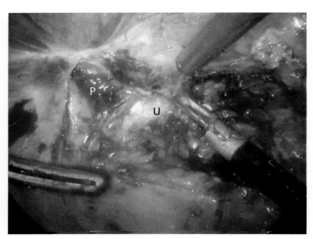

Fig. 26.**12**   Fixation of the left uterus horn (*U*) on the left lateral pelvic wall (*P*) following previous resection of the left ovary. Deep infiltrating recurrent endometriosis.

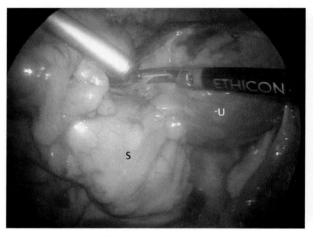

Fig. 26.**13**   Deep infiltrating endometriosis between sigmoid colon (*S*) and uterus (*U*). The uterus is dissected from the colon sharply with the 5 mm CS shears.

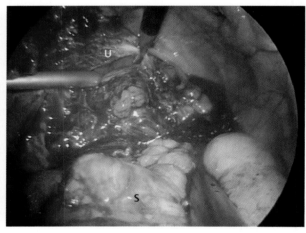

Fig. 26.**14**   The infiltrated obstructed sigmoid colon (*S*) can only sharply be dissected from the uterus (*U*).

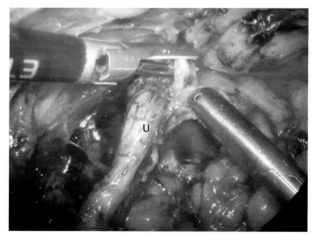

Fig. 26.**15**   White endometriosis around the left ureter (*U*) has to be dissected in fragments in order not to impair the ureter wall.

Not infrequently the endometriosis also affects the tissue around the distal ureter (Fig. 26.**15**). The lesions are dissected from the ureter (Fig. 26.**16**) with the UltraCision shears.

The mesorectum is transected down to the pelvic floor (Fig. 26.**17**) and all endometriosis is carefully removed. The rectum is transected with the Linear Cutter EZ45 blue (Fig. 26.**18**). The splenic flexure of the colon is completely dissected in order to avoid length problems when the anastomosis is established.

The colon is guided out through a mini-laparotomy and bowel resection performed. The resected specimen is prepared for histological examination (Fig. 26.**19**). The anvil of the ILS CH29 stapler is introduced externally into the proximal part of the colon, the purse string suture is closed (Fig. 26.**20**), the bowel repositioned, the incision closed so that the 312 port can be inserted without air leakage, and the pneumoperitoneum is reestablished.

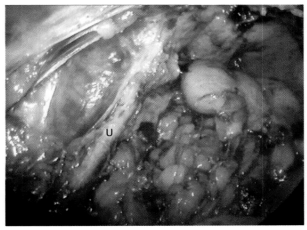

Fig. 26.**16** The left ureter (*U*) has been splinted preoperatively. However, the ureter looks unhealthy after it had been dissected out from an obstructive endometriosis with the UltraCision shears. Ureter function proved to be excellent in the long-term follow-up.

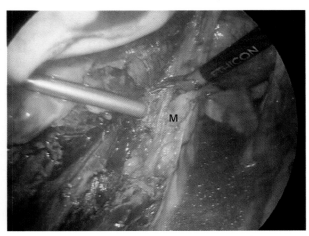

Fig. 26.**17** If not only the sigmoid colon but also the proximal rectum are affected by deep infiltrating endometriosis, a low anterior rectum resection has to be performed. The mesorectum (*M*) is transected with the 5 mm CS shears.

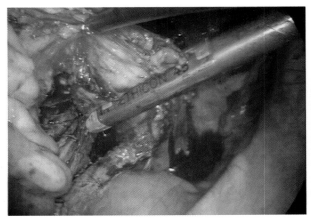

Fig. 26.**18** The distal rectum is transected with the Endo-Linear Cutter EZ45 (*blue*).

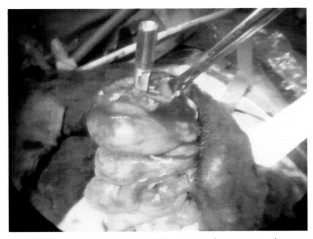

Fig. 26.**19** Macroscopic view to a specimen of deep infiltrating endometriosis in the sigmoid colon.

The ILS CDH 29 is inserted transanally (Fig. 26.**21**) and connected to the anvil with the EH41L clamp (Fig. 26.**22**). The anastomosis is checked by transanal instillation and the donuts are examined. A drainage is inserted into the pelvis and the incisions are closed.

⚠ Hints and Pitfalls

- If bowel resection turns out to be unnecessary, three 5 mm ports and one camera port are adequate. If bowel resection is performed, the 5 mm port in the right quadrant is changed to a 512 port for the stapling device and, after bowel resection, for the introduction of the EH41L introducer clamp.
- When sigmoid resection is necessary it is recommended to transect the mesentery first and identify the left ureter and proceed with the resection of the

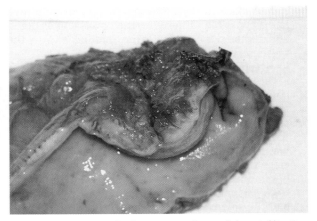

Fig. 26.**20** The anvil of the ILS CDH 29 stapler is inserted externally into the colon.

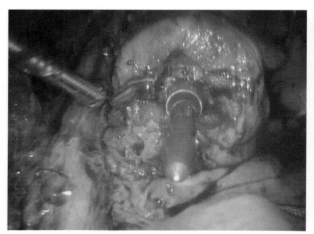

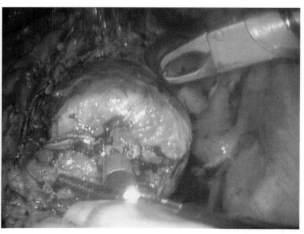

Fig. 26.**21** The splint of the ILS CDH 29 stapler is guided through the staple row of the rectum stump.

Fig. 26.**22** The stapler is connected with the EH41L clamp and anastomosis is performed.

mesentery as far as necessary. The sigmoid colon can be left fixed to the lateral pelvic wall (the more it is attached the better) and is dissected laterally as late as possible. Otherwise, the bowel comes down and reduces the sight to the midline and to the mesentery.

- In all types of sigmoid colon and rectum resection it is recommended to dissect the left colonic flexure completely in order to have enough colon for the anastomosis. This procedure may be tedious in obese patients when the access to the splenic flexure is taken from the descending colon upwards. It is easier to incise the gastrocolic ligament close to the colon, left from midline, and open the bursa omentalis. Then, the transverse colon distal from the colica media vessels can be pulled down and the splenic flexure is easier to be dissected.
- The safest way to be sure that the colon is long enough for a laparoscopically assisted anastomosis is to perform a subcutaneous "Pfannenstiel" incision as a mini-laparotomy. When the colon is guided out here and is long enough after resection to bring in the anvil without tension, the anastomosis should also work without tension. If the mini-laparotomy is placed at other locations (e.g., in the scar of an appendectomy) it is recommended to be sure that the splenic flexure is totally mobilized.
- It is more than annoying to recognize that the colon is too short when the pneumoperitoneum has already been reestablished, since the anvil is positioned on the promontory and cannot be moved down in the pelvis without tension and everybody is assuming that the operation is to be finished in next 20 minutes.

 Personal Experience

Whereas "regular" endometriosis surgery is performed by the gynecologist, all cases of deep infiltrating endometriosis are performed by the visceral surgeon together with the gynecologist. It is mandatory for these patients to undergo a tedious preoperative examination protocol at the gynecologist, who carries the main treatment responsibility, and the surgeon, who is in charge of the visceral resection.

Here, a series of 18 teamwork cases can be reported. All these operations were performed laparoscopically; there were no conversions. In 11 patients, bowel resection with anastomosis was necessary; in seven patients, segmental wall resections were performed. In two patients, parts from the bladder had to be resected. In all patients, the left ureter was affected by endometriosis; in one case, a ureter lesion had to be fixed laparoscopically. One patient developed a late rectovaginal fistula following segmental wall resection from the rectum. She was reoperated and an open low rectum resection, closure of the fistula, and an omentum plug were performed successfully. One patient developed obstruction of the right ureter postoperatively and was dilated. In all other patients, the postoperative course was uneventful.

 Discussion

This small series shows that laparoscopic treatment of deep infiltrating endometriosis with extension of the resection to the bladder and to the colon (sigmoid colon and rectum) and desobliteration of an obstructed ureter can be performed safely by a visceral surgeon and a gynecologist in teamwork.

The use of UltraCision is a *conditio sine qua non* for this type of surgery. The mobilization of the sigmoid colon and of the rectum, the desobliteration of the ureter, the resection of lesions in the bladder wall and any other resection of endometriosis are a clear domain for the 5 mm CS shears.

When deep infiltrating endometriosis is suspected (e.g., from ultrasound), a series of preoperative investigations is necessary. A CT scan gives further information about the disease and can also show a possible ureter obstruction. In these cases, preoperative splinting is highly recommended.

Patients with bowel obstruction can often present results of a barium enema from previous investigations. However, each patient has to undergo flexible sigmoidoscopy in order to detect intramural infiltration and to gather further information about a possible obstruction. A typical situation is that patients with deep infiltrating endometriosis involving the sigmoid colon present not only with an endometriosis-typical history but frequently have a history of bowel obstruction and bowel-associated problems. In these cases it is usual that flexible sigmoidoscopy cannot proceed higher than the proximal rectum without pain because the sigmoid loop is closely attached to the pelvic wall.

In cases of severe endometriosis, the only way to get the patient free from trouble is surgical treatment. The aim of surgery is to perform the operation in such a way that all the conspicuous lesions are totally removed. Radical surgery is the only way to achieve the best result for the patients who suffer from pain and infertility.

 Suggested Reading

Canis M, Bouquet De Jolinieres J, Wattiez A, Pouly JL, Mage G, Manhes H, Bruhat MA. Classification of endometriosis. Baillieres Clin Obstet Gynaecol 1993; 7: 759–74.

Chapron C, Guibert J, Fauconnier A, Vieira M, Dubuisson JB. Adhesion formation after laparoscopic resection of uterosacral ligaments in women with endometriosis. J Am Assoc Gynecol Laparosc 2001; 8: 368–73.

Chapron C, Dubuisson JB, Fritel X, Fernandez B, Poncelet C, Beguin S, Pinelli L. Operative management of deep endometriosis infiltrating the uterosacral ligaments. J Am Assoc Gynecol Laparosc 1999; 6: 31–7.

Cornillie FJ, Oosterlynck D, Lauweryns JM, Koninckx PR. Deeply infiltrating pelvic endometriosis: histology and clinical significance. Fertil Steril 1990; 53: 978–83.

Donnez J, Nisolle M. Advanced laparoscopic surgery for the removal of rectovaginal septum endometriotic or adenomyotic nodules. Baillieres Clin Obstet Gynaecol 1995; 9: 769–74.

Donnez J, Nisolle M, Casanas-Roux F, Bassil S, Anaf V. Rectovaginal septum, endometriosis or adenomyosis: laparoscopic management in a series of 231 patients. Hum Reprod 1995; 10: 630–5.

Fedele L, Piazzola E, Raffaelli R, Bianchi S. Bladder endometriosis: deep infiltrating endometriosis or adenomyosis? Fertil Steril 1998; 69: 972–5.

Keckstein J, Wiesinger H, Schwarzer U. Endometriose. In: Die endoskopischen Operationen in der Gynäkologie. Eds.: J Keckstein, J Hucke. Urban & Fischer, Munich, 2000, pp. 189–213.

Koninckx PR, Oosterlynck D, D'Hooghe T, Meuleman C. Deeply infiltrating endometriosis is a disease whereas mild endometriosis could be considered a non-disease. Ann N Y Acad Sci 1994; 734: 333–41.

Koninckx PR, Martin D. Treatment of deeply infiltrating endometriosis. Curr Opin Obstet Gynecol 1994; 6: 231–41.

Koninckx PR, Martin D. Surgical treatment of deeply infiltrating endometriosis. In: Endometriosis. RW Shaw. editor. London: Blackwell Science; 1995. pp. 264–81.

Nezhat F, Nezhat C, Pennington E. Laparoscopic proctectomy for infiltrating endometriosis of the rectum. Fertil Steril 1992; 57: 1129–32.

Vercellini P, Trespidi L, De Giorgi O, Cortesi I, Parazzini F, Crosignani PG. Endometriosis and pelvic pain: relation to disease stage and localization. Fertil Steril 1996; 65: 299–304.

27 The UltraCision Shears in Major Breast Surgery

G. Lesti, F. Ciampaglia, C. Lanci, A. L. Sardellone

The surgical treatment of breast cancer, which had remained basically unchanged for almost a century, has changed dramatically during the last twenty years. It has passed from radical surgical operations in all of the cases, to conservative operations in the majority in the patients.

The role of surgery is to guarantee the local control of the disease, to supply all the information necessary to establish the adjuvant therapies, and to allow an adequate esthetic result. The surgeon has to direct his attention not only to the disease, but even and especially to the patient, to whom he/she has to offer the best quality of life. In this perspective, the preservation of the breast must be one of the primary goals, being understood within the framework of the necessary oncological radicality.

The role of axillary dissection needs to be discussed separately. For more than one-hundred years, it has been an integral part of breast carcinoma surgery. As a therapeutic measure, axillary dissection modifies the loco-regional control of the disease. The impact on the rate of survival is still controversial.

In fact, it is known that axillary dissection *per se* does not significantly improve the prognosis of the patient, but allows the physician to collect all the information necessary to plan a proper adjuvant treatment. When histological examination of the axillary lymph nodes shows negative results, dissection does not bring any therapeutic benefit, but renders the patient more susceptible to possible complications or collateral effects such as lymphoedema, neuralgia, paraesthesia, infections, hematoma, and functional limitations of the limb. For this reason the possibility to perform the axillary dissection only in those patients with positive lymph nodes is under study. In this way we obtain information about the lymph-node status. Sentinel lymph node detection is predictive for the axillary lymph node invasion in early breast cancer.

Indication and Preoperative Management

Many possible surgical operations for breast carcinoma have been described; herein emphasis is placed on our therapeutic approach.

- In the case of tumors less than 2 cm in diameter, and unifocal in the mammography, tumorectomy is performed with a margin of 2 cm into healthy tissue, including the sentinel lymph node, and intraoperative radiotherapy.

- In the case of tumors larger than 3 cm in diameter, a radical Patey's mastectomy is performed with immediate reconstruction and remodeling of the contralateral breast, all in a single sitting.
- For tumors with dimensions between 2 and 3 cm, the surgical choice depends on the size and shape of the breast, and on the tumor's location.
- In tumors bigger than 3 cm, we sometimes subject our patients to neoadjuvant treatment, in order to reduce the tumor dimensions and to allow application of a conservative therapy.

In our experience with 3000 breast operations (1600 for malignant pathology and 1400 for benign pathology), we believe that the UltraCision shears have taken on important an important role in lymphectomy of the axillary cavity and in the preparation of the muscle pocket for the immediate reconstruction.

Operation

We describe here the radical mastectomy according to Patey, with immediate reconstruction.

The first step is to make a skin incision. The knife must not plunge down to the level of the superficial fascia; this delicate but distinct fascia can be seen under the dermis, and is the right plane. We follow a dissection with the UltraCision 5 mm LCS shears of 14 cm length at power level 5.

The preparation of the skin flaps lasts no more than 15 minutes, after which hemostasis is performed without either ligature or electric current (Fig. 27.1).

The flaps are retracted with light, sharp single or double elastic hooks created for this special purpose. These hooks do not injure the flaps as much as happens with the various types of forceps, or with the toothed hooks generally used. Maintaining such a level of dissection of the flap is fundamental from the viewpoint of a good cancer surgery. First, we make the superior flap, and subsequently the inferior and the lateral ones. The line of dissection of the lateral flap reaches the latissimus dorsi muscle. As the dissection of this flap is carried out cephalad, the operator must never lose sight of the latissimus muscle, particularly in obese patients. The dissection of the axillary portion of the lateral skin flap is the final step; in this phase of the process, the good plane of the dissection is superficial to the surface layer of the superficial fascia. The apocrine glands are placed in the inner flap and act as an excellent guide for the surgeon. This plane is made quickly and safely with UltraCision at power level 5.

Editor's tip: Preservation of intercostobrachial nerves avoids sensitivity disorders of the axilla, the internal aspect of the arm, and the thoracic wall.

Following the edge of the latissimus muscle, the thoracodorsal vessels and the nerve are isolated and the axillary content is retracted medially. The vessels and the nerve are dissected until reaching the axillary vein; the dissection of the lymph nodes and the fat from the vessels is performed using the UltraCision power level 2. The dissection is rapid, without bleeding, and nerve stimulation as would be the case with electric current. The next step is the localization and the dissection of the long thoracic nerve, which is placed on the serratus anterior muscle (Fig. 27.**2**).

Even this phase is made easy, rapid, and safe by the UltraCision shears at power level 5. Then, the mammary gland is detached from the major pectoralis muscle, the fascia of the muscle is removed together with the breast, and the plane is easily displayed by UltraCision at level 5.

After having reached the lateral edge, the pectoralis major is lifted up and the minor pectoralis is displayed. We do not cut the pectoralis minor next to the coracoid process but 3 or 4 cm below caudad to the medial thoracic nerve branches, so intersecting the minor pectoralis muscle. This procedure, carried out with the UltraCision level 5 is safe, very rapid, and without any bleeding.

It is mandatory to pay particular attention to the medial thoracic nerve in the breast reconstruction, as this nerve supplies the lateral edge of the major pectoralis muscle that represents the most important part of the muscle's pocket. The major pectoralis muscle is retracted and lifted up, and the attention is turned to the apex of the axilla. The fat and the lymphatic tissue are dissected from the medial portion of the axillary vein, up to the point where it passes beneath the subclavian muscle. The reflection of the costocoracoid fascia onto the chest wall, opposite the upper portion of the vein, is then dissected from the chest wall to the apex of the axilla. UltraCision at level 2 is placed across the apex of the mass as high as possible, in order to coagulate and

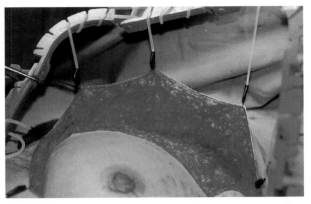

Fig. 27.**1** The superior flap made by UltraCision. Care is taken to carry the skin incision only down to the level of the superficial fascia.

to avoid back-flow of lymph into the wound and to secure the small blood vessels (Fig. 27.**3**). The pyramidal mass of fat and lymph nodes are cut and put into separate specimen bottles for the pathologist, and is marked as level III. The next step in the operation is to continue laterally the dissection of the areolar tissues in the cleft between the chest wall and the axillary vein. A number of small vessels and lymphatics are coagulated and cut with UltraCision at level 5. The dissection is carried out laterally and caudad towards the lateral thoracic artery and vein, which are coagulated separately with the UltraCision at level 2. The axillary content is separated from the serratus muscle. At this point the thoracodorsal nerve and the Bell's nerve are again identified, so as to avoid damaging them. The next step is to separate the pectoralis minor fibers from serratus digitations which are placed under them and which do not have to be cut.

The final step is the preparation of the muscle pocket for the positioning of the Becker's prosthesis. We first start dissection of the major pectoralis muscle from the 5-6-7 ribs, and subsequently proceed caudad under the fascia of the rectus, finishing with the dissection of the anterior serratus, laterally. Particular attention has to be paid to elevating only the fascia and not the

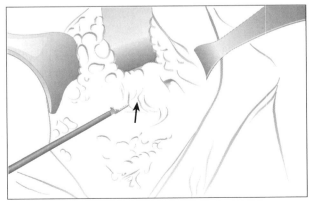

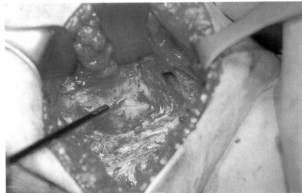

Fig. 27.**2** Dissection of the long thoracic nerve (Bell's nerve) is made by UltraCision at level 2.

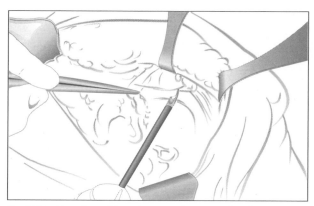
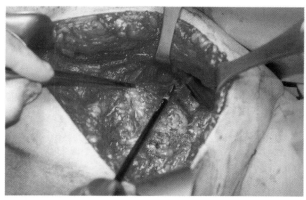

Fig. 27.**3**   Vessels and lymphatic at the apex of axilla are coagulated and cut with UltraCision at level 2.

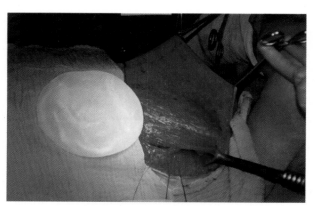

Fig. 27.**4**   Preparation of the muscle pocket is made by UltraCision. The Becker's prosthesis is inserted at the end procedure.

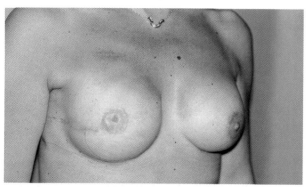

Fig. 27.**5**   Breast reconstruction after six months.

muscle fibers of the rectus. The whole preparation of the muscle pocket is made by UltraCision at level 2 and no bleeding points are observed. The Becker's prosthesis is inserted and the pocket is sutured with Vycril 00 (Fig. 27.**4**).

Editor's tip: Recent studies illustrate that cosmetic results could be enhanced using Mac Ghan-style anatomic prothesis.

The Jackson Pratt No. 7 drainage is positioned to drain the pocket and the axilla simultaneously. A second similar drainage is positioned under the skin flap which is sutured with running non-absorbable suture. The contralateral breast can be reduced or augmented, in order to have the same shape and volume as the reconstructed breast (Fig. 27.**5**). We usually need three months to obtain symmetry of both the breasts.

The reconstruction of the nipple and areola is made after six months in local anesthesia when the valve is removed.

⚠ Hints and Pitfalls

- The axillary dissection in conservative surgery is performed through the above-mentioned technique.
- Whenever possible the cutaneous incision of 5–6 cm is made in the axillary cavity and executed from the lateral edge of the major pectoralis to the edge of the latissimus dorsi muscle.
- The use of UltraCision is very helpful with such a short incision, because the fine vessels can be prepared, coagulated, and transected in a single step without instrument changes and without the application of clips or electric current.

Personal Experience

One of the most frequent complications encountered in breast surgery is the development of an axillary seroma. The rate of this occurrence ranges from 18% to 59% following operations for breast carcinoma: seromas may become infected, cause flap necrosis, and increase the likelihood of lymphoedema of the arm. Traditionally, it is thought that seroma formation occurs as a consequence of both lymphatic disruption and oozing of capillary beds following axillary node dissection. Interference with this response should decrease the amount of wound drainage and thus minimize the formation of seromas.

Furthermore, any technique that could potentially obliterate the dead space associated with axillary dissection also might lessen the incidence of this complication. Because of this, we have always performed an accurate axillary dissection with large use of metallic clips and locating a high vacuum drain. In August 1997 we started using the UltraCision shears to minimize blood loss during breast surgery procedures, and to reduce postoperative seroma.

We have compared the mastectomies with immediate reconstruction performed from January to December 1998 using UltraCision with the same breast operations performed from September 1996 to August 1997 without UltraCision. From January to December 1998, 68 patients with known carcinoma of the breast were submitted to modified Patey radical mastectomy with contemporary reconstruction and a contralateral plastic procedure (nodes: N+: 44; N–: 24). The procedures included dissection of the 1st, 2nd, and 3rd axillary lymph node levels, as well as resection of the pectoralis minor muscle, saving the medial nerve. Medial nerve conservation is essential to perform a better reconstruction and to obtain a good trophic muscular pocket. The UltraCision 10 mm LCS 14 cm shears were used for axillary dissection and muscular pocket preparation in all patients in this study.

This first group was compared with another group which was composed of 63 patients who, from September 1996 to August 1997, underwent the same surgical treatment for known breast carcinoma (Nodes: N+; 42; N–: 21) without UltraCision. All operations were performed by the same surgeon. Operating time, blood loss, wound lymphatic drainage, and early complications up to 60 days after surgical procedures were monitored.

In all patients the Becker prosthesis (Siltex Becker Expander Prosthesis, Mentor, Leiden, The Netherlands) was employed and was covered using a muscular pocket consisting of the major pectoralis muscle, anterior serratus muscle, and the rectum fascia. The wound was then sutured over two closed suction drains (Jackson–Pratt 7 mm wide silicone flat drain, Baxter, Deerfield, USA), one in the axilla, passing through the muscular pocket, and the other under the skin flaps. The drains were connected to a high vacuum system, in which there was a drain bottle with negative pressure (720 mmHg), without valves. In this system the vacuum remained largely unchanged with the increasing filling of the container. Both drains were brought out through separate stab wounds. No attempts were made to close the dead space in the axilla or the breast wound by additional measures. Full range of motion exercises were performed 24 hours after the operation. Drainage volumes were registered daily. The skin flap drain was removed after two days and the pocket and axillary drain after 5 days, at the time of discharge.

Each patient was seen one week after discharge and weekly thereafter or more frequently as needed. After drainage removal, a fluid collection in the axilla was removed by percutaneous aspiration with a short Abocath No. 16. The total drainage volume and the number of aspirations were recorded.

Variables recorded included patient weight, age, and breast weight. Also the total number of lymph nodes removed and the total number of positive nodes per patient were recorded. The results are summarized in Tables 27.1–4.

Table 27.**1** Characteristics of the UltraCision group patients (68) versus the control group (63)

Characteristics	UltraCision group (*n*=68)	Control group (*n*=63)
Age (mean)	52.7	54.1
Weight (kg)	64.8	63.9
T1	13	8
T2	53	52
Double localization	2	3
Patients N⁺	44	42
Patients N⁻	24	21

Table 27.**2** Surgical characteristics of the UltraCision group (68) versus control group (63)

	UltraCision group	Control group
Radical mastectomy	68	63
Time of procedure (min)	196	161
Blood loss (g Hb)	1.2	3.4
Breast weight (g)	682.1	639.4
Becker prosthesis (g)	400	400

Table 27.**3** Values of drainage

	UltraCision group (*n*=68)	Control group (*n*=63)
Total volume	612	824
Skin flap volume (2 days)	85	174
Axillary+pocket volume (5 days)	527	650

Table 27.**4** Seroma

Seromas	12	25
One aspiration	0	0
Less than 5	10	14
More than 5	2	11
Wound complication	0	0

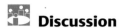 **Discussion**

Surgery of the axillary space is associated with numerous postoperative fluid collections (seromas). Multiple studies have been performed, aimed at preventing seromas, some with encouraging results. Arm immobilization, closed suction drainage, and flap tacking sutures have all been shown to decrease this incidence; however, it remains a significant complication. The exact etiology of seroma formation remains controversial. Some cite the surgical disruption of lymphatics and capillaries, coupled with the creation of dead space; others maintain that postmastectomy fluid collections are not real "seromas" or lymphatic collections, but are actually inflammatory exudates that accumulate in this dead space.

The UltraCision shears system is able to coagulate all lymphatic vessels with deep accuracy and the blunt dissection is abolished and substituted by coagulation and cutting using the shears.

During isolation and section of arteries and veins, the UltraCision shears grip the periadventitial surface too, decreasing lymphatic escape. The dissection is precise, accurate, and quick: no suture is necessary during axillary dissection.

We think that the seroma reduction of about 50% and the possibility to resolve the few cases with less than 30 days of therapy are important results.

In the modified Patey radical mastectomy with concomitant reconstruction and contralateral plastic procedure, the use of UltraCision permits a significant reduction of blood loss.

The use of UltraCision shears in major breast surgery reduces the main complications and does not significantly prolong the operation time.

 Suggested Reading

Becher H. Breast reconstruction using an inflatable breast implant with detachable reservoir. Plast Reconstr Sur 1984; 70: 678.

Bonadonna G, Valagussa P, et al. Primary chemotherapy in operable breast cancer: eight-year experience at the Milan Cancer Institute. I. Clin Oncol 1998; 16: 93–100.

Bridges M, Morris D, Hall JR, Deitch EA. Effect of wound exudates on in vitro immune parameters. J Surg Res 1987; 43: 133–8.

Cataliotti L, Pacini P, et al. Terapia delle neoplasie precliniche. In: Cataliotti L., Ciatto S., Luini A. editors. Le neoplasie precliniche della mammella, Milano: Sorbona; 1990. p. 31.

Cataliotti L. La terapia demolitiva. In: Senologia Oncologica di U. Veronesi. Milano: Masson; 1999. pp. 368–74.

Dawson I, Stam L, Heslinga JM, Kalsbeek HL. Effect of shoulder immobilization on wound seroma and shoulder dysfunction following modified radical mastectomy: a randomized prospective clinical trial. Br J Surg 1989; 76: 311–2.

Haagensen CD. Diseases of the breast. 3rd ed., Philadelphia: W.B. Saunders Co.; 1986.

Lesti G. Il carcinoma della mammella. Roma: De Feo Editore; 1983.

Lesti G. Reduction of blood loss and seroma after surgery for breast cancer using ultrasound dissection. Supplement to Surgical Rounds 2000; 3: 10.

Kameron AE, Ebbs SR, Wylie F, Boum M. Suction drainage of the axilla: a prospective randomized trial. Br J Surg 198; 75: 1211.

Madden JL. Modified radical mastectomy. Surg Gynecol Obstet 1965; 121: 1221–30.

Nava M, Quattrone P, Riggio E. Focus on the breast fascial system: a new approach for inframammary fold reconstruction. Plast Reconstr Surg 1998; 1020–31.

Patey DH, Dyson WH. The prognosis of carcinoma of the breast in relation to the type of operation performed. Brit J Cancer 1948; 2: 7–13.

Tejler G, Aspegren K. Complications and hospital stay after surgery for breast cancer: a prospective study of 385 patients. Br J Surg 1985; 72: 542–4.

Urban JA. Management of operable breast cancer: the surgeon's view. Cancer 1978; 42: 2066–77.

Veronesi U, Salvadori B. Breast conservation is a safe method in patient with small cancer of the breast. Long-term results of three randomized trials on 1,973 patients. Eur J Cancer 1995; 31(10): 1574–9.

West IP, Ellison IB. A study of the causes and prevention of edema of the arm following radical mastectomy. Surg Gynecol Obstet 1959; 109: 359–63.

28 Axillary Lymphatic Node Dissection in Breast Surgery

F. Quenet

Axillary node status remains the most important prognostic factor in breast cancer, and enables the elaboration of an adjuvant postoperative strategy. Axillary lymphatic node dissection was, until recently, carried out systematically on patients with invasive breast cancer; in spite of recent progress, this dissection brings with it a significant morbidity risk.

The introduction of the UltraCision shears is part of an evolution in surgical techniques and thinking, generally aimed at reducing the morbidity associated with axillary lymphatic node clearance, and particularly aimed at diminishing postoperative lymphorrhea and damage resulting from dissection in the immediate proximity of the nerves in the axilla.

> Editor's tip: Although sentinel node biopsy seems a promising approach in order to obtain information on axillary staging, axillary dissection remains the standard of care for many breast cancer patients.

Indication and Preoperative Management

Within the axilla, the lymph nodes are arranged in five groups: the axillary vein, subscapular, external thoracic vein, central, and axillares apicales groups. There are also three levels, known as Berg levels, according to their position: under, behind, or above the pectoralis minor muscle.

The boundaries of the pyramidal form of the axilla are defined (a) to the front, by the pectoralis major and minor muscles (b) to the rear, by the teres major and subscapularis muscles (c) on the flank, by the latissumus dorsi muscle (d) and below, by the clavipectoroaxillary aponeurosis.

The critical elements most at risk in lymphatic node dissection are above, the axillary pedicle and the brachial plexus, the thoracodorsal pedicle and the thoracodorsalis nerve to the rear, the thoracicus longus nerve within, and above and within, the ansa pectoralis. In addition, sensitivity within the inside arm is governed by the intercostobrachialis nerve that runs through the axilla, both before and after its division.

Operation

The patient is positioned in a dorsal decubitus position, the arm laid at 90°. It is important not to strain the brachial plexus during the procedure.

Except in the context of modified radical mastectomy, we proceed via a horizontal incision located two finger-widths below the axillary fold; the incision runs from the rear of the pectoralis major muscle and as far as the latissimus dorsi muscle, and is generally not connected with the lumpectomy incision.

Once within the subcutaneous wall, progress is restricted to the avascular tracts that run close to the axillary muscular wall. From the rear of the pectoralis major, the clavipectoroaxillary aponeurosis is easily incised using the cutting edge of the curved blade of the dissector, giving access to the serratus major muscle, where the thoracicus longus nerve is identified and left in place on the muscular wall.

Without recourse to the UltraCision generator, the inherent geometry of the curved blade of the dissector is such that delicate and precise dissections can be carried out in contact with vascular and nervous networks at no risk. Blood vessels can be cleanly skeletonized with no ancillary damage by gentle combing movements on neighboring fat tissues, enabling them to be laid aside and isolated.

At the summit of the axilla, and now using the curved blade of the dissector in the ultrasonic (US) mode, the aponeurosis is incised to look for the axillary vein. The lymph nodes located to the front of and above the vein are left intact. Using the vein wall as a guide, a progressive separation along the underside enables the identification of the external thoracic vein, together with the thoracodorsal pedicle, located below and generally in a more external position.

At this point, while the external thoracic vein can still be put under tension, it is advisable not to divide it immediately but first to uncross and separate the intercostobrachial nerve running behind (Fig. 28.1). With the curved blade of the dissector in the neutral, non-US setting, the sharp edge enables the separation of the respective matrices and skeletonization of the nerve as far as the thoracic wall.

The coagulation and cutting of the vein are carried out with the instrument in the live US mode on level 5, in most cases without recourse to clips.

The group of lymph nodes that lies between the thoracodorsal and thoracicus longus nerves is now isolated, coagulated, and divided at the summit of the axillary pyramid. There is generally a further branch running down from the ansa pectoralis which requires coagulation and division.

The dissection continues towards the base of the pyramid, arriving at and then following the limits of the thoracodorsal pedicle, the lymphatic elements contained within being folded below and aside to improve access.

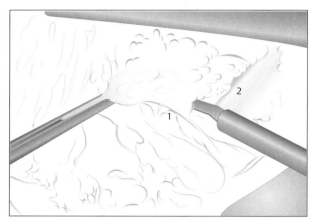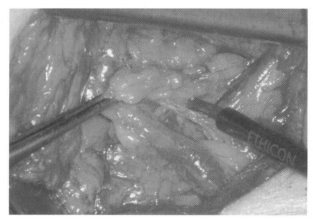

Fig. 28.**1**   Dissection of external thoracic vein with identification of the intercostobrachial nerve. *1* intercostobrachial nerve, *2* external thoracic vein.

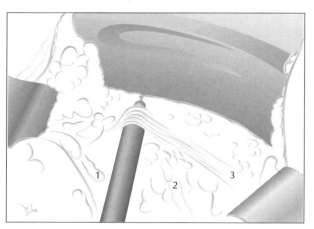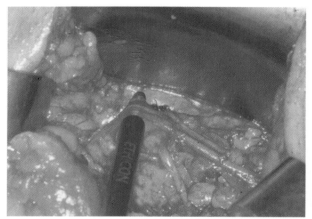

Fig. 28.**2**   Removal of axillary tissue at top of the pyramid, exposing the axillary vein. *1* external thoracic vein, *2* intercostobrachial nerve, *3* axillary vein.

The base of the pyramid can then be sectioned, using level 5, and the lower section of the external thoracic vein coagulated and divided (Fig. 28.**2**).

The condition of the axillary vein, thoracodorsal pedicle, the thoracicus longus nerve, and the intercostobrachial branches will now be clear.

The vacuum drain on the axilla should be left in place until the drainage rate falls below 30 ml/day.

⚠ Hints and Pitfalls

- It is essential to remove completely the lower scapular and lower external thoracic lymph nodes, these having been confirmed by recent sentinel lymph node analysis as being the most critical sites for node metastases (8, 9). In order to better identify and protect the intercostobrachial nerve, two aspects should be considered:
  1. During dissection of the external boundary of the axilla, care must be taken not to damage the external section of the intercostobrachial nerve, between the external thoracic vein and the external wall of the axillary pyramid.
  2. In the case of obese patients, it is advisable to skeletonize the intercostobrachial nerve via a vertical dissection along the alignment of the nerve, having first identified its external and internal sections. Thus, the nerve path can be followed with precision, and the separation of the intercostobrachial nerve and the external thoracic vein becomes easier.
- The use of the UltraCision shears permits dissection in close proximity to venous and nervous systems as a consequence of the inherent low thermal diffusion. In the region of the thoracodorsal pedicle, however, the division of an arterial branch requires that the hemostasis be carried out at an adequate distance from the thoracodorsal pedicle, to avoid any unintentional damage—particularly given the critical importance of the latter as regards breast reconstruction.

Personal Experience

Between December 1998 and July 1999, we have operated on 49 patients using the UltraCision shears with an average age of 57 years, all having invasive breast cancer. Lymphatic node dissection was carried out within the first two Berg levels. The average number of nodes harvested was 14.

> Editor's tip: At least 10 lymph nodes are necessary to obtain an accurate axillary staging.

The mean operating time was 72 minutes (including histological analysis) and 20 minutes for the lymphatic node dissection itself. The mean hospital stay was seven days, ranging between four and 13 days. In 43 patients, the UltraCision shears were used exclusively; on the remaining six patients clips were necessary, either for small vascular branches in close proximity to nerves, or where larger diameter blood vessels precluded the use of pure UltraCision scalpel methods. In none of these cases were there any postoperative hemorrhages.

The integrity of the sensitive intercostobrachial nerve was maintained in 44 cases. If the nerve is sectioned, there is increasing anesthesia in the armpit and hypoesthesia on the posterointernal face of the arm, while for the patients in whom the intercostobrachial nerve remains intact, these alterations are less intense and not so long-lasting (6, 7). The incidence of permanent, postoperative sensitivity dysfunction will be difficult to quantify accurately until the results of a longer-term analysis are known. This problem could be lessened or resolved on follow-up assessment (5).

Average daily lymph-drainage rates were 47 ml with a mean drain time of just over five days. Once the vacuum drain had been removed, five of the patients required supplementary lymph evacuation but in no case were there any lymphodema or upper-limb invalidity.

Discussion

Although we have not carried out a phase III analysis, which would compare in a prospective and randomized trial the use of the UltraCision shears and traditional methods, we have been able to evaluate the advantages of UltraCision in the dissection of axillary lymph nodes.

Use of the UltraCision shears involves a fairly rapid learning curve of approximately 10 axillary dissections, after which there is no difference in the length of the operation. This learning curve is largely due to a initial impression of a slow cutting speed, dictated by the coagulation performance; however, since no changes of instrument (clips, shears, etc.) are required, the time effectively necessary is quite similar to that required using conventional devices.

The UltraCision shears do not generally require the use of hemostatic clips. Even so, the hemostasis produced is of good quality, both immediately and in the long-term, even when applied to vessels of larger diameter like the axillary vein.

As regards lymphorrhea, the results using UltraCision are quite comparable with those obtained by traditional methods. The figure of only five patients requiring supplementary drainage is of some interest.

UltraCision's simultaneous capacity for coagulation and cutting means that the entire dissection requires only one instrument. Furthermore, the absence of electric current means that the risk of thermal injury to nerve or venous structures is much reduced.

In general terms, the use of systematic and complete axillary dissection is being called into question, and the evolution of surgical practice is towards lower rates of morbidity.

The feasibility of lymphatic mapping, involving the identification of the sentinel lymph node, is now well established. (1, 2, 3, 4).

The principle is to develop a technique that retains the advantages of previous approaches yet:
- Tends towards being less traumatic,
- Furnishes a precise axillary staging without any risk of neoplastic dissemination,
- Carries no risk of early lymphatic relapse.

It has recently been shown that the analysis of the sentinel lymph node enables the prediction of the condition of the axilla in 97.5% of the cases (8). This technique is used as an alternative to complete axillary dissection when faced with smaller tumors where the axilla is not clinically involved.

There remain, however, several problems:
- The complexity of the isotopic identification and its relative cost,
- The false-negative rate inherent in frozen-section analyses (17%).

The reduction in the number of complete axilla dissections, together with the use of new technologies such as the UltraCision scalpel, will allow a considerable reduction in the morbidity associated with lymph node dissections and, as a consequence, in a significant improvement in the quality of life as experienced by women suffering from breast cancer.

Acknowledgements

The authors would like to thank Mr. R. Simpson for his valuable help.

References

1. Brenin DR, Morrow M, Moughan J, Owen JB, Wilson JF, Winchester DP. Management of axillary lymph nodes in breast cancer: a national patterns of care study of 17,151 patients. Ann Surg 1999; 230: 686–91.

2. Flett M, Going J, Stanton P, Cooke T. Sentinel node localization in patients with breast cancer. Br J Surg 1998, 991–3.
3. Giuliano A, Dale P, Turner R, Morton D, Evans S, Krasne D. Improved axillary staging of breast cancer with sentinel lymphadenectomy. Ann Surg 1995; 222: 394–401.
4. O'Hea B, Hill A, El-Shirbiny A, Yeh S, Rosen P, Coit D, et al. Sentinel lymph node biopsy in breast cancer: Initial experience at Memorial Sloan-Kettering Cancer Center. Surg 1998; 186: 423–7.
5. Roses DF, Brooks AD, Harris MN, Shapiro RL, Mitnick J. Complications of level I and II axillary dissection in the treatment of carcinoma of the breast. Ann Surg 1999; 230: 194–201.
6. Temple WJ, Ketcham AS. Preservation of the intercostobrachial nerve during axillary dissection for breast cancer. Am J Surg 1985; 150: 585–8.
7. Paredes JP, Puente JL, Potel J. Variations in sensitivity after sectioning the intercostobrachial nerve. Am J Surg 1990; 160: 525–8.
8. Veronesi U, Luini A, Galimberti V, Marchini S, Sacchini V, Rilke F. Extent of metastatic axillary involvement in 1446 cases of breast cancer. Eur J Surg Oncol 1990; 16: 127–33.
9. Veronesi U, Paganelli G, Galimbrti V,Viale G, Zurrida S, Bedoni M, et al. Sentinel-node biopsy to avoid axillary dissection in breast cancer with clinically negative lymph nodes. The Lancet 1997; 349: 1864–67.

29 Tonsillectomy with the UltraCision Scalpel

H. Löppönen

Tonsillectomy is a very common otolaryngological and pediatric surgical operation. We present our two-year experience with the UltraCision scalpel in tonsillectomy.

Indication and Preoperative Management

The indications for tonsillectomy are chronic tonsillitis, recurrent acute tonsillitis, peritonsillar abscess, and upper airway obstruction due to obstructive tonsils (3). Periodic fever and suspected malignant disease of the tonsil are rare indications.

An untreated known bleeding disease is a contraindication to surgery. Atrophic rhinitis and pharyngitis may also aggravate after tonsillectomy. The surgeon should consult a phoniatrician or speech therapist before operating a patient with a cleft palate.

Operation

The following choice of instruments is recommended:
- Mouth gag with tongue blade
- Tonsil-seizing forceps
- UltraCision 5 mm sharp-pointed blade (SH105 or SH145),
- Suction tube

The following instruments may be used additionally or alternatively:
- Elevator "Hurd"
- Freer

- Electrocautery
- 4/0 Vicryl sutures

After premedication, general anesthesia with orotracheal intubation is induced. The patient is placed in a supine position on the operating table. The patient's head is slightly extended but excessive extension should be avoided. The surgeon sits on a chair on the frontal side of the patient's head. A mouth gag is introduced and opened, with the tongue blade in the midline, to provide a good view of the patient's throat and palatine tonsils. Tonsillectomy forceps are used to grasp the palatine tonsil. The tonsil is drawn in a medial direction to visualize the anterosuperior part of the tonsil through the mucosa of the anterior faucial arch.

The whole operation is done with the UltraCision blade (SH105). At first, an incision is made by cutting the mucosa down to the surgical "capsule" of the tonsil (level 2–3). The incision begins from the lower pole at the base of the tongue, following the lateral edge of the tonsil to the upper pole just laterally to the uvula (Fig. 29.1).

When the capsule has been reached, the dissection should follow the surface of the tonsil. It is usually easiest to start the dissection from the superior pole of the tonsil. The superior vessels are identified and coagulated with the blunt side of the blade (level 3). When the superior pole of the tonsil has been separated from the surrounding peritonsillar tissues, the dissection proceeds downwards between the tonsil and the constrictor muscle layer. Care must be taken to keep the blade as close as possible to the capsule throughout the dissection. "Digging" into the fossa may cause bleeding and excessive postoperative scarring. Gripping the tonsil by its upper pole, the surgeon continues the dissec-

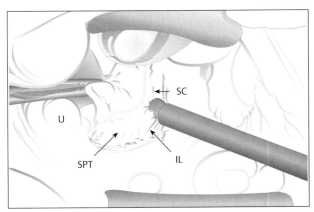
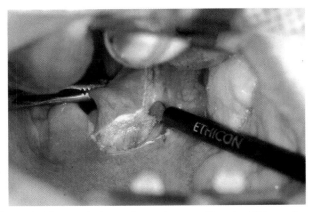

Fig. 29.**1** The incision from the base of the tongue laterally to the uvula. The surgical capsule can be seen. *U* uvula, *SPT* superior pole of tonsil, *SC* surgical capsule, *IL* incision line.

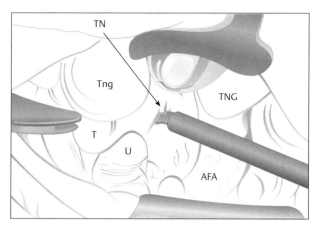
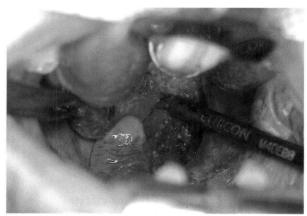

Fig. 29.**2**   The tonsil has been dissected and the "neck" is cut near to the tonsillolingual sulcus. *TN* tonsil neck, *Tng* tounge, *T* tonsil, *U* uvula, *AFA* anterior faucial arch.

tion with the blunt side of the blade (level 3–5) by separating the peritonsillar tissues from the capsule until the lower pole is approached.

Towards the lower pole of the tonsil there is a firm, fibrous triangular fold which tends to hold up the dissection at this point. This fold can be easily cut with the sharp side of the blade (level 3), however, and the dissection is then carried on to the base of the tongue. When the lower pole has been dissected, the "neck" of the tonsil, which passes from the lower pole of the tonsil to the tonsillolingual sulcus, is cut close to the sulcus with the sharp side of the blade (level 3) (Fig. 29.**2**). Normally, there are no bleeding problems when this surgical technique is used.

> Editor's tip: Control over bleeders is excellent with the UltraCision blade, as long it is possible to compress the bleeding vessel to underlying tissue or structures in order to weld the vessel walls together. If this is not possible, the new 5 mm shears (curved tip) can be recommended as the instrument of choice.

Hemostasis can be controlled with the flat side of the blade (level 2–3). Very rarely is vessel ligation needed.

 Hints and Pitfalls

- Dissect the superior pole of the tonsil first to find the surgical capsule and follow this anatomic landmark throughout the dissection.
- Keep the level at 2 or 3 during the dissection. Although you may feel that you do not proceed fast enough, you will minimize the total operation time by ensuring good hemostasis during the dissection already.
- Avoid pulling hard on the tonsil and ensure hemostasis as soon as you detect even a small vessel.

> Editor's tip: Pulling too hard also means that the blade cuts too quickly, because the tissue reaches its elastic limits before the vessels are sealed properly.

 Personal Experience

We have two years of experience of use of the UltraCision scalpel in tonsillectomies. After the normal learning period, all of our surgeons have found this device very easy to handle. At the beginning, the dissection takes longer compared to the blunt or electrocautery technique. However, there is practically no need for extra hemostasis with the UltraCision technique, which reduces the operation time to equal to or less than with the other methods. According to our experience, the control of hemostasis is the best benefit of this surgical method.

In our pilot study of 30 tonsillectomy patients, we compared UltraCision to the blunt dissection technique. In this randomized prospective and single-blinded study, no differences were found regarding postoperative complications. The amount of intraoperative bleeding and the total operation time were significantly less with UltraCision.

Discussion

Tonsillectomy is typically done under general anesthesia as an in-patient procedure with one-night postoperative follow-up at hospital. However, there is more and more pressure towards day-case surgery for economic reasons (4). According to our experience, this may be problematic because postoperative complications, including hemorrhage, pain control, poor oral intake, nausea and vomiting, may indicate a longer follow-up at the hospital.

Several surgical techniques have been introduced for tonsillectomy, including blunt and sharp dissection, electrocautery, ultrasonic aspiration, and different laser techniques (2, 5, 8). The aim of all these techniques is safe surgery with minimal complications. Local anesthetics have also been infiltrated to the tonsillar fossa to reduce postoperative pain (6).

The UltraCision scalpel can offer a number of advantages over lasers and electrosurgery in tonsillectomy. With this technique, cutting and coagulation are possible with decreased thermal damage to tissue (1, 7). Because no electrical current is delivered to the tissue, nerve and muscle stimulation may be reduced, leading to less postoperative pain for the patient. Our experience with this technique is encouraging and the UltraCision scalpel can be well applied to tonsillectomy in day-case surgery.

 References

1. Amaral JF. Depth of thermal injury: ultrasonically activated scalpel vs. electrosurgery. Surg Endosc 1995; 9: 226.
2. Auf I, Osborne JE, Sparkes C, Khalil H. Is KTP laser effective in tonsillectomy? Clin Otolaryngol 1997; 22: 145–6.
3. Bluestone CD. Current indications for tonsillectomy and adenoidectomy. Ann Otol Rhinol Laryngol 1992; 101: 58–64.
4. Drake-Lee A, Harris S. Day case tonsillectomy: what is the risk and where is the economic benefit? Clin Otolaryngol 1999; 24: 247–51.
5. Isaacson G, Szeremeta W. Pediatric tonsillectomy with bipolar electrosurgical scissors. Am J Otolaryngol 1998; 19: 291–5.
6. Jebeles JA, Reilly JS, Gutierrez JF, Bradley EL, Kissin I. The effect of pre-incisional infiltration of tonsils with bupivacaine on the pain following tonsillectomy under general anesthesia. Pain 1991; 47: 305–8.
7. McCarus SD. Physiologic mechanism of the ultrasonically activated scalpel. J Am Assos Gyn Lap 1996; 3: 601–8.
8. Weingarten C. Ultrasonic tonsillectomy: rationale and technique. Otolaryngol Head Neck Surg 1997; 116: 193–6.

30 Tonsillectomy and UltraCision

G. Bates, N. Steventon

 ## Indication and Preoperative Management

Tonsillectomy is one of the most common procedures performed in otolaryngological practice. Tonsillectomy is indicated in patients presenting with a history of recurrent acute tonsillitis, chronic tonsillitis, and obstructive sleep apnea syndrome, where the procedure may be combined with adenoidectomy, removal of the tonsil for suspected malignancy, or to gain access to structures lying deep to the tonsil.

Operation

The anaesthetized patient is placed supine on the operating table. A sandbag is inserted under the shoulders to facilitate extension of the head on the body. Historically, this position was adopted to allow blood to pass into the postnasal space rather than entering the unprotected airway. The use of a cuffed endotracheal tube or the laryngeal mask protects the airway today, but the patient position affords a good view and access to the tonsils.

> Editor's tip: When a laryngeal mask is used to deliver anesthetic to the patient rather than an endotracheal tube, the increased diameter of the tube can cause difficulties inserting the Boyle Davis gag. Using a size smaller tongue blade for the gag helps to overcome this problem.

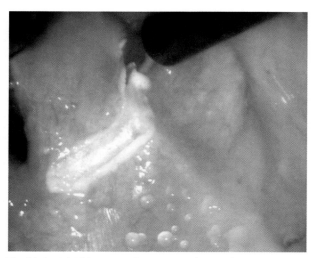

Fig. 30.1 Initial incision of mucosa, right tonsil.

The following instruments are recommended:
- Boyle Davis gag
- Draffin bipod to suspend the gag
- Lucs or Dennis Brown forceps to grasp the tonsil
- UltraCision blade DH105
- Mollison's anterior pillar enucleator
- Yankauer sucker

Additional equipment may occasionally be required to help with additional hemostasis such as bipolar diathermy using 1–2 mm width forceps and a 20 W current setting.

The tonsil is grasped with the Luc's forceps and medialized. Traction applied to the tonsil in this way defines the lateral extent of the tonsil and facilitates dissection by placing the tissue around the capsule of the tonsil under tension. The back of the UltraCision blade is applied to the mucosa of the anterior tonsillar pillar to begin the dissection (Fig 30.1).

> Editor's tip: Use power level 3 throughout the dissection which offers the perfect balance between coagulation and cutting.

Cutting through the mucosa in the region of the upper pole enables the peritonsillar space to be entered. Dissection then continues as close to the capsule of the tonsil as is possible without breaching the capsule itself (Fig. 30.2). The aim is to leave the large plexus of veins known as Dennis Brown's plexus undisturbed. Copious bleeding during tonsillectomy usually occurs from these veins. UltraCision, with its defined cutting accuracy, is able to avoid these veins, or if they are closely applied to the tonsil capsule, coagulate them with ease. The dissection proceeds to separate the tonsil from the tonsillar fossa. Extra care is needed at the apex and the tail of the tonsil. Blood vessels in these areas can cause troublesome bleeding. The lower pole of the tonsil and its covering mucosa runs into the tongue base. Excessive dissection into the tongue base can lead to bleeding and postoperative otalgia due to referred pain from the glossopharyngeal nerve. When the tonsil has been removed entirely, a few small vessels may produce a minor amount of bleeding. A mastoid swab placed in the tonsillar fossa while dissecting the opposite tonsil will achieve hemostasis.

Once all bleeding has stopped, the tension is released on the Boyle-Davis gag. After 30 seconds the gag is then reopened. This maneuver will reveal any bleeding points occluded by the gag tension. The final stage is to pass the Yankauer sucker into the postnasal space to remove any retained clot. This clot is known as the "coroner's clot" as failure to remove the clot can lead to it's aspiration as the patient wakes up from the anesthetic.

⚠ **Hints and Pitfalls**

- The dissection process is facilitated by medializing the tonsil. This places the tissues in the dissection plane under tension and makes the procedure more manageable.
- When the UltraCision blade first comes into contact with the mucosa, there is a blanching of the tissues up to 2 cm away from the cutting area. This is disconcerting when first seen, but represents no tissue damage.
- UltraCision is a fantastic dissecting tool and cuts this particular tissue with ease. It is possible to dissect the tonsil free from its bed in a matter of seconds. However, this often provokes unnecessary bleeding. Active bleeding is much more difficult to stop if it occurs and can disrupt the field of view. It is far better to proceed slowly, making sure the tissues are coagulated prior to division. Total dissection time is reduced compared with conventional techniques. Experience with the technique allows a bloodless dissection
- The dissection process is carried out with the broad surface area back of the dissecting hook. The inside curve of the blade is particularly useful at the lower pole of the tonsil where the tissue is more fibrous as it joins the tongue base (Figs. 30.**3**, 30.**4**). Prior coagulation with the back of the blade facilitates division with the sharp inside curve, which is better for simple dissection.
- At the end of the procedure (Fig. 30.**5**) Bupivicaine local anesthetic can be infiltrated into the tonsillar pillars. Even in the absence of local anesthetic, the postoperative pain scores are low.

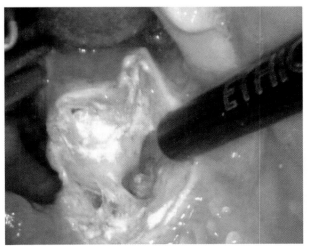

Fig. 30.**2**   Dissection in the peritonsillar plane.

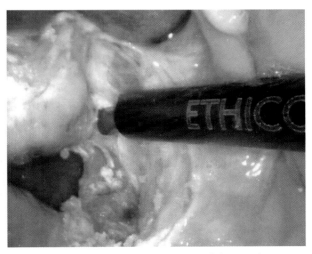

Fig. 30.**3**   Coagulation at the lower pole of the tonsil.

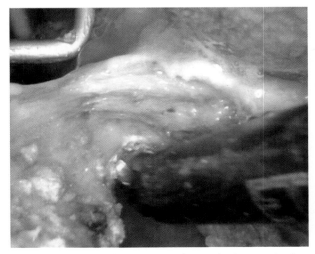

Fig. 30.**4**   Using the sharp curve to dissect the lower pole after coagulation.

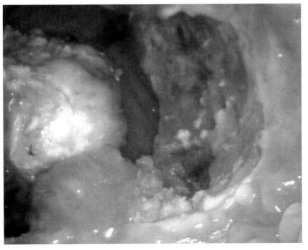

Fig. 30.**5**   The tonsillar fossa at the end of dissection.

Personal Experience

We have carried out over 200 procedures on both adults and children with this technique. We have evaluated the instrument in a randomized, double blind, controlled trial comparing UltraCision tonsillectomy with bipolar dissection tonsillectomy. In this trial and in our continued experience, we found the technique to be safe and reliable. In the trial, 100 patients were randomized to receive a tonsillectomy by UltraCision or bipolar dissection. Their pain scores were collected daily for 14 days. In the early postoperative period the patients who had an UltraCision tonsillectomy ate food significantly more quickly than those who had a bipolar tonsillectomy. The pain scores were low and the incidence of complicated secondary hemorrhage was approximately 1%. All patients in the study returned to school and were pain free at two weeks following surgery. The need for additional hemostatic methods during surgery were of the order of 2%. Similar results have been reported in the literature(1–5).

 Discussion

Tonsillectomy is a commonly performed procedure in otolaryngology. The ideal method removes the tonsil from the tonsil bed carefully and with minimal intraoperative bleeding. Postoperatively, the patient should have minimal discomfort, be able to eat a normal diet and have an acceptable rate of secondary hemorrhage. UltraCision is the ideal instrument to achieve these aims. The ability of UltraCision to cut and coagulate enables careful, bloodless dissection of the tonsil minimizing intraoperative bleeding. The main advantage of the instrument is the minimal lateral thermal injury caused by the instrument during coagulation and cutting. The temperature at the instrument tip is only 60° C which is far less than that produced by electrosurgical techniques. In the UK there have been concerns about the emergence of variant CJD and its possible spread by using reusable instruments. In this regard the disposable nature of UltraCision is an invaluable advantage.

 References

1. Metternich FU, Sagowski C, Wenzel S, Jakel K. [Tonsillectomy with the ultrasound activated scalpel. Initial results of technique with ultracision harmonic scalpel]. Hno 2001; 49(6): 465–70.
2. Sood S, Corbridge R, Powles J, Bates G, Newbegin CJ. Effectiveness of the ultrasonic harmonic scalpel for tonsillectomy. Ear Nose Throat J 2001; 80(8): 514–6, 518.
3. Walker RA, Syed ZA. Harmonic scalpel tonsillectomy versus electrocautery tonsillectomy: a comparative pilot study. Otolaryngol Head Neck Surg 2001; 125(5): 449–55.
4. Wiatrak BJ, Willging JP. Harmonic Scalpel for Tonsillectomy. Laryngoscope 2002; 112(8 Pt 2): 14–6.
5. Willging JP, Wiatrak BJ. Harmonic scalpel tonsillectomy in children: a randomized prospective study. Otolaryngol Head Neck Surg 2003; 128(3): 318–25.

31 Orthopedic Exposure for Total Hip Replacement

T. Heier

Total hip replacement is the most commonly performed adult reconstructive hip procedure in orthopedic surgery. The modern hip arthroplasty started with Sir John Charnley around 1960. There are numerous types of implants manufactured by several companies (10), but the surgical approach to the hip joint does not vary much. The majority of primary hip replacements in Norway is done through a direct lateral approach. In revision arthroplasties the approaches may vary more and may also be more extensive.

Indication and Preoperative Management

Indications for total hip replacement are many. The aim of the procedure is to relieve pain and improve function in patients with disease in the hip joint. Degenerative arthritis, rheumatoid arthritis, arthritis secondary to trauma, avascular necrosis, and slipped capital femoral epiphysis are among the more common reasons for arthroplasty. Pain, reduced range of movement, and reduced function in the hip joint are the main symptoms. The diagnosis must be confirmed by an X-ray examination.

Operation

For both primary and revision hip procedures, the patient is positioned in a lateral position. The operation is done almost without exception in a lumbar spinal anesthesia using a combination of marcaine and morphine. Standard instruments for hip arthroplasty are used. The UltraCision scalpel with the short, sharp hook dissector (5 mm DH or SH 105 or 405) is used for the first part of the operation, and left in place when full access to the hip joint is reached.

A modified Hardinge technique with a direct lateral approach to the hip is used. The dermal part of the skin is incised with an ordinary knife. The incision starts lateral, is continued over the tip of trochanter major, and curved slightly dorsally in a proximal direction. The incision is deepened down to the fascia lata using UltraCision with the curved sharp hook (Fig. 31.1). The fascia is split in the direction of the fibers with scissors and the muscular tissue of the tensor fascia lata is split with UltraCision. The 3 proximal centimeters of the anterior part of the musculus vastus lateralis, musculus gluteus medius and minimus are detached from the trochanter major with an omega-shaped incision. The UltraCision scalpel is used for this part of the procedure, taking care that all the muscles are kept together in one continuous unit (8). The muscular tissue is retracted anteriorly and the joint capsule is exposed, incised, and partially excised (Fig. 31.2). Dislocation of the hip is then carried out by flexion, adduction, and external rotation. The soft tissue around the

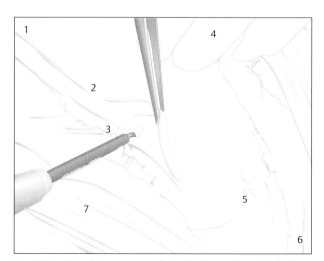
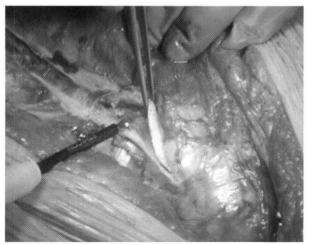

Fig. 31.**1** Detaching m. vastus lateralis. Desection with the flat part of the hook. *1* distal, *2* divided facia of m. vastus lateralis, *3* linea aspera, *4* anterior, *5* trochanter major, *6* proximal, *7* posterior.

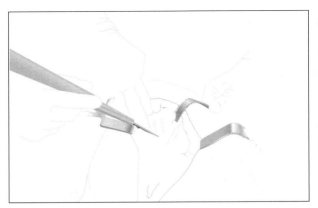
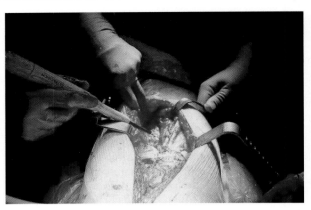

Fig. 31.**2** Surgery with UltraCision.

acetabulum is removed to enhance reaming and fixation of the acetabular component. This capsular tissue may sometimes be very thickened and tough, and it can sometimes be difficult to use UltraCision all the way. This is often the case in obese patients when the structures are situated deep, or if variations in the anatomy of the patient make the access difficult. The operation is completed by fixation of the prosthetic components according to our standard procedure.

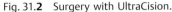 **Hints and Pitfalls**

- Until now UltraCision has not been used very extensively in orthopedic surgery. There are some reasons for this that are obvious. It is not possible to use the UltraCision in bone, and fibrous connective tissue also offers some problems. Also, when the tendinous part of the gluteal musculature is detached from trochanter major there may be some difficulties.

  > Editor's tip: Cutting of extremely "dry" tissue like tendinous structures may be difficult with UltraCision. In these cases, cutting with a regular steel scalpel or shears can be recommended, as bleeding is not a problem in these situations.

- The main problem is that the dissector sticks in the tissue. This compromises the vibration and the function of the scalpel. A continuous beep is then heard instead of the interval beep. To overcome this problem, it is necessary to carry out the dissection in a part of the tissue that is a few millimeters from the insertion to the bone. It is also important to work smoothly and let the UltraCision scalpel decide the pace and not try to force it through the tissue.

 Personal Experience

We have performed about 30 primary total hips with UltraCision dissection of the soft tissues. Twenty of these have been included in a prospective ongoing randomized trial, where the operating time, preoperative blood loss, and postoperative wound problems are compared with 20 hips operated using our standard technique with scalpel and electrosurgery. The usefulness of UltraCision cannot be emphasized enough in revision hip surgery with an extensive exposure of the upper femur. This often requires release of up to 25 cm of vastus lateralis to expose the bone for a longitudinal osteotomy. Also in fracture surgery that requires major exposure of the distal femur we have found UltraCision to be very useful for minimizing blood loss from the vessels penetrating the fascia at the linea aspera. To transect these vessels the broad side of the dissecting hook is used, letting it slowly work itself through the vessel.

 Discussion

UltraCision has been widely used in abdominal surgery, laparoscopic surgery, surgery of solid parenchymatous organs, and in endocrine surgery (1, 2, 3, 4, 5, 6, 7, 9, 11, 12, 13). The publications regarding ultrasonic dissection are mainly from these fields. Both experimental and clinical studies have been carried out, and the documentation is quite extensive. The equipment and tools are primarily designed for this type of surgery. Some orthopedic surgeons have found the technology and principles of UltraCision to be very interesting and have gained some experience. More experience with it is required to define its place in orthopedic surgery. New designs of tools and equipment need to be developed to make the ultrasonic dissection technology more suitable for orthopedic surgical procedures.

Editor's tip: The new 5 mm, 14 cm or 23 cm long "Metzenbaum"-like shears are also be a suitable instrument for soft tissue dissection and preparation in orthopedic surgery.

Randomized prospective trials should be encouraged, and collection of the experience should be recorded in a systematic manner.

 ## References

1. Amaral JF. Laparascopic application of an ultrasonically activated scalpel. Gastrointestinal Endoscopy Clinics of North America 1993; 3: 381–92.
2. Amaral JF. Laparoscopic cholecystectomy in 200 consecutive patients using an ultrasonically activated scalpel. Surg Laparosc Endosc 1995; 5: 255–62.
3. Castaing D, Garden OJ, Bismuth H. Segmental liver resection using ultrasound-guided selective portal venous occlusion. Ann Surg 1989; 210: 20–3.
4. Erian M, McLaren GR, Buck RJ, Wright G. Reducing costs of laparoscopic hysterectomy. J Am Assoc Gynecol Laparosc 1999; 6: 471–475.
5. Ferland RJ, Rizk Y. Ultrasonically activated coagulating shears versus bipolar electrosurgery in laparoscopic-assisted vaginal hysterectomy. J Am Assoc Gynecol Laparosc 1995; 2: S15–S16
6. Hashizume M, Tanoue K, Akahoshi T, Morita M, Ohta M, Tomikawa M, Sugimachi K. Laparoscopic splenectomy: the latest modern technique. Hepatogastroenterology 1999; 46: 820–4.
7. Kusunoki M, Shoji Y, Yanagi H, Ikeuchi H, Noda M., Yamamura T. Current trends in restorative proctocolectomy: introduction of an ultrasonically activated scalpel. Dis Colon Rectum 1999; 42: 1349–52.
8. Learmonth ID, Allen PE. The omega lateral approach to the hip. Journal of Bone & Joint Surgery – British Volume 1996; 78-B: 559–61.
9. McCarus SD, Miller CE. Tissue effects of ultrasonic cutting and coagulation in gynecologic laparoscopic surgery. J Am Assoc Gynecol Laparosc 1995; 2: S73.
10. Murray DW, Carr AJ, Bullstrode CJ. Which primary total hip replacement? Journal of Bone & Joint Surgery – British Volume 1995; 77-B: 520–7.
11. Sawaizumi M, Maruyama Y, Onishi K, Iwahira Y, Okada E. Endoscopic extraction of lipomas using an ultrasonic suction scalpel. Ann Plast Surg 1996; 36: 124–8.
12. Stanton CJ. Laparoscopic splenectomy for idiopathic thrombocytopenic purpura (ITP). A five-year experience. Surg Endosc 1999; 13: 1083–6.
13. Tazaki H, Baba S, Murai M. Technical improvements in laparoscopic adrenalectomy. Tech Urol 1995; 1: 222–6.

32 Miscellaneous Knee and Spine Surgery

R. Eyb

Surgical approaches to the knee and spine are standard in orthopedic surgery. For the implantation of artificial knee joints, usually indicated in cases of osteoarthrosis, a median anterior approach is chosen. If the lower limb is in varus deformity, the knee joint is opened by a medial parapatellar cut, in valgus deformity a lateral parapatellar cut is used. Some variations are described such as osteotomy of the tibial tuberosity or the cut through the mid-vastus, to name some examples. The approach to the knee joint and the cuts of the femoral condyles and the tibial plateau are essentially independent of the implants used.

In spine surgery the number of the approaches is much more varied, according to the nature of the surgical pathology. In general, one can distinguish between anterior and posterior as well as mono- or multisegmental exposures. Most frequently, the dorsal midline approach is utilized since it is the easiest way to reach the spine but, compared with anterior approaches, the blood loss is higher.

Indication and Preoperative Management

Knee Surgery

The indication for the use of the UltraCision harmonic scalpel in knee surgery is any approach in which soft-tissue surgery plays the major role compared to the bone surgery. This is the case in synovectomy due to rheumatoid or other arthritis in which the entire synovialis has to be removed as well as for the removal of Baker's cysts. In both techniques, bone and cartilage, which cannot be cut using UltraCision, are not touched. The most frequent indication for knee surgery is exposure of the knee joint for implantation of a total joint replacement. Preoperatively, function and stability should be documented with knee scores and X-rays with the patient in a standing position should be performed.

Spine Surgery

UltraCision is indicated for a number of approaches to the spine. Only for disc surgery, either open or endoscopic, is the incision minimized so that bleeding as a complication of the approach is very rare. In these cases, UltraCision would not decrease the blood loss significantly. For spinal instrumentation and fusion, larger approaches are necessary, especially when de-

formities have to be corrected and a number of segments have to be exposed. Reduction of spondylolisthesis, fusion of segmental instability, scoliosis and kyphosis correction, as well as tumor surgery are the most frequent indications for the use of the UltraCision scalpel.

For mono- and oligosegmental spinal instrumentation and fusion, the preoperative management contains a number of investigations. Pain assessment, neurological examination, and controlled conservative treatment are mandatory: X-ray in the standing position, function exposures in side bending or anteposterior bending, MRI of the spine, and in cases of presumed instability bracing of the spine complete the information that is necessary to select the right number and levels of the segments which have to be decompressed and fused. In cases of multisegmental instrumentation, segment selection is essential and can be obtained by the same X-ray and MRI investigations as mentioned above, together with the orthopedic and neurological status.

Operation

Exposure of the knee joint for total knee replacement The patient is positioned supine with exposure 20 cm proximally and distally of the joint level. A tourniquet is not applied. After a median skin incision reaching 5 cm proximal of the patella to the tibial tuberosity, the UltraCision scalpel is used. The rectus femoris tendon, the medial or lateral aspect of the patella, and the insertion of the patella tendon at the tibial tuberosity are exposed (Fig. 32.**1**). Afterwards, the longitudinal cut of the rectus tendon and the peripatellar cut are performed with the sharp side of the UltraCision scalpel. With this cut, the two layers of the tendon can be clearly separated and the inserting vessels at the proximal and distal medial edges of the patella transected and coagulated (Fig. 32.**2**). The next step is the dissection of the synovialis and the opening of the joint. The knee is flexed, the patella everted, and the Hoffa fat pad resected to the patella tendon (Fig. 32.**3**).

In cases of synovialitis, the plica synovialis is resected with the UltraCision scalpel at this stage of the operation. The suprapatellar recess can be resected in one piece. For the synovectomy of the cruciate notch and subligamental recess of the collateral ligaments, it is still easier to work with conventional instruments. The subsequent bone cuts are performed according to the implants used.

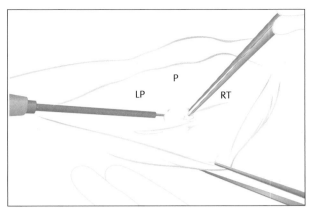
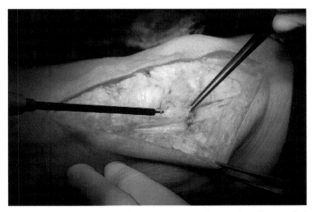

Fig. 32.**1**   Preparation of the medial retinaculum. The rectus tendon (*RT*) is being split, the further cut is performed at the medial rim of the patella (*P*) and ends medial of the ligamentum patellae (*LP*).

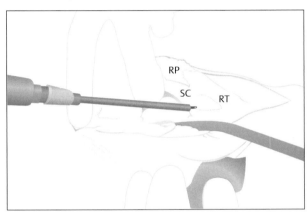
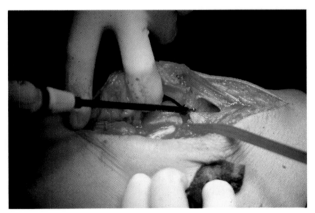

Fig. 32.**2**   With further preparation, the joint capsule (*JC*) is opened. The layers of the retinaculum patellae (*RP*) and of the rectus tendon (*RT*) are separated.

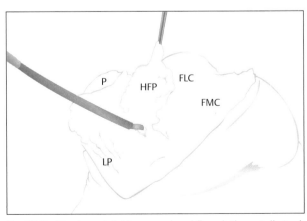
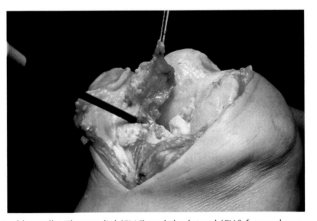

Fig. 32.**3**   The knee joint is opened and flexed; the patella is elevated laterally. The medial (*FMC*) and the lateral (*FLX*) femoral condyles are exposed. After resection of the Hoffa fat pad (*HFP*), the preparation of the knee joint is completed.

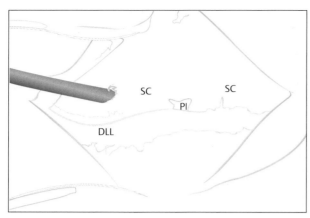
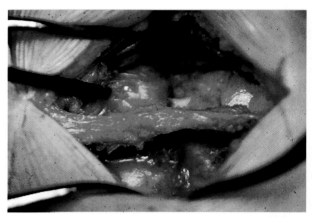

Fig. 32.**4**   Preparation of the dorsal lamina for monosegmental spondylodesis. The joint capsules (*JS*) are still intact. With the UltraCision scalpel, the joints are exposed and the pars interarticularis (*PI*) is visible. The dorsal longitudinal ligament (*DLL*) is still intact.

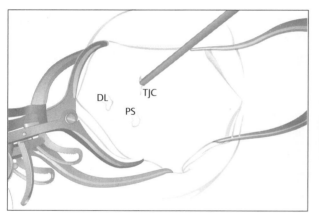
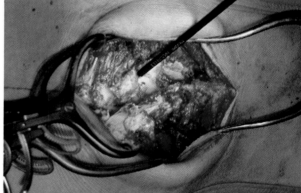

Fig. 32.**5**   Preparation of multiple dorsal lamina (*DL*) for instrumentation of a scoliotic deformity. At this step, the thoracic joint capsules (*TJC*) are opened with the UltraCision scalpel. The dorsal longitudinal ligament is removed and the procesus spinosi (*PS*) are exposed.

Dorsal approach to the spine for transpedicular and intercorporeal spondylodesis For the dorsal approach to the spine, it is mandatory to have the patient's abdomen free when lying in a prone position. This helps to reduce the blood loss especially after opening the spinal canal.

The skin incision is performed in the median line over two segments. The subcutaneous layer, the muscle fascia, and the paraspinous muscles are detached with the UltraCision scalpel; bleeding can be immediately coagulated with the blunt side of the blade.

On reaching the joint capsules, the muscles can easily be retracted further laterally to allow a good exposure of the joint (Fig. 32.**4**). At this stage of the operation X-ray control should be performed to ensure that the correct level is chosen operatively. Then the joint is opened and the distal two-thirds of the facets of the superior segments are osteotomized (Fig. 32.**5**). The ligamentum flavum is resected with a Kerrison and the dura exposed. Cauterization of the epidural veins may

be performed with the blunt side of the blade. After dissection of the coagulated veins, the posterior ligament of the disc is exposed.

> Editor's tip: Preparation close to the dura mater and the nerve roots is an excellent argument for the use of the UltraCision scalpel. As there is no electric current and tissue temperature is not exceeded, the risk of injury to the nerve root is minimized.

After insertion of the transpedicular screws and distraction of the segment with the transpedicular instrumentation, the dorsal ligament is resected. Further steps of the operation are performed with conventional instruments. The disc material is removed, the endplates of the vertebral bodies are opened, and intervertebral spacers are inserted. The transpedicular instrumentation is brought to compression and posterolateral spondylodesis is performed.

⚠ Hints and Pitfalls

Knee Surgery

- Since the approach to the knee joint with the UltraCision scalpel is performed as an open procedure, there are no differences to standard knee expositions with scalpels and electrocautery. There are no pitfalls regarding the use of UltraCision.
- The preparation with UltraCision allows a more anatomic dissection leaving the musculature in a very healthy condition. For cutting and coagulation the surgeon uses only one instrument which increases the comfort of exposure of the knee joint.

Spine Surgery

- Coagulation of epidural veins can sometimes not be managed by UltraCision. Therefore, it is useful to have bipolar cautery at hand. Typical limitations for the use of UltraCision are confluent veins that cannot be separated for coagulation; sometimes the veins are simply too big. In these cases, coagulation can only be obtained by using a blunt pincers and carefully coagulating these veins between the open branches.
- Veins below the facet cannot be reached by UltraCision. In these cases, the medial rim of the facet has to be removed with a small Kerrison. Care should be taken not to open the epidural veins beneath. After removal of the bone, coagulation can be performed by gently pressing the blunt side of the blade against the veins.
- For the removal of the disc material, conventional instruments are used since it is necessary to cut the endplate of the vertebral bodies. Bone cutting with UltraCision is not possible.

Personal Experience

Knee Surgery

Seventy-two approaches to the knee joint for implantation of total endoprosthesis have been performed in our department to date. Since we expected to reduce the blood loss with the UltraCision technique we designed a randomized study in 40 cases comparing operating time, blood loss during the exposure of the knee, during the whole operation, as well as postoperatively. We also compared the number of blood units the patient needed during the hospital stay.

The operations were all performed by the author; all patients had general anesthesia and a tourniquet was never used. Blood loss was measured by suction with a cell saver. Swabs were not used. As result, we did not find a significant difference between the operating time in both groups. The same was true for the overall blood loss, postoperative blood loss, and the blood units needed. For the preparation and exposure of the joint, the difference was highly significant (see Table 32.1).

Until now, we have not found any complications such as wound healing problems, infections, or postoperative bleeding. Patients could be mobilized as usual from the second postoperative day on. Suction drains were removed after the second or third postoperative day. We do not expect any late complications related to UltraCision since the bone cuts were performed with conventional instruments.

Spine Surgery

We started using UltraCision for the dorsal approach to the spine for scoliosis surgery. These are extensive exposures over six to 15 motion segments with muscle detachment from the spinous processes and the dorsal laminae. With conventional techniques the mean blood loss is 1100 ml in our cases. Comparing our first six cases performed with UltraCision with our previous operation we already found a significantly decreased blood loss of 685 ml. With these results it was not justified to perform a randomized comparison. Since then we have performed every scoliosis approach using UltraCision.

Table 32.1 UltraCision in total knee arthroplasty

	Operating time	Blood loss: exposure of the knee	Blood loss: intraoperative implantation of the arthroplasty	Blood loss: postoperative	Blood units
Group 1 (UltraCision) n=20	133 min	4 ml	345 ml	575 ml	1.5
Group 2 (control) n=20	126 min	23 ml	390 ml	605 ml	1.7
P	0.18	0.000	0.09	0.27	0.23

Table 32.**2**   UltraCision in spine surgery (monosegmental spondylodesis with transpedicular screws and interbody cages)

	Operating time	Blood loss intraoperatively	Blood loss postoperatively	Blood units
Group 1 (UltraCision) *n*=20	253 min	267 ml	440 ml	0.5
Group 2 (control) *n*=20	275 min	459 ml	445 ml	1.1
P	0.03	0.006	n.s.	0.01

Meanwhile, the number of our scoliosis patients exceeds 18 consecutive patients. Further reduction of blood loss could not be achieved since two patients with Duchenne scoliosis had to be operated. These are long-lasting procedures with additional fixation of the spine to the pelvis, usually with an exposition from the second thoracic vertebra to the sacrum. The two patients had a blood loss of 2000 ml and 1400 ml, respectively. These were the only patients where homologous donation of blood units was necessary postoperatively. All other patients were managed with the intraoperative cell saver and their blood units. Seven patients did not need any additional blood postoperatively.

With the experience of scoliosis surgery we started to use the UltraCision scalpel for mono- and oligosegmental approaches with removal of the posterior lamina and surgery in the spinal canal. All patients were candidates for transpedicular and intercorporeal spondylodesis. This requires a wide decompression of the nerve roots to get space for the insertion of the intercorporeal implants. To achieve this, the epidural venous plexus has to be coagulated. We could not manage this step of the operation with UltraCision techniques in all cases. Sometimes the veins reach a diameter of 3 mm or show a confluent pattern. In these cases coagulation can only be achieved with the use of pincers but until now pincers can only work with electro-coagulation. To compare the blood loss of our UltraCision cases with our previous cases we investigated 40 patients. Twenty of them were operated conventionally; the other 20 had their approach performed with the UltraCision scalpel. Operation time was even shorter in the UltraCision group; the intraoperative blood loss was significantly reduced. Additionally, the need of blood units postoperatively was decreased significantly as well (see Table 32.**2**). Since we have found a significantly decreased blood loss, even in our early cases, we did not start a randomized trial to compare UltraCision with conventional techniques; rather, we used the UltraCision scalpel consecutively. The number of our cases to date with the use of UltraCision amounts to 34. Preparation of epidural veins in the direct vicinity of the nerve roots and the dura did not reveal any complications. Especially, the nerve roots did not cohere with the surrounding tissue when ultrasonic energy was applied beneath the nerve structures.

Discussion

The use of the UltraCision scalpel in orthopedic surgery has not been reported so far. Its main indication can be seen in laparoscopic visceral techniques (2). But the new technology with the possibility to reduce or avoid the risks of electrocautery, the atraumatic way of cutting and thus the possible reduction of blood loss seems to be an attractive application also for open orthopedic approaches.

For the implantation of total knee replacements, tourniquets have been advocated but on the other hand the risks of tourniquets have been reported (1, 3, 4, 5). With the use of UltraCision, the blood loss could be significantly reduced for the approach to the knee joint in our series, so that the use of a tourniquet was not necessary. On the other hand, most of the blood was lost during the implantation of the knee arthroplasty and not when the joint was exposed. Thus, bleeding from the bone cuts will remain the most significant origin of blood loss in knee arthroplasty.

To date, we see the advantage of UltraCision in the preparation of the soft tissue with the use of only one instrument, allowing a dry and clear exposure of the operated knee.

In spine surgery it is essential to have a dry operating field during the procedure. Since the patient is lying in a prone position, blood will remain in the wound. For transpedicular instrumentation, one has to detach the paraspinous muscles far laterally across the spinal joints until the transverse processes. UltraCision makes these steps of the exposure much easier than the preparation with a scalpel and electrocautery. Since there are no comparative studies in the literature we investigated the intraoperative blood loss and found a significantly smaller amount of blood loss in the group of patients who where operated with UltraCision.

The only limitation for the use of UltraCision was epidural veins which could not be reached beneath the facet joints as well as veins with a diameter of more than 3 mm.

We started to use the UltraCision scalpel in a few indications to have the possibility of comparison with conventional techniques. The advantage of UltraCision preparation encouraged us to use it for any approach to the spine in open as well as in endoscopic techniques, in tumor surgery of the spine, and in any open knee surgery such as synovectomy and removal of Baker's cysts.

References

1. Bradford EMW; Haemodynamic changes associated with the application of lower limb tourniquets, Anaesthesia 1969; 24: 190.
2. Feil W.; Novi G; Laparoskopische Fundoplication: Indikation, Strategie, Technik; Acta Chir. Austriaca Suppl 1999; 153: 36.
3. Matulli N, Testa V, Capasso G; Use of a tourniquet in the internal fixation of fractures of the distal part of the fibula: A prospective and randomised trial; J Bone Jt Surg 1993; 75-A: 700.
4. Salam AA, Eyres KS, Cleary J, El-Sayed HH; The use of a tourniquet when plating tibial fractures; J Bone Jt Surg 1991; 73-B: 86.
5. Salam AA, Eyres KS; Effects of tourniquet during total knee arthroplasty; J Bone Jt Surg 1995; 77-B: 250.

33 Anterior Endoscopic Approach for the Spine

J. Burgos, F.J. Lozano, S. Amaya Alarcon

Thoracoscopy has become a frequently used technique in anterior thoracic spine surgery and is, in many cases, replacing open procedures because of enhanced visualization, reduced incisional pain, lower respiratory complications, shorter hospitalization, lower medical costs, shorter recovery time, and a more cosmetic scar (1, 2, 3, 4, 5, 6).

The thoracolumbar spine approach represents a challenging combination of thoracoscopy and retroperitoneum dissection (7). The endoscopic approach is much less aggressive than open thoraco-lumbotomy.

Endoscopy of the anterior lumbar spine has developed due to advances in urology and general surgery (8, 9). We can choose between retroperitoneal and transperitoneal approaches. The retroperitoneal approach needs to create a virtual space with the use of CO_2. Laparoscopic surgery is almost limited to the L5–S1 space and technically follows the rules for laparoscopy.

Indication and Preoperative Management

Indications for these procedures are the same as those for the anterior approach to the spine. We use endoscopic surgery as a diagnostic (biopsies, collections, drainage) or as a therapeutic tool (deformities, disk surgery, infections, tumors, neurologic decompression) (6, 9, 10, 11, 12, 13, 14, 15, 16, 17, 18, 19).

Thoracoscopy could be contraindicated in patients with severe respiratory insufficiency, intolerance to lung exclusion with a double-lumen tube, and high pressure in the airway (1, 6). By using thoracoscopy, combined with a mini-thoracotomy, we can perform surgery without lung exclusion, as described later.

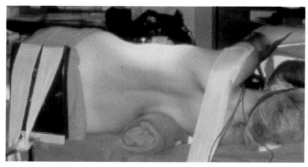

Fig. 33.1 Positioning of the patient for thoracoscopic spine surgery.

Retroperitoneal and laparoscopic approaches are contraindicated in patients with abdominal adhesions due to previous procedures and in those with severe heart or lung pathologies where insufflation with CO_2 can be dangerous (1, 6).

Preoperative management depends on the level to be reached. In thoracoscopy, anesthetic assessment is mandatory in order to do a double-lumen tube intubation (3, 20). The preparation of the digestive tract before surgery is necessary in laparoscopic patients (19, 21).

Thorascopic Spine Surgery

 Operation

Surgery is carried out under general anesthesia with a double-lumen tube.

We place the patient in lateral decubitus position with the side to be operated up (Fig. 33.1). We prefer the right side up to avoid the aortic artery on the left side. The arm at the side to be operated on has to be placed at the same level as thorax, and there must be nothing overhanging proximally. The reason for this is that we have to incline the telescope next to the chest wall in order to see the caudal thoracic spine or to introduce distal trocars.

If two monitors are available they must be placed proximally at both sides, in front of the surgeon and the assistant. If there is only one, it must be placed at the head of the operating table and the anesthetist is displaced laterally.

The surgeon can be in front or behind the patient. The assistant and the nurse (more distally) are in front of the surgeon. Operating table and patient positioning must allow fluoroscopy to be used. Finally, a thoracotomy set must be ready in case of conversion to an open procedure.

The following instruments are used in thoracoscopy:

- Imaging system: The standard telescope is 0°end viewing scope. Thirty degree scopes are useful to visualize deep structures at different levels of the entry point.
- Trocars: We prefer rigid 10.5 mm trocars. They are twisted and stay fixed to chest wall once they are introduced.
- Retractors: They must be used with caution and not for a long time because they can be aggressive. The Endopath-Ethicon 18 mm trocar axis is an easy-to-use and safe retractor.

- Suction-irrigation devices
- Graspers and scissors
- Clip appliers
- UltraCision 10 mm/5 mm LES shears
- Hemostatic cotton balls
- Specific instruments for endoscopic spine surgery: they are longer and thinner so they can be introduced through the portals.

Every point has to be reached over the superior rib edge to avoid intercostal nerve and vessel injuries. The first portal is placed on the middle axillary line, at the same level as the vertebra to be treated, never bellow the 8 th space because diaphragm and abdominal viscera can be damaged. Two other portals are positioned under sight, two spaces above or below the first one and one, or two small extra portals (with or without trocars) on the posterior axillary line for suction and electrocautery. Finally, we use a small incision on the anterior axillary line on the 10 th space at the diaphragm insertion. Through this small incision we place the retractor as distal as possible, and without a trocar because this is a narrow space that makes it stable.

To expose the thoracic spine, the parietal pleura is incised with UltraCision and retracted to reach the bone or disk. Segmental vessels must be preserved. In the following situations a wide exposure is mandatory: bone resection, drainage of collections, vertebral instrumentation, release and arthrodesis in young and small patients, surgery on the left side where the aorta must be pushed aside. In these cases, the pleura must be incised and opened with UltraCision, coagulating segmental vessels and exposing most of the vertebral body until the other side is reached.

> Editor's comment: Bone and cartilage cannot be cut with UltraCision, but dissection of all soft tissue structures close to it is feasible.

In cases of anterior release of scoliosis, discectomies are started with UltraCision to prepare the edges of the vertebral bodies and finished with the rongeur. The rib head is dissected from vertebra and ligaments until it can be easily moved.

Hints and Pitfalls

- When double-lumen intubation is not possible or not tolerable for the patient, we perform a minithoracotomy in connection with the thoracoscopy. A small incision on the anterior axillary line allows lung retraction and exposure of the spine (22). Thoracoscopy can then be performed as usual. This approach can be made as a routine in low weight or very young patients, as well as in curves over 90° (Fig. 33.**2**).
- Long Ethicon trocars are very useful above the fifth rib, where short trocars are hard to introduce due to the chest wall thickness at that level.

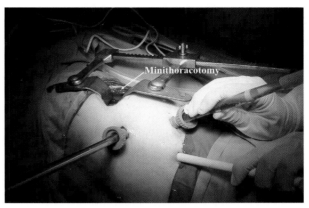

Fig. 33.**2** Thoracoscopically assisted surgery. An additional minithoracotomy facilitates exposure of the spine.

- An entry point above the fourth rib entry point on the posterior axillary line is difficult because of the scapula that must be retracted on its distal angle.
- Endoscopic anatomy changes in thoracic spine proximal to T4 at the right side due to intercostal veins. At the left side one must notice the subclavian artery next to T1 and T2.

Personal Experience

We have performed 96 thoracoscopies: 60 for scoliosis (anterior release and arthrodesis), eight for hyperkyphosis, three for congenital lordosis, 10 for thoracic disk herniation, eight for infections, four for tumors, and three for fractures. In 15 patients we also performed vertebral instrumentation and in three of them a structural bone graft. Mean surgical time was 3 hours (range 0.6–12 hours) and mean bleeding was 230 ml (range 100–2000 ml).

Three cases were converted to open thoracotomy (one for bleeding and two for lung exclusion intolerance). All these cases were performed before the minithoracotomy had been developed. In the last few years, the minithoracotomy was used in 15 cases due to low weight patients, intolerance to lung exclusion, or impossibility of double-lumen intubation. Endoscopic thoracoplasty of more than five ribs was used in eight patients. We no longer use thoracoplasty because of the high incidence of pleural effusion (75%).

In 64 patients with a minimum follow-up of two years, the complications were: five cases of intercostal neuralgia (7%) that resolved within a few weeks, four of atelectasis (5.7%), one in the contralateral lung, five of pleural effusion (7%), and one case of azygos tear treated with endoscopic clippage. No neurological complication was found.

Discussion

Endoscopic approaches to the spine are now one of the best options for the spine surgeon. Many reports emphasize the learning curve and the human and technical equipment aspects (20, 23, 24).

Endoscopic surgery needs a bloodless field so it is very important to coagulate all small vessels. UltraCision represents a very useful tool in this regard. It enables a bloodless exposure of the spine—with less smoke—and this means better working conditions and time saving.

The first thing to do with hemorrhage is compression using a hemostatic ball on a clamp, and then coagulation with UltraCision or clip appliers. Bone wax is useful for bone bleeding.

When bleeding from a major vessel occurs, it is necessary to convert to an open thoracotomy or minithoracotomy to repair the tear.

Complications due to thoracoscopy are rare (1, 20), with mortality ranging between 0–4%. Minor complications are intercostal neuralgias, pleural effusions, and atelectasis. Major complications include vessel or lung damage. Conversion to an open thoracotomy ranges between 5–24% in the literature.

As an advantage, compared with open thoracotomy, thoracoscopy reduces postoperative pain, hospitalization and does not compromise lung function (25).

Thoracolumbar Anterior Endoscopic Surgery

 Operation

Below the 10th thoracic level the operation is feasible. Patient positioning, room set-up, and imaging system are the same as for thoracoscopy (Fig. 33.**1**).

Exposure is started with a conventional thoracoscopy using four portals: the first above the 7th rib in the posterior axillary line; the second above the 6th rib in the anterior axillary line; the third above the 10th rib in the anterior axillary line, and the last one exactly above the diaphragmatic insertion for the retractor. The parietal pleura of the thoracic column is sectioned endoscopically from the level required to the diaphragm, preferably with UltraCision. Following the pleural opening, half of the hemidiaphragm is superficially disinserted in its costal union with UltraCision or scissors.

Now, a conventional retroperitoneal approach is carried out with a balloon inflation method.

The psoas is sectioned from its lateral edge and pushed medially, allowing complete exposure until L4 (Fig. 33.**3**). The diaphragm is closed with separate sutures and one chest tube and a Redon drain are placed.

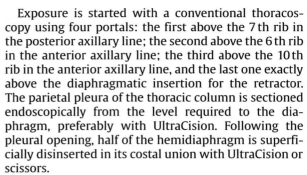 **Hints and Pitfalls**

- If the peritoneum is opened during the dissection, we recommend conversion to an open procedure because endoscopic closure of the peritoneum is very difficult.
- The initial diaphragmatic desinsertion, made from the thorax, should not be deep distally because the peritoneum could be perforated. The diaphragm must not be sectioned centrally because peritoneum ruptures are then frequent.
- To reach the retroperitoneum from a lateral incision and distal to 12th rib, we make a small opening with scissors on the fascia transversalis (this is a very hard fascia) and introduce a finger. Once we reach the retroperitoneum we can make the dissection.
- To complete diaphragmatic desinsertion on the balloon, we empty it to half of its original volume. In this way the dissection can be completed.

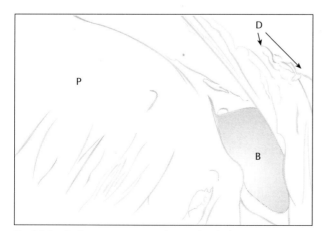

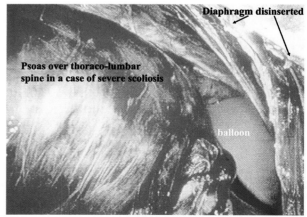

Fig. 33.**3** Endoscopic anterior thoracolumbar surgery. Retroperitoneal approach and exposure of L4 by balloon inflation. *P* psoas over spine in a case of scoliosis, *D* diaphragm, *B* balloon.

Personal Experience

We have performed 23 thoraco-lumbar endoscopic approaches: 16 for scoliosis (anterior release and arthrodesis—two were instrumented), three for infections (drainage and culture), two for fractures, and two for tumors. Five cases were done without lung exclusion. No conversion to open surgery was needed in any case. Six patients were approached from the left side. The mean surgical time was 4.6 hours (range 2.4–8.3 hours), including cases with instrumentation that take longer. Mean bleeding was 250 ml (range 150–1850 ml).

Complications were: two cases of postoperative atelectasis (one associated with pneumonia in the other lung); one minimal lung tear in a patient with pleural adhesions; and one intercostal neuralgia that was resolved within two months. We did not observe any neurological or vascular complications.

 ## Discussion

In this approach, use of UltraCision is of great utility for diaphragmatic desinsertion and psoas release to the other side. Using UltraCision we can reduce bleeding and save operating time. If we consider the high incidence of pathologies in this area, this technique is very useful with low complication rates (27). The open procedure is very aggressive, with higher mortality and morbidity rates and unsightly scars. We also avoid CO_2 and complications related to it (1, 6, 7).

Retroperitoneal Endoscopic Approach to the Lumbar Spine

 ## Operation

It is necessary to clarify that this approach is really a retroperitoneoscopy, creating real spaces where, anatomically, they only exist hypothetically (8, 26, 28).

The patient must be placed in a lateral decubitus position with the side to be operated on up. The "jack-knife" position allows a better exposure. We also use fluoroscopy to confirm the correct vertebral level. The anatomic space runs from the posterior kidney fascia to the transversalis fascia, distally limited by the pelvis and proximally by the diaphragm (Fig. 33.**4**).

The retroperitoneal space can be reached endoscopically through a closed or an open approach. The closed approach starts by introducing a Verres needle in the lumbar or the Petit triangle. The retroperitoneum is insufflated with CO_2 until it reaches a pressure of 15 mm Hg. When the needle is extracted, we place a trocar, generally 12 mm, through the same incision where we introduce the optics. Through the same trocar, a semi-rigid bladder probe is inserted and inflated with saline to 1200 ml volume. An artificial cavity is formed in which the other trocars can be placed.

The open technique starts by making a small incision of 3–4 cm at the posteroinferior level at the point of the 12th rib. The subsequent structures are dissected to the retroperitoneum and we start making the cavity with the index finger. The dilatation balloon can then be passed directly into the retroperitoneum and finish creating the space.

Once the balloon is withdrawn, the first Hasson trocar is introduced to which the CO_2 insufflator is connected, reaching 14 mm Hg of pressure. In this way, we keep the cavity distended and the intraperitoneal organs out of the way. Now, under direct vision, the other working trocars of 5 and 10 mm diameter, respectively,

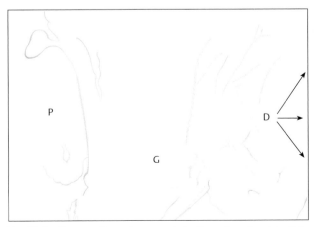 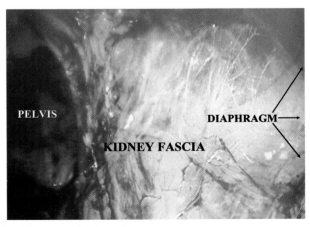

Fig. 33.**4** Retroperitoneal approach to the spine. *P* pelvis, *G* fascia of Gerota, *D* diaphragm.

are introduced. For this technique they can be placed in the medioaxillary line.

The first step consists of identifying the psoas muscle and freeing it from fatty and fibrous tissues. The psoas muscle, genitofemoral nerve, and ureter are dissected. Spinal exposure on the right side can be made between the cava vein and the iliopsoas muscle. On the left side, we dissect between the iliopsoas and the aorta.

By using this approach, the large vessels stay in front and, therefore, we can avoid their dissection and thus their possible damage.

Finally, the intervention is exteriorized, under direct vision, the three trocars are removed, and the incision is closed with silk or staples.

 ## Hints and Pitfalls

- Before introducing the balloon, we dissect the peritoneum with the finger between the psoas and the kidney, which is gently pushed anteriorly.
- On occasion, a small hemorrhage can be seen during the distension of the balloon in the retroperitoneal space; in such a case, the only precaution is to keep the balloon inflated for approximately 5 minutes. and the resulting pressure will produce hemostasis of the bleeding point.

 ## Personal Experience

We have performed this approach in six patients: four anterior fusions in degenerative spine (cages were used in three of them), one extraforaminal L2–L3 disc herniation, and one infectious collection at the L3–4 level. Mean surgical time was 255 minutes (range 150–430 minutes), and mean bleeding was 210 ml (range 110–820 ml). One patient developed a deep venous phlebitis, and another had a ureter section as a major complication that was repaired with an open lumbotomy.

 ## Discussion

The retroperitoneal endoscopic approach is technically demanding and in the first cases we recommend that it be assisted by a urologist (1, 8, 26, 28). The dissection must be done very carefully to avoid lesions to the many structures in this anatomic region. Conversion to open procedure (lumbotomy) must be done in difficult cases or if a major complication arises.

Transperitoneal Endoscopic Approach

 ## Operation

General anesthesia is necessary and the patient is placed in a Trendelenburg position. This position moves the abdominal content upward and enhances spine visualization. A roll is place under lumbar spine to facilitate exposure. Instruments needed are:

- C-arm image intensifier
- 0° or 30° endoscope
- CO_2 insufflation equipment
- Insufflator needle
- Laparoscopic trocars with 10 mm adapters
- Fan retractors
- UltraCision
- Specific spinal endoscopic instruments

We introduce an insufflating needle and create a 12 mm Hg. pneumoperitoneum. Then, through a periumbilical incision, the first trocar is placed and we introduce the 30° endoscope. Under direct endoscopic vision, two other 5 mm trocars are introduced lateral to the epigastric vessels at the level of the spine to be worked on. Intestines are pushed proximally and the sigmoid colon laterally with the retractor. Now, we must look forward to see the promontory. It is always necessary to make another portal on the middle line for suction/irrigation devices.

> Editor's tip: Preparation is facilitated by the use of the 5 mm curved shears. The instrument can be used as a grasping device, for blunt dissection, and for single-step coagulation and cutting.

To reach the L5–S1 disk space we incise the peritoneum to reach the anterior aspect of disc. Now we can identify the sacral vein and artery which are transacted with the UltraCision shears. The rest of exposure must be done with blunt dissection to avoid injury to the hypogastric plexus. After exposure, we perform surgery on the bone or disc (Fig. 33.**5**).

To reach the L4–L5 disc we incise the right side of mesocolon. In this way, we can take it apart to the left side. The aortic bifurcation is carefully dissected, separating the iliac artery and vein. To complete the exposure, we coagulate segmental vessels with UltraCision and then perform surgery on the disc.

For this step, an extra trocar must be introduced in front of the spine. We first place a fluoroscopy-guided Steimann pin to confirm the correct level and introduce the trocar.

Bone grafts, if needed, can be obtained from iliac crest. Before closure we irrigate well and finally close the peritoneum over the spine.

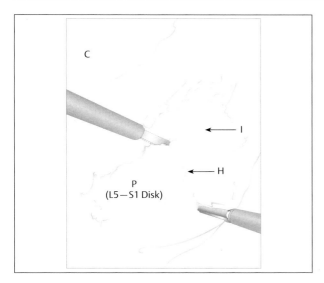

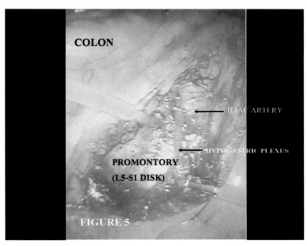

Fig. 33.**5**   Transperitoneal endoscopic approach to the spine (L5–S1). *C* colon, *I* iliac artery, *H* hypogastric plexus, *P* promontory.

 ## Hints and Pitfalls

- As preoperative management, we recommend a CT or MRI scan in order to exactly observe the anatomy, especially the location of the great vessels.
- Blunt dissection on the promontory is recommended to avoid injury to the plexus. Retrograde ejaculation is a rare complication but may occur.
- If, during L4–L5 exposure, the great vessels cannot be retracted properly, it is better to perform open surgery because a vessel injury at this level can be dramatic.
- To retract vessels, we use plastic-protected Kirschner wires at both sides on the vertebral bodies.

 ## Personal Experience

A total of 12 patients have been treated with this technique: nine for degenerative conditions and three for spondylolisthesis. Arthrodesis was done in all cases. Nine were L5–S1 and three were L4–L5 approaches. All but two were female. In three cases of L5–S1, a laparotomy was needed to finish the procedure due to technical difficulties. One case of L4–L5 was also converted for the same reason.

Mean surgical time was 230 minutes (range 150–370 minutes) and mean bleeding was 340 ml (range 210–950 ml).

One case of retrograde ejaculation resolved spontaneously. There was one muscular herniation through a portal incision that needed surgical repair.

 ## Discussion

We recommend the assistance of a general surgeon with experience in laparoscopy for the first cases.

The L5–S1 approach in cases of severe spondylolisthesis may be very hard because the sacrum is placed horizontally. In this situation, laparoscopy can be assisted with a minilaparotomy through a Pfannestiel incision.

The L4–L5 approach is not easy endoscopically. Vessel retraction can be difficult and dangerous. For this reason we use retroperineoscopy for this vertebral level.

 ## References

1. Reagan JJ, Guyer RD. Endoscopic techniques in spinal surgery. Clin Orthop 1997; 335: 122–39.
2. Kaisser LR. Video assisted thoracic surgery. Current state of the art. Ann Surg 1994; 220: 720–34.
3. Rusch VW. Toracoscopia. Suplementos de técnica quirúrgica II. 1993–1994, Scientific American Inc.
4. Allen MS, Trastek VF, Daly RC, Deschamps C, Pairolero PC. Equipment for thoracoscopy. Ann Thorac Surg 1993; 56: 620–23.
5. Landreneau RJ, Mack MJ, Keenan RJ, Hazelrigg SR, Dowling RD, Ferson PF. Strategic planning for video assisted thoracic surgery. Ann Thorac Surg 1993; 56: 615–19.
6. Reagan JJ. Endoscopic spine surgery. Mapfre Medicina 1996; 7(Suppl. II): 13–15.
7. Burgos J, Rapariz JM, Hevia E, González-Herranz P. Anterior endoscopic approach to toracholumbar spine. Mapfre Medicina 1996; 7(Suppl. II): 37–43.
8. Gasman D, Saint F, Barthelemy Y, Anthipon P, Chopin D, Abbou CC. Retroperitoneoscopy: A laparoscopy approach for adrenal and renal surgery. Urology 1996; 47: 801–06.
9. Coltharp WH, Arnold JH, Alford WC, Burrus GR, Glassford DM, Lea JW et al. Videothoracoscopy: Improved technique and expanded indications. Ann Thorac Surg 1992; 53: 776–79.

10. Mack MJ, Reegan JJ, Bobechko WP, Acuff TE. Application of thoracoscopy for diseases of the spine. Ann Thorac Surg 1993; 56: 736–38.
11. Dickman CA, Mican C. Thoracoscopic approaches for the treatment of anterior thoracic spinal pathology. BNI Quarterly, 1995; I: 3.
12. Horowitz MB, Moossy JJ, Julian T, Ferson PF, Huneke K. Thoracic discectomy using video assisted thoracoscopy. Spine 1994; 19: 1082–86.
13. Landreneau RJ, Mack MJ, Hazelrigg SR, Dowling RD, Acuff TE, Magee MJ et al. Video assisted thoracic surgery: Basic technical concepts and intercostal approach strategies. Ann Thorac Surg 1992; 54: 800–07.
14. Mehlman CT, Crawford AH, Wolf RK. Endoscopic thoracoplasty technique. Spine 1997; 22: 2178–82.
15. Dickman CA, Mican C. Multilevel anterior thoracic discectomies and anterior interbody fusion using a microsurgical thoracoscopic approach. J Neurosurg 1996; 84: 104–09.
16. McAfee PC, Reegan JR, Fedder IL, Mack MJ, Geis WP. Anterior thoracic corpectomy for spinal cord decompression performed endoscopically. Surg Laparoscopy Endoscopy 1995; 5: 339–48.
17. Rosenthal D, Marquardt G, Lorenz R, Nichtweis M. Anterior decompression and stabilization using a microsurgical endoscopic technique for metastatic tumors of the thoracic spine. J Neurosurg 1996; 84: 565–72.
18. Parker LM, McAfee PC, Fedder IL, Weis JC, W. Geis P. Minimally invasive surgical techniques to treat spine infections. Orthop Clin North Am 1996; 27: 1–11.
19. Zucherman JF, Zdeblick TA, Bailey SA, Mahvi D, Hsu KY et al. Intrumented laparoscopic spinal fusion. Spine 1995; 20: 2029–35.
20. Mulder DS. Pain management principles and anesthesia techniques for thoracoscopy. Ann Thorac Surg 1993; 56: 630–32.
21. Reagan JJ, Yuan H; McAfee P. Laparoscopic fusion of the lumbar spine: Minimally Invasive Spine Surgery. Spine 1999; 24: 402–11.
22. Lozano FJ, Burgos J, Amaya S, Gonzalez-Herranz P, López Mondejar JA. Minithoracotomy combined with video thoracoscopy in scoliosis surgery. Presented at the "Scoliosis Research Society" Meeting. San Diego, CA. 1999.
23. Wain JC. Thoracoscopy training in a residency program. Ann Thorac Surg 1993; 56: 799–800.
24. Jancovici R, Lazdunski LL, Pons F, Cador L, Dujon A, Dahan M et al. Complications of video assisted thoracic surgery: a five year experience. Ann Thorac Surg 1996; 61: 533–37.
25. Landreneau RJ, Hazelrigg SR, Mack MJ, Dowling RD, Burke D, Gavlick J et al. Postoperative pain related morbidity: video assisted thoracic surgery versus thoracotomy. Ann Thorac Surg 1993; 56: 1285–89.
26. Gaur D. Laparoscopic operative retroperitoneoscopy: Use of a new device. J Urol 1992; 148: 1137.
27. McAfee PC, Regan JR, Zdeblick T, Zuckerman J, Picetti GD, Heim S et al. The incidence of complications in endoscopic anterior thoracolumbar spinal reconstructive surgery. Spine 1995; 20: 1624–32.
28. Himpens J, Van Alphen P, Cadière GD, Verroken R. Ballon dissection in extended retroperitoneoscopy. Surg Laparoscopy Endoscopy 1995; 5: 193–96.

34 The UltraCision Scalpel in Thoracic Surgery

R. Jancovici, L. Lang-Lazdunski, X. Kerangal, F. Pons

Thoracoscopic Sympathectomy

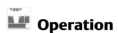 Indication and Preoperative Management

Upper limbs hyperhidrosis is a disabling condition affecting predominantly women. This condition often constitutes a social and psychological handicap (9, 11, 18).

Palmar axillary hyperhidrosis depends on the hyperactivity of the vasomotor nervous fibers going along the thoracic sympathetic chain and going through the stellate ganglion to finally reach the brachial plexus (19). The principle of radical upper thoracic sympathectomy consists in a resection of the sympathetic chain between the inferior border of the second rib to the inferior border of the fifth rib. The procedure is usually performed on both sides because almost 100% of the patients suffer bilateral hyperhidrosis (4). Upper thoracic sympathectomy is also performed for reflex sympathetic dystrophy and causalgia (14).

Operation

The following instruments are used:
- 2 × 5 mm ports (camera and UltraCision)
- 1 × 5 mm port (grasper)
- 1 × 0° camera
- 1 chest tube (20 Fr)

Under general anesthesia and with a double-lumen tracheal tube allowing one-lung ventilation, the patient is placed in the appropriate lateral decubitus position with the upper limb abducted 90° and raised to expose the axilla.

The first 5 mm port is inserted on the mid-axillary line in the fourth intercostal space. A 0° camera is inserted. The second and third ports (5 mm) are placed in the third anterior and fourth anterior intercostal spaces. The entire pleural cavity is visualized and the sympathetic chain localized beneath the parietal pleura at the junction of the transverse processes of the spine and ribs. The UltraCision scalpel is introduced through the second port. The subclavian artery is used as a landmark for the first rib. The second, third, fourth, and fifth ribs are marked and the parietal pleura overlying the sympathetic chain from T2 to T5 is incised using the UltraCision scalpel (Fig. 34.1). The sympathetic chain is divided using UltraCision on the inferior border of the second rib and it is grasped on its

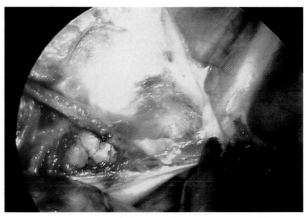

Fig. 34.**1** Incision of the parietal pleura using the UltraCision scalpel.

superior extremity. Progressively, all communicating branches are divided from the second to the fifth rib (Fig. 34.**2**). Finally, the sympathetic chain is divided on the superior border of the fifth rib (Fig. 34.**3**). Care is taken not to injure intercostal arteries and veins during all these maneuvers. Then, the nervous chain is exteriorized and sent to the pathologist, and the bodies of the second, third, fourth, and fifth ribs are coagulated over 4 cm using a power setting level 4 to destroy accessory branches of the sympathetic chain (nerve of Kuntz). After verification of hemostasis, a chest tube (20 Fr) is inserted through an anterior port and the two other incisions are closed in layers.

⚠ Hints and Pitfalls

- It can be helpful to bring the patient into a 110° lateral decubitus position by rolling the operation table, to make the lung fall anteriorly and improve exposure to the sympathetic chain.
- There is usually no need to retract the aorta on the left side. Vascular wounds to the aorta of the left subclavian artery have been reported with electrocautery during these procedures; making use of UltraCision is an excellent alternative to minimize the risk of major arterial injury.
- Intercostal vein wounds are not exceptional, particularly on the right side, and can be controlled by using either UltraCision on its maximum power level (4 or 5) or surgical endoclips.

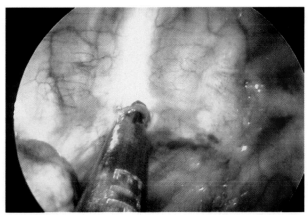

Fig. 34.**2**   Transection of the rami communicantes with UltraCision.

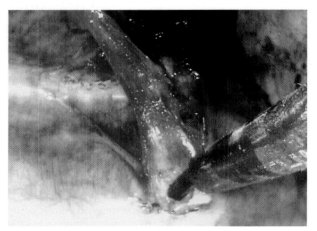

Fig. 34.**3**   Division of the rami communicantes of the sympathetic trunk.

 Personal Experience

Since 1995 we have operated more than 150 patients using exactly the same technique. The UltraCision scalpel is used for all video-assisted thoracic sympathectomies.

There was no intraoperative bleeding and no conversions to open thoracotomy. We had only one postoperative complication (hemopneumothorax) over 5 years.

Discussion

Video-assisted thoracic sympathectomy has become standard therapy for upper limb hyperhidrosis when medical therapy and ionophoresis have failed (5, 9, 11, 18, 19).

Success rates for this procedure range between 94% and 98% in most series (1–5). The rate of complication is very low (2.7%) in a recent series of 412 consecutive patients (17). Most patients are satisfied initially. Some investigators reported late recurrences of hyperhidrosis (5, 6, 9, 11, 18, 19). The rami communicantes are also divided and coagulated over the body of the second, third, fourth, and fifth ribs. The goal of this technique is to prevent recurrences due to the persistence of small accessory nervous branches of the sympathetic chain, which are present in about 10% of patients and that may be overlooked (5). We used UltraCision to dissect the sympathetic chain on the inferior border of the second rib to prevent thermal injury to the stellate ganglion. UltraCision was used for the division and section of all other parts of the sympathetic chain. We never attempted to include the T1 ganglion in our resection, because the division between T1 and the lower cervical sympathetic ganglion (C7–C8) within the stellate ganglion is ill-defined. Thus, inclusion of T1 may result in Horner's syndrome. Only the T2, T3, and T4 + T5 ganglia are resected.

No patient has complained of interscapular pain since we have been using UltraCision. We postulate that interscapular pain may be due to thermal injury related to the use of monopolar or bipolar diathermy. The risk of thermal injury to the nerves or stellate ganglion is significantly lowered. In addition, lethal arrhythmia has been reported with electrocautery and may be prevented by the use of UltraCision(3).

Thoracoscopic Splanchnicectomy

 Indication and Preoperative Management

Many techniques and methods have been advocated for the control of chronic pain during pancreatic cancer, ranging from the use of morphinomimetic drugs to celiac plexus block (12). Recent publications stated that videothoracoscopic splanchnicectomy represents a very safe and effective technique for pain relief during pancreatic cancer (13, 20). We and others have recently reported our experience with this technique (13).

 Operation

The following instruments are used:
- 2 × 5 mm ports (camera and UltraCision)
- 1 × 5 mm port (diaphragm retractor and grasper)
- 1 × 0° camera
- 1 chest tube (20 Fr)

Under general anesthesia and with a double-lumen tracheal tube, the patient is placed in the right lateral decubitus position. We currently make three small incisions for working instruments and a 0° camera. The

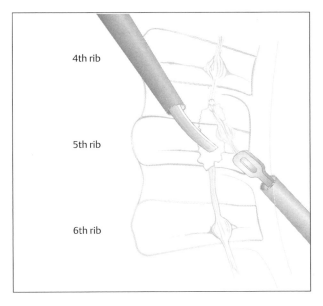

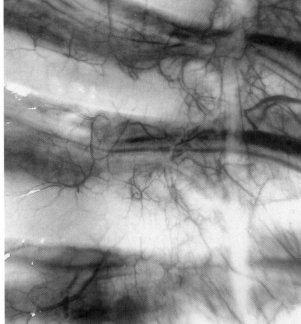

Fig. 34.**4** Video-assisted thoracic sympathectomy. The sympathetic trunk is seen crossing the ribs and intercostal bundles.

first port is inserted on the mid-axillary line in the sixth intercostal space and the camera is introduced into the pleural cavity. Then, two additional ports are placed anteriorly in the fifth and eighth intercostal spaces. The sympathetic chain and the left greater splanchnic nerve are visualized under the parietal pleura. Usually, we use a 5 mm instrument to retract the diaphragm inferiorly. The pleura is incised and the sympathetic chain is divided using the UltraCision scalpel just above the first root of the left greater splanchnic nerve (T7) (Fig. 34.**4**). Then, the sympathetic chain is grasped and all rami communicantes are divided to the T10 ganglion. At this level, the chain is divided just below the inferior root of the greater splanchnic nerve. The divided sympathetic chain is then retracted internally and all roots are dissected free to the greater splanchnic nerve trunk, and the trunk divided. This technique has been proposed by us and called "radical sympatho-splanchnicectomy".

Other techniques can be easily performed by just dividing the greater splanchnic nerve itself or by dividing its roots from the T7 to the T10 ganglion.

Additional resection can be performed as well, i.e., division of the lesser splanchnic nerve itself or its roots up to T12 (those may arise from below the diaphragm and may not be accessible by videothoracoscopy), or division of the posterior vagus nerve.

During the entire procedure, special care must be taken not to damage intercostal arteries that are in close contact with the sympathetic chain and the nervous roots. Thus, the Adamkiewicz artery arises from a left-sided intercostal artery situated between T9 and T12 in approximately 70% of patients, and in-

jury to one of these arteries may result in postoperative paraplegia (2, 10).

At the end of each procedure, a chest tube (20 Fr) is inserted through an anterior port and the two others are closed in layers.

Hints and Pitfalls

- It can be helpful to bring the patient into a 110° lateral decubitus position combined with a Trendelenburg position to make the lung fall superiorly and improve exposure to the lower sympathetic chain and splanchnic nerves. Division of the pulmonary ligament may also be a helpful maneuver.
- Two instruments can usually be passed through an anterior port. One is used for diaphragm retraction. The other one can be used to grasp the sympathetic chain.
- The presence of tight adhesions or the presence of fibrohyaline plaques on the pleura may preclude access to the sympathetic chain and make a minithoracotomy necessary for adequate exposure and splanchnic nerve division.

Personal Experience

We have operated 20 patients with this technique, all patients had a left splanchnicectomy, nine had an associated posterior vagotomy, six had an associated right splanchnicectomy. All patients recovered un-eventfully. Three patients with associated vagotomy suffered postoperative transitory diarrhea. Pain was totally relieved and drug addiction stopped in 77 % of patients. Partial relief of pain was obtained in 11 % of patients. Only 12 % of patients had an intermediate or poor result of pain relief.

 ## Discussion

Unilateral left splanchnicectomy provides excellent results in terms of pain relief in the majority of patients (13, 20). In those with incomplete relief of symptoms, an associated right splanchnicectomy can be performed (4, 15). However, side effects such as transient orthostatic hypotension or intermittent diarrhea have been reported with bilateral procedures and have been related to the suppression of the physiological sympathetic tonus (13, 15).

> Editor's tip: UltraCision may be of special interest for the performance of splanchnicectomies. It can easily replace two instruments: grasper and scissors. It minimizes the risk of intercostal vessel injury, which may be extremely vulnerable in this area (T7–T12) where segmental intercostal arteries provide the arterial blood supply to the lower thoracic and lumbar spinal cord. It can also be used safely to divide the pulmonary ligament if required.

Thoracoscopic Pericardial Window

 ## Indication and Preoperative Management

During the past eight years, videothoracoscopy has become a useful tool in performing a pericardial window in patients with pericardial effusion (7, 8).

The use of UltraCision was recently reported in this indication. It allows for the rapid and safe performance of this procedure (16).

 ## Operation

After general anesthesia with a double-lumen endotracheal tube, the patient is placed in the appropriate lateral decubitus position (referentially the left one). The first port is placed in the fifth intercostal space under the tip of the scapula, to introduce the camera. The second and third ports are placed anteriorly in the fourth and sixth intercostal spaces. The pericardium is grasped using a grasping instrument and the UltraCision scalpel is introduced through an anterior port.

> Editor's tip: The first incision for creating the window can be made with the jaws of the shears open by just puncturing the pericardium.

The tip of the blade is pressed against the distended pericardium for a few seconds with the highest power level (4 or 5) to make a perforation, then the pericardium is hooked in traction and a large piece of it is excised (4–5 cm in diameter). One chest tube (24 Fr) is inserted and the small incisions are closed in layers.

 ## Hints and Pitfalls

- The phrenic nerve and the diaphragmatic pedicle should be visualized before choosing the site for the pericardial window.
- Pericardial vessels should be transected with UltraCision as they may be a source of secondary bleeding.

 ## Discussion

The main advantage of using UltraCision for this procedure is that no grasper is necessary since the pericardium has been opened. Thus, only two ports may be required. Moreover, the risk of electrocautery-induced arrhythmia is virtually eliminated (16).

 ## References

1. Amaral JF. Depth of thermal injury: ultrasonically activated scalpel vs. electrosurgery. Surg Endosc 1995; 9: 226.
2. Cheshire WP, Santos CC, Massey EW, Howard JF. Spinal cord infarction: etiology and outcome. Neurology 1996; 47: 321–30.
3. Chow TC, Tan CT, Hwang YS, Ting MC, Cheu YP, Lin JC, Lin CC. Sudden cardiac arrest during left thoracoscopic T1 sympathectomy. Ma Tsui Hsueh Tsa Chi 1992; 30: 277–82.
4. Cuschieri A, Shimi SM, Crosthwaite G, Joypaul V. Bilateral endoscopic splanchnicectomy through a posterior thoracoscopic approach. JR Coll Surg Edinb 1994; 39: 44–7.
5. Gossot D, Toledo L, Fritsch S, Celerier M. Thoracoscopic sympathectomy for upper limb hyperhidrosis looking for the right operation. Ann Thorac Surg 1997; 64: 975–8.
6. Hashmonai M, Kopelman D, Kein O, Schein M. Upper thoracic sympathectomy for primary palmar hyperhidrosis: long-term follow-up. Br J Surg 1992; 79: 268–71.
7. Hazelrigg SR, Mack MJ, Landreneau RJ, Acuff TE, Seifert PE, Auer JE. Thoracoscopic pericardiectomy for effusive pericardial disease. Ann Thorac Surg 1993; 56: 792–5.
8. Hazelrigg SR, Numchuck SK, Lo Cicero J. Video assisted thoracic surgery group data. Ann Thorac Surg 1993; 56: 1039–44.
9. Herbst F, Plas EG, Függer R, Fritsch A. Endoscopic thoracic sympathectomy for primary hyperhidrosis of the upper limbs: a critical analysis and long-term results of 480 operations. Ann Surg 1994; 220: 86–90.

10. Koshino T, Murakami G, Morishita K, Mawatari T, Abe T. Does the Adamkiewicz artery originate from the larger segmental arteries? J Thorac Cardiovasc Surg 1999; 117: 898–905.

11. Kux M. Thoracic endoscopic sympathectomy palmar in and axillary hyperhidrosis. Arch Surg 1978; 113: 264–6.

12. Lebovits AH, Lefkowitz M. Pain management of pancreatic carcinoma: a review. Pain 1989; 36: 1–11.

13. Le Pimpec Barthes F, Chapuis O, Riquet M, Cuttat JF, Peillon C, Mouroux J, Jancovici R. Thoracoscopic splanchnicectomy for control of intractable pain in pancreatic cancer. Ann Thorac Surg 1998; 65: 810–3.

14. Mc Fadden PM, Hollier LH. Thoracoscopic sympathectomy in Haimavici's vascular surgery. Haimavici. editor, 4 th edn., London: Blackwell science; 1996. pp. 1118–26.

15. Maher JW, Johlin FC, Pearson D. Thoracoscopic splanchnicectomy for chronic pancreatitis pain. Surgery 1996; 120: 603–10.

16. Ohtsuka T, Wolf RK, Wurnig P, Park SE. Thoracoscopic limited pericardial resection with an ultrasonic scalpel. Ann Thorac Surg 1998; 65: 855–6.

17. Plas EG, Függer R, Herbst F, Fritsch A. Complications of endoscopic thoracic sympathectomy. Surgery 1995; 118: 493–5.

18. Shachor D, Jedeikin R, Olsfanger D, Bendethan J, Sivak G, Freund U. Endoscopic transthoracic sympathectomy in the treatment of primary hyperhidrosis. Arch Surg 1994; 129: 241–4.

19. Wittmoser R. Thoracoscopic sympathectomy and vagotomy. In: Cuschieri A, Buess G, Perissat J. editors. Operative manual of endoscopic surgery. New York: Springer; 1992. pp. 110–33.

20. Worsey J, Ferson PF, Keenan RJ, Julian TB, Landreneau RJ. Thoracoscopic pancreatic denervation for pain control in irresectable pancreatic cancer. Br J Surg 1993; 80: 1051–2.

35 Radical Laparoscopic Prostatectomy

H. Mignot

Radical laparoscopic prostatectomy has become a standard treatment for localized prostate cancer. The development of laparoscopy offers the hope of less complicated surgical recovery and decreased morbidity, particularly concerning urinary incontinence and sexual dysfunction.

This technique was developed by Dr. Richard Gaston (Bordeaux, France), whose technical innovations and simplifications include an initial transperitoneal approach of the seminal vesicles and vasa deferentia. Based on his experience, the technique has spread throughout France and the world.

Indication and Preoperative Management

The diagnosis of prostate cancer is based on rectal palpation and PSA levels. Confirmation is provided by an anatomical pathology examination of biopsies.
If the PSA is <10 and the Gleason score <7 (no element > or = 4), evaluation for extracapsular extension is not necessary. If this is not the case, an abdominopelvic CT scan and bone scintigraphy may be required. In general, prostatectomy is indicated for patients in excellent health, under 70 (survival >10 years) with tumors believed to be localized. Antibiotic therapy is initiated two hours before the procedure. Deep vein thrombophlebitis prophylaxis is routine.

When new to the procedure, bowel preparation as for colonic surgery is advised, due to the risks of rectal perforation described by several authors. With increasing expertise, bowel preparation will no longer be absolutely necessary, except for constipated patients.

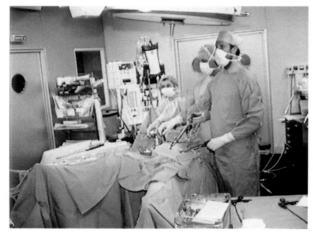

Fig. 35.**1**　Position of surgeon during operation.

> Editor's tip: Patients scheduled for laparoscopy should undergo bowel preparation preoperatively in order to ameliorize intra-abdominal visualization, reduce intra-abdominal gas pressure and also in order to prevent massive fecal contamination if there is accidental injury to the colon that may be sutured laparoscopically.

Operation

The patient is placed in supine position, with his left arm along the body and right arm extended (the right arm may also lie along the body, to avoid any tension on the plexus when an assistant stands to the right of the patient). The legs are slightly abducted to allow access to the perineum for urinary catheterization and, if necessary, rectal palpation. After establishment of pneumoperitoneum, Trendelenburg's associated with left lateral position is required to move the bowel away.

> Editor's tip: It is advisable to avoid shoulder supports, as this may cause painful, long-term disorders of the shoulder function and can also be responsible for severe nerve injuries.

Shoulder supports are not used. The video monitor is placed either at the patient's right foot (55 cm screen) or between the patient's legs (36 cm screen). The surgeon stands on the patient's left side, the assistant at the head or right side. The second assistant, possible though not essential, stands to the left of the surgeon. The patient's head is covered with a sterile drape to protect the assistant. The anesthetists, therefore, stand to the right of the assistant (Fig. 35.1). The use of a high-quality camera (if possible a 3-CCD) with 0° or 30° lenses is recommended.

The following trocars must be available:
- 1 ×10 mm trocar
- 3 or 4 5 mm trocars
- 1 × 12 mm trocar when automatic forceps or a 5/8 circle needle are used

In addition to the usual laparoscopic instruments, certain specialized instruments may be used:
- 5 mm UltraCision blade or shears
- Bipolar grasping forceps
- 2 × grasping forceps
- 1 pair of mono- or bipolar scissors
- 1 × aspiration-lavage tube, 5 mm diameter

- Linear vascular-type stapler
- 2 × needle holders permitting a strong grip
- Monofilament or braided absorbable sutures, needles 26, 3 or 5/8

After establishment of pneumoperitoneum with a pressure of 12, the camera is inserted through a 10 mm umbilical trocar.

Under camera control, the following are then inserted:
- 1 × 5 mm trocar at the lateral third of the right umbilicoiliac line
- 1 × 5 mm trocar at the medial third of the right umbilicoiliac line
- 1 × 5 mm trocar at the lateral third of the left umbilicoiliac line
- 1 × 5 mm or 12 mm trocar at mid-distance on the umbilicopubic line

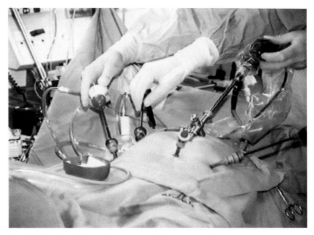

Fig. 35.**2** Position of trocars during operation.

If the sigmoid colon is large and obtrusive, it may be attached by a transparietal suture to the left flank using an epiploic fold to free the Douglas' pouch (Fig. 35.**2**).

The vasa deferentia are identified through the peritoneum at the lower fold of Douglas' pouch, which is incised transversally. The upper fold corresponds to the ureters. The inner aspects of the vasa deferentia are dissected down to the ampullae, where they are sectioned.

When new to the operation, it is easier and more reassuring to locate the vasa deferentia along the pelvic wall. It is not then essential to make a circular dissection of these ducts, but only to dissect their inner surfaces to the level of the ampullae, where they are then sectioned. The deferential stump must be kept short so that it does not interfere with later dissections of the posterior area.

Traction on the ductus deferens permits the identification and dissection of the homolateral seminal vesicle. Dissection, down to the level of the latter using the UltraCision blade, and bipolar coagulation of the two transverse arteries (one at the base, the other at the bottom of the vesicle) saves the neurovascular bundles.

These bundles are located near the bottom of the seminal vesicles. Particular care must be taken with hemostasis as the seminal vesicles are highly vascularized (Fig. 35.**3**).

The simultaneous upwards traction of both vasa deferentia brings Denonvillier's aponeurosis into view. It is incised to expose the pre-rectal fat below the vesicoprostatic junction (Fig. 35.**4**).

The rectum is gently pushed to the back in order to free it from the posterior aspect of the prostate, as low as possible towards the apex and the anterior face of the rectum. The presence of pre-rectal fat indicates that dissection is in the correct plane. The dissection of the outer lobes of the prostate will depend, in part, on the quality of the dissection of the posterior aspect.

Using a 30° lens can assist in visualizing the posteroinferior plane towards the apex, especially when the prostate is large. In some cases the bladder neck may be identified posterior, however this dissection requires the greatest care to avoid injuring the ureters.

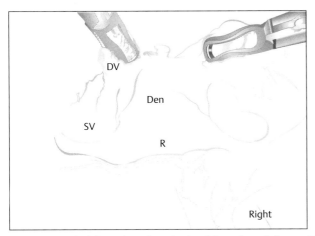

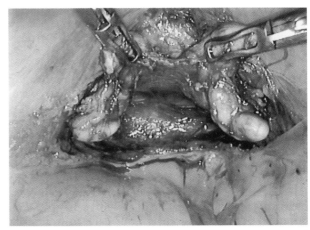

Fig. 35.**3** End of dissection of seminal vesicle and vas deferens. *DV* vas deferens, *Den* Denonvillier's aponeurosis/incision, *SV* seminal vesicle, *R* rectum.

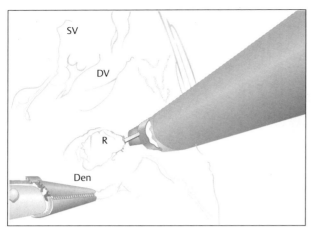

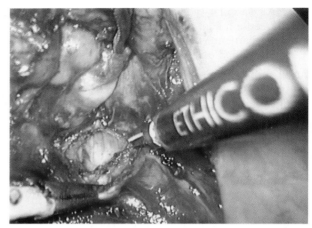

Fig. 35.**4**   Dissection of aponeuosis anorectal. *DV* vas deferens, *Den* Denonvillier's aponeurosis/incision, *SV* seminal vesicle, *R* rectum.

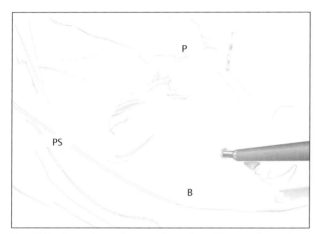

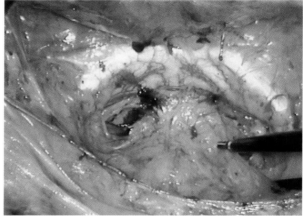

Fig. 35.**5**   Preperitoneal space dissection. *PS* preperitoneal space, *P* pubis, *B* bladder.

The supravesicular parietal peritoneum is sectioned transversally. The section must be perpendicular to the muscle wall to avoid becoming lost in the layer of fat, which is much denser than in females. In males, the bladder is located higher than in females. If in doubt, the bladder may be inflated with CO_2 gas (Fig. 35.**5**), enabling the visualization of the dome and the peritoneal incision zone.

Once the muscle is visualized, vesicoparietal dissection is performed downwards to the puboprostatic ligament and laterally to the perineal aponeurosis and Cooper's ligaments. The correct dissection plane is practically avascular. Dissection can, therefore, be performed between two forceps by dilaceration, with some coagulation if necessary.

The perineal aponeurosis is opened front to back, starting at the foramen obturatum, once the area has been cleared of all fat. This operation seems to be easier with a blade, but may be done with scissors. Some authors cut the aponeurosis from back to front. The lateral lobes of the prostate are tilted back while also pushing the elevator muscles aside (Fig. 35.**6**).

The puboprostatic ligaments are sectioned as close to the pubis as possible. Attention should be paid to collapse of the veins of Santorini's plexus (venous compression due to pneumoperitoneum and traction on the prostate alters their appearance and color so they become nacreous white like ligaments). Lessening the traction on the prostate permits modification of vein color and thus prevents very troublesome venous trauma (Fig. 35.**7**).

The section and hemostasis of Santorini's plexus can be accomplished by a ligature (0 gauge absorbable braided thread) or by pinching-off with a linear vascular-type stapler inserted through the 12 mm subumbilical trocar (Figs. 35.**8**, 35.**9**).

Dissection of the prostate may be continued retrograde using the standard technique with section of the urethra, but forward dissection is preferable for two reasons:

- Absence of urethral bleeding. Such bleeding can be heavy and very troublesome during the remainder of the dissection.

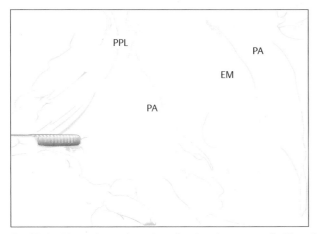
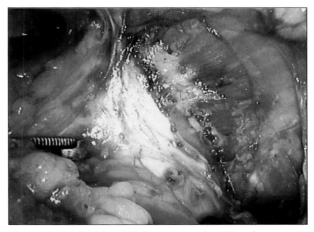

Fig. 35.**6**   Dissection and section of perineal aponeurosis. *PA* perineal aponeurosis/incision, *EM* elevator muscles, *PPL* puboprostatic ligaments.

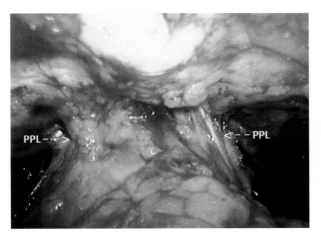
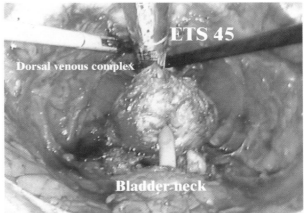

Fig. 35.**8**   Stapling of dorsal venous complex.

- Dissection in the direction of the visual field of the lens.

Dissection along the intervesicoprostatic line most often preserves the bladder neck (except when the prostate is very large or its median lobe is hypertrophied). This procedure is sometimes difficult because there are no clearly defined anatomic limits. It may be performed transversally with an UltraCision blade. The bladder neck can be located using:

- The superior staple line,
- The fat which adheres to the bladder but is removed easily from the prostate, delineating the cutting line of the neck,
- The Foley catheter balloon under traction (Fig. 35.**10**).

The vesical pedicles located at two and 10 o'clock must be carefully coagulated with bipolar forceps. After section of the anterior part of the neck, traction on the Foley catheter (with balloon inflated) exposes the posterior aspect of the neck and vesical trigone.

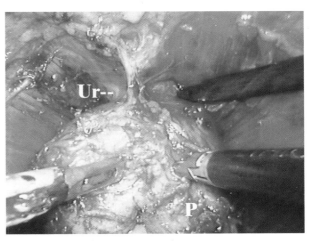

Fig. 35.**9**   Urethral section. *Ur* urethra

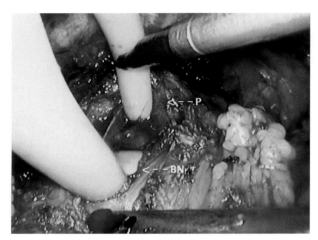

Fig. 35.**10** Section of bladder neck. *P* prostate, *BN* bladder neck.

Once the posterior side of the neck has been sectioned, at some distance from the trigone, the vasa deferentia and the seminal vesicles may be pulled into the incision forming a pedicle with the lateral bladder neck and lobes (Fig. 35.**11**).

The section of the lateral lobes may be performed with the UltraCision shears or bipolar coagulation and section with an UltraCision blade. The upper part of the lateral lobes is very dense and highly vascularized. The bottom part is much more slender, but close to the neurovascular bundles.

Special care must also be taken of the posterior aspect of the apex, the second high risk site of the neurovascular bundles (Figs. 35.**12**, 35.**13**).

The urethra is sectioned below the apex of the prostate, with a cold scalpel or a monopolar hook. This step may be facilitated by inserting a Béniqué catheter in the urethra. Once the front half has been sectioned, the Béniqué catheter is pulled out as far as the edge of the incision (Fig. 35.**14**).

The final delicate step in the excision of the prostate consists in sectioning the posterior half, which involves:

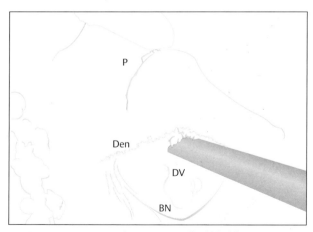

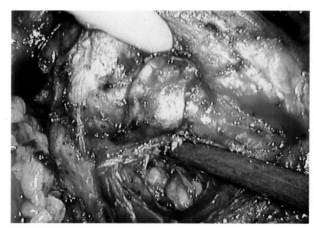

Fig. 35.**11** Dissection of posterior wall of bladder neck. *P* prostate, *DV* vas deferens, *Den* Denonvillier's aponeurosis/incision, *BN* bladder neck.

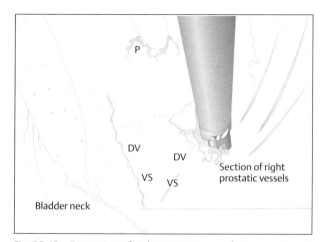

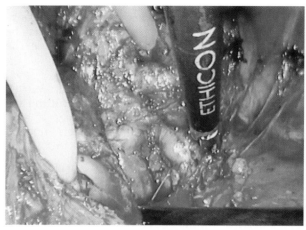

Fig. 35.**12** Dissection of right prostatic vessels. *P* prostate, *DV* vas deferens, *SV* seminal vesicle, *BN* bladder neck.

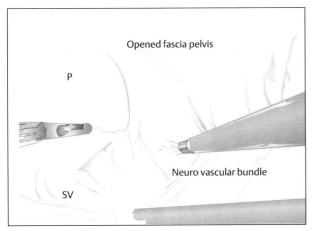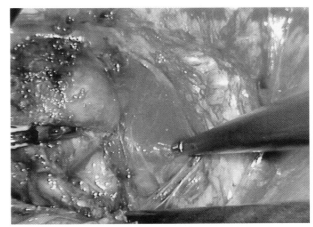

Fig. 35.**13**   Sparing of neurovascular bundle. *P* prostate, *SV* seminal vesicle.

- The posterior part of the urethra,
- Denonvilliers' fascia,
- The two lateral prolongations of this fascia (rectourethral muscles). The latter are thick and located interior to the neurovascular bundles. Rectal palpation or the introduction of an endorectal bougie can permit better verification of the various anatomic planes.

The specimen is thus totally mobilized, placed in a plastic sack, and left in the right iliac fossa (Fig. 35.**15**).

The suture consists of a circumferential, monofilament running suture with a 26, 3/8 or 5/8 needle. 5/8 needles seem to be the easiest to use, particularly for the recapture of the needle point after passage. The suture begins at three o'clock then continues on the posterior aspect. A Foley or Béniqué catheter facilitates the positioning of the urethral sutures (Figs. 35.**16**, 35.**17**).

As soon as the posterior sutures are finished, the catheter is passed into the bladder. The anterior suture completes the anastomosis. The suturing can also be done with:

- Two hemicircumferential sutures (anterior and posterior),
- Separate sutures (usually eight sutures),
- A tennis-racket-type closure when the bladder neck is very wide.

Using two needle-holders facilitates positioning of the various sutures. Knowledge of the different suturing techniques ensures the quality of the anastomosis and, therefore, shortens the recovery period. Impermeability can be controlled by injection of physiological saline with methylene blue.

As soon as the dissection is finished, the specimen is placed in a plastic sack in order to avoid any contamination by neoplastic cells, and left in the right iliac fossa. After suture, the whole is brought out by enlarging the subumbilical trocar port, or from the right iliac fossa.

Lymph adenectomy can be associated at the beginning of the procedure. An approach using two lateral

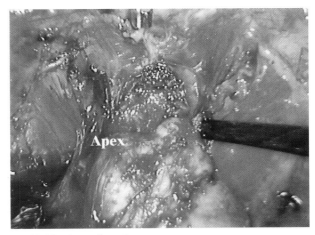

Fig. 35.**14**   Apex dissection.

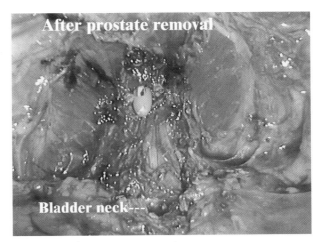

Fig. 35.**15**   After prostate removal.

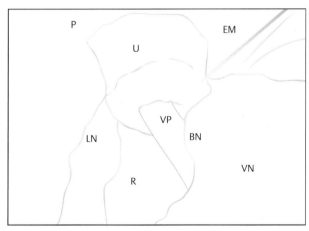 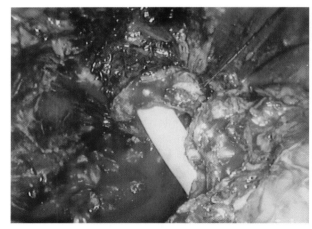

Fig. 35.**16**   Beginning of posterior continuous suture. *P* pubis, *Ur* urethra, *EM* elevator muscles, *BN* bladder neck, *VP* vesical probe, *LN* left neuro-vascular bundle, *R* rectum, *VN* vesical neck.

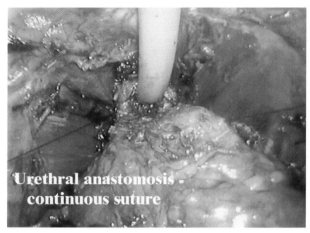

Fig. 35.**17**   Posterior continuous suture with urethral anastomosis.

peritoneal incisions enables dissection without lowering the bladder, which would make dissection of the posterior plane impossible. Lymph adenectomy can also be carried out at the end of the procedure, using the opening above the bladder.

Redon drains are used, one anterior to the bladder, and possibly another posterior.

The procedure can take from 2 to 6 hours, depending upon the difficulty, with an average of 2 1/2 hours for experienced teams. Intestinal function usually resumes after about 48 hours.

Depending on the surgical team, the Foley catheter is removed between 4 to 10 days after operation. The patient may be discharged as early as the third postoperative day if there are no complications. The patient returns for catheter removal.

Hints and Pitfalls

Radical laparoscopic prostatectomy is the most difficult and time-consuming operation in urology. It requires familiarity with both excision and reconstruction techniques. This surgery can be greatly facilitated early in the learning curve if two surgeons can replace each another in case of fatigue or technical difficulties.

Bleeding is generally slower and lighter than with laparotomy. Damage to the epigastric arteries usually occurs during insertion of the trocars. Video monitored insertion avoids this complication, which can be treated by bipolar coagulation or by a transparietal X suture.

Bipolar coagulation of the vascularization of the seminal vesicles has to be carried out with great care, and flush with the vesicles. Secondary hemostasis is difficult because the arterioles retract rapidly, and present a major risk for the neurovascular bundles.

Damage to Santorini's plexus may be controlled temporarily by bipolar coagulation or compression with a hemostatic swab. The latter must always be accompanied by a suture or mechanical stapling.

Sectioning the urethra last avoids troublesome bleeding or oozing while dissecting the neck and lateral lobes.

Rectal damage may go unnoticed or may be the result of the loosening of a coagulation (particularly monopolar) scab. Though damage to the rectum is rare, it can be detected by rectal palpation or methylene blue test, when there is the slightest doubt. The wound must be sutured immediately.

Damage to the bladder occurs mainly when the incision of the anteroparietal peritoneum is too low and horizontal. Care must be taken to make the incision of the peritoneum sufficiently high. When in doubt, filling the bladder with saline solution enables location of the bladder dome before incising the peritoneum. If bladder damage occurs, it should be repaired with an extramucosal running suture.

Damage to the ureter can occur when sectioning the bladder neck and may require laparoscopic reimplantation.

Surgical conversion is required for any complication not managed rapidly, depending on the surgeon's experience.

Catheter obstruction may cause urine leakage in the drain. This is treated by lavage or catheter change—if necessary under radiographic or cystoscopic control.

A urinoma, resulting from urethrovesical anastomotic leakage and drainage failure, may require laparoscopic intervention for lavage.

Throughout anastomosis, care must be taken to create a watertight anastomosis and avoid eversion of one of the ureteral orifices.

Discussion

Technical difficulty increases mainly with prostate size (over 70 g) and, to a lesser degree, with the patient's weight and adiposity. Furthermore, a hypertrophied middle lobe increases dissection difficulty in the posterior vesicoprostatic plane due to proximity of the ureters. Usually conservation of the bladder neck is impossible. Small or resected prostates (under 20 g) do not provide clear margins for excision.
We totally avoid any preoperative hormone therapy.

The number of young patients with small prostatic tumors will probably increase. Prostatectomy morbidity should the lowest possible, particularly concerning sexual function. Coagulation, whether by mono- or bipolar bistouries, runs the risk of damage to the neuromuscular bundles. UltraCision dissection can avoid distant lesions by thermal diffusion, thus preserving the neurovascular bundles, and in doing so, erectile function.

Laparoscopic vision permits precise dissection and, with experience, should enable the reduction of:

- Sexual dysfunction rate,
- Urinary incontinence rate,
- Bleeding during surgery.

The minimally invasive procedure shortens hospital stay.

Suggested Reading

Abbou CC, Doublet JD, Gaston R, Guillonneau B. Rapport du Congrès 1999 de l'Association Française d'Urologie.

Abbou CC, Antiphon P, Salomon L, Hoznek A, Bello J, Lefrere-Belda MA, Chopin DD.Laparoscopic radical prostatectomy: preliminary results. J Endourol, 1999, 13 (suppl. 1), A 45.

Raboy A, Ferzli G, Albert P. Initial experience with extraperitoneal endoscopic radical retropubic prostatectomy. Urology, 1997, 50: 849–853

Schluesser W., Kavoussi LR, Clayman R, Vancaille TH. Laparoscopic radical prostatectomy : initial case report. J Urol, 1992, 4: 246 A

Guillonneau B., Vallancien G. Laparoscopic Radical Prostatectomy : the Montsouris experience. J Urol, à paraître

Guillonneau B, Cathelineau X, Barret E, Rozet F. Vallancien G. Prostatectomie radicale coelioscopique. Première évaluation après 28 interventions. Presse Med., 27: 1570, 1998

Rassweiler J, Seemon O, Abdel-Salam Y, El Quran M, Lanz E, Frede T. Laparoscopic radical prostatectomy ; the Heilbron Technique. J Endourol, 1999, 13 (suppl. 1), A 46

Teichman JM, Reddy PK, Hulbert JC. Laparoscopic pelvic lymph node dissection, laparoscopically assisted seminal vesicle mobilization, end total perineal prostatectomy versus radical retropubic prostatectomy for prostate cancer. Urology, 1995, 45: 823–829.

Schluesser W., Schulam P, Clayman R, Kavoussi L. Laparoscopic radical prostatectomy: initial short-term experience. Urology, 1997, 50: 854–857.

Guillonneau B., Vallancien G. Laparoscopic Radical Prostatectomy : Initial experience and preliminary assessment after 65 operations. The Prostate, 1999, 39: 71–75.

Index

Numbers in *italics* indicate figures.